Lange Review:
MRI Clinical Concepts and
Imaging Applications Manual with
Registry Review

Lange Review:
MRI Clinical Concepts and Imaging Applications Manual with Registry Review

Authors

W. Zachary Rich, JD, MBA, MS Ed., RT(R)(CT)(MR)
Attorney/Senior Conflict Analyst
MRI Technologist

Michael L. Grey, Ph.D, RT(R)(MR)(CT), FASRT
Former Professor of Radiologic Sciences
Former Program Director MRI/CT Specialization
Southern Illinois University
Carbondale, Illinois

McGraw Hill

New York   Chicago   San Francisco   Athens   London   Madrid   Mexico City
Milan   New Delhi   Singapore   Sydney   Toronto

Lange Review: MRI Clinical Concepts and Imaging Applications Manual with Registry Review

1 2 3 4 5 6 7 8 9   DSS   28 27 26 25 24 23

ISBN 978-1-264-63279-4
MHID 1-264-63279-7

This book was set in Minion Pro Regular by KnowledgeWorks Global Ltd.
The editors were Sydney Keen and Christie Naglieri.
The production supervisor was Rick Ruzycka.
Project management was provided by Nitesh Sharma, KnowledgeWorks Global Ltd.
The cover designer was W2 Design.
This book is printed on acid-free paper.

Library of Congress Cataloging-in-Publication Data

Names: Rich, W. Zachary, author. | Grey, Michael L, author.
Title: Lange review : MRI clinical concepts and imaging applications manual
    with registry review / authors: W. Zachary Rich, Michael L Grey.
Other titles: Lange review (Rich) | MRI clinical concepts and imaging
    applications manual with registry review
Description: New York : McGraw Hill, [2023] | Includes bibliographical
    references and index.
Identifiers: LCCN 2022024398 (print) | LCCN 2022024399 (ebook) | ISBN
    9781264632794 (paperback ; alk. paper) | ISBN 9781264634149 (ebook)
Subjects: MESH: Magnetic Resonance Imaging—methods | Patient Care—methods
    | Examination Questions
Classification: LCC RC386.6.M34 (print) | LCC RC386.6.M34 (ebook) | NLM
    WN 18.2 | DDC 616.07/548—dc23/eng/20220817
LC record available at https://lccn.loc.gov/2022024398
LC ebook record available at https://lccn.loc.gov/2022024399

Contents

Contributing Authors

Dr. Jagan Mohan Ailinani
CT and MRI Contrast Agents

Neal Weston Langdon, M.D.
Premier Radiology

Preface

The purpose in writing the *MRI Clinical Concepts and Imaging Applications Manual with Registry Review* textbook is to provide a clinically oriented book for individuals entering into the medical imaging field of magnetic resonance imaging. This book is designed with the learner in mind and is laid out in three main sections. The first section focuses on topics like patient care and preparation, contrast media and medicolegal issues.

The second section addresses common imaging applications performed in MRI today. Each imaging application includes concise information on patient/part positioning, slice alignment, scan range, general sequences, and suggested protocol variations. In addition, MR images are provided to support each application.

Finally, the third section is comprised of 250 multiple-choice questions covering a wide range of topics to help the learner prepare for the American Registry of Radiologic Technologists (ARRT) examination. Of those 250 questions, 50 are image based. Finally, an answer explanation sub-section is used as an answer key and resource to better understand the correct answer.

The intent of this textbook is to be used as a supplement during either a classroom lecture or to assist the student while attending their clinical internship.

W. Zachary Rich
Michael L. Grey

Acknowledgments

In reflecting on the journey in the development of the *MRI Clinical Concepts and Imaging Applications Manual with Registry Review*, I would like to say thank you to the editorial staff at McGraw-Hill, especially Ms. Sydney Keen. The many tasks involved in writing one book can be challenging, however, working on two books (*CT Clinical Concepts and Imaging Applications Manual with Registry Review*) simultaneously is crazy insane. To those who encouraged me to finish these books, you made the journey easier – thank you!

Finally, to Zach Rich, an individual with many titles and a lot of letters behind his name. To me, he was a student, a teaching assistant, and now an author. I have seen this young man accomplish much. Thank you.

Michael – a.k.a. "the Tutelar"

I want to start off by thanking my wonderful wife, Madelaine, and my parents, Jeff and Carol. You were incredibly supportive and understanding of the countless hours it took to put together not only one textbook, but two (*MRI Clinical Concepts and Imaging Applications Manual with Registry Review* and *CT Clinical Concepts and Imaging Applications Manual with Registry Review*). I would like to also thank Jack Bryant, Judd Hill, and Anwar Hanna for their help. You were the best technologists and people I have had the pleasure of working with. Jack, I appreciate your friendship and support over the many years we worked together and also your help with this project.

To my co-author, Michael Grey (a.k.a. "the Tutelar"), thank you so much for your guidance and encouragement over the years. We began this textbook project many years ago and it is such a relief to finally see it through. Thank you for pushing me to do more, both professionally and personally. Simply put, from the Tutelee to the Tutelar, thank you. I would like to also thank the publishing team. I appreciate your work taking rough drafts and molding them into amazing final manuscripts. Finally, thank you Lord for your guidance, answered prayers, and healing.

Zach

Nuclear Magnetic Resonance Imaging (NMRI)

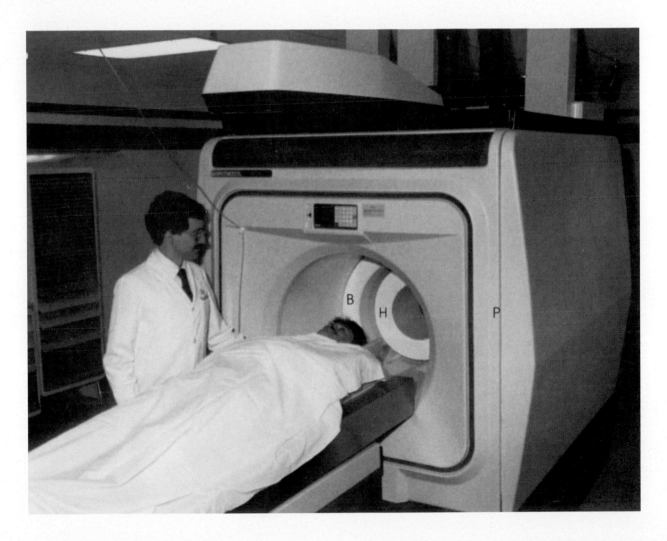

This is a photo of the first commercially made nuclear magnetic resonance (NMR) imaging unit in the world. NMR imaging is commonly referred to today as magnetic resonance imaging (MRI).

This photo shows the head coil (H), the body coil (B) in the center of the bore, and the plastic housing (P). This NMR unit was a Technicare 0.15 T Resistive system. As a show site to the world, visitors were frequent, and many tours were given to introduce this new technology to the world.

This photo was taken in the mid-1980s. By that time, several companies had also begun producing their own NMR units. The gentlemen posing for this photo are Michael Grey (standing) and the service engineer (positioned on the patient couch).

Source: Reprinted from Grey ML, Alinani JM. CT and MRI Pathology: A Pocket Atlas. 3rd ed. New York, NY: McGraw-Hill; 2018, with permission from The McGraw-Hill Professional.

PART I

Introduction to Imaging Applications

MRI Patient Care and Preparation

INTRODUCTION

The role of an MRI technologist is multifaceted and requires them to be versatile in the performance of their job. In addition to performing the specific examination ordered by the referring physician, the technologist must be sensitive to the needs of the patient. In this section, discussion topics will focus on various aspects surrounding the actual examination being performed.

FACTORS INFLUENCING EFFECTIVE COMMUNICATION

Effective communication is very important when relating to patients. When meeting and preparing the patient for their examination, realize that each person is uniquely different in how they understand, communicate, and function. With this in mind, the technologist should be sensitive to these differences and adjust the conversation accordingly. These differences may vary depending on many factors such as the individual's values, development, gender, age, sociocultural background, and perceptions. To better communicate with individuals and, more specifically, to help the patient successfully complete the examination ordered and have a positive experience in an imaging facility, the technologist should consider these factors.

The values of an individual are based on the things they consider important in life. The values of an individual define their beliefs, ideals, and desires and have a major influence on their behavior and attitude. Listening to an individual and what they talk about will usually provide a sense of their values, interests, and previous experiences.

The personal development of an individual varies depending on their age, experiences, education, various abilities and disabilities, and maturity. Age alone cannot determine maturity. Some children may be very mature for their age, whereas some young adults may appear childish in their behavior. The level of education an individual has achieved may influence their level of understanding. The technologist should choose their words wisely to improve their communication with their patients.

Gender differences between men and women may be seen in their communication style and how each hears or listens to what is being discussed. Cultural differences when working with individuals from other countries may also affect the communication process. Being knowledgeable and respectful of these differences will be greatly appreciated and benefit the outcome of the examination.

While patients come in all ages, being cognizant of whether the patient is understanding the content of the conversation is foundational to the successful experiences of the individual. Modifying communication skills to the needs and level of understanding of the patient will be much appreciated. For children and patients under the legal age, communication needs to be flexible and also include parents or legal guardians.

The patient's values and sociocultural background are based on their general understanding and preconceptions surrounding their world and their personal experiences. Sociocultural differences may be seen in the individual's language skills, such as in their accent, the gestures they make, and the attitudes they demonstrate.

An individual's perceptions, which may be based on their physical senses such as gut feelings, observations, or hearsay, can affect how they understand and interpret information and their surrounding environment. Trying to communicate better with individuals, accepting them as they are, and trying to better understand their concerns, fears, and previous experiences will help the patient complete the exam. The successful outcome of the examination being performed and the individual's experience rest largely on the initial care, skills, and character demonstrated by the technologist. As part of the health care team and as a health care professional, technologists should always conduct themselves in a professional manner. This includes addressing individuals with honorific titles (eg, Mr., Mrs., Ms., Dr., Sir, and Ma'am), maintaining eye contact during conversation, answering questions clearly and at a level the individual can understand, maintaining good personal hygiene, and dressing in modest attire. Ideally, the manner in which a technologist is seen in their workplace is also demonstrated in the public setting.

STYLES OF COMMUNICATION

In all basic forms of communication, there are at least two individuals involved, a sender and a receiver. As communication occurs, there is a message, such as an instruction, given by the sender and feedback from the receiver. Interpersonal communication is performed verbally and nonverbally. While conversing with the patient, it is important for technologists to be aware of the nonverbal actions being projected by both the patient and themselves. Points to consider in verbal communication include vocabulary, denotation and connotation, pacing, intonation, clarity, and timing. Points to consider in nonverbal communication include appearance, posture, facial expression, eye contact, body gestures, touch, sounds, and personal space (Table 1–1).

Verbal Communication

Verbal communication includes the spoken and written word. Choosing words wisely and appropriately and pronouncing them clearly at an understandable level will help to assure good communication. In addition, the manner in which these words are spoken can also assist in the communication process. The technologist should also realize that some words can have several meanings and be careful as to how these words may be interpreted to avoid any misunderstanding or confusion regarding what is said.

One example of a word that has a variety of meanings is *sports* (eg, baseball or basketball). When using the word *sports*, one person may be thinking of baseball, while another may be

thinking of basketball. In a more practical example, the use of the word *okay* or the phrase "you are doing fine" may communicate the wrong message to an individual. For example, image how embarrassing it was for the following radiography student working alongside a technologist as the technologist was telling the patient what to do while positioning the patient for a posteroanterior upright chest exam. Several times during the instructions, the technologist said the word *okay*. After the patient was positioned for the upright chest exam, the technologist and student turned and walked back to the operator console to select the technique to use. During their walk back to the console, the technologist said the word *okay* again. As they rounded the corner to the console and looked through the window, they noticed that the patient was not at the upright chest board; instead, the patient was right behind them in the x-ray control area. Shocked and confused, the technologist asked the patient why he had followed them. The patient responded that he had heard them say "okay" and thought the exam was complete and that he was supposed to follow them out of the exam room. As a habit, the overuse of the word *okay* misled the patient to think the exam was finished because the technologist used the word *okay* to transition to performing the next step of the exam and then again before asking the patient to take a deep breath. Likewise, using the phrase "you're doing fine" with a patient may communicate the message that the patient does not need the examination or that the examination appears to be normal. A better and more specific phrase would be, for example, "You are doing a good job holding still." Miscommunication can lead the patient to question the doctor's report, especially if the report is found to be pathologically positive.

Pacing or talking too fast may inhibit the individual's ability to clearly understand or remember what is being said. It is important to speak slowly so that words are processed clearly and understood. In addition, elderly patients may not hear as well as younger patients, and others with a hearing impairment may better understand what is being said by reading lips. Printing short instructions on a note pad and letting the patient read the message can be very helpful for patients with hearing impairments.

The tone or intonation of the communication can also be misleading. The technologist's emotions, feelings, or fatigue may influence the way they express what they are saying to the patient. The technologist must always be aware of how they are expressing the communication and how it is being perceived by the patient. Is the patient perceiving anger, frustration, or joy? What is the technologist perceiving about the patient? Sometimes, it is helpful to empathize with the patient and try to understand what the patient may be going through or other issues in their life. As a word of caution, an expression such as, "I know what you're dealing with" may not be ideal. For example, if the patient has been diagnosed with cancer and the technologist has never had cancer, how could the technologist

TABLE 1–1 • Key Points of Verbal and Nonverbal Communication	
Verbal	**Nonverbal**
• Vocabulary	• Appearance
• Denotation and connotation	• Posture and gait
• Pacing	• Facial expression
• Intonation	• Eye contact
• Clarity	• Body gestures
• Timing	• Touch
	• Sounds
	• Personal space

possibly know what the patient is dealing with? Further, if the technologist has personally experienced cancer, how could they fully know the degree of pain and suffering the patient is experiencing. As a suggestion, the technologist could say, "I understand what it was like when they had cancer."

The clarity of what is being communicated will help in reducing confusion. Technologists should try to choose their words and sentences so they are short and to the point. Their words should be clearly enunciated (especially for those with difficulty hearing) to improve communication.

Small adjustments by technologists in how they communicate may have a big effect on how well patients understand what is being said and will demonstrate the technologist's concern and care for them. The patient's experience will greatly affect how they view the imaging facility. If it is a good experience, the imaging facility will be highly thought of and much appreciated.

Nonverbal Communication

An individual's appearance is the first thing noticed in an interpersonal encounter. Many physical characteristics, such as clothing, grooming, and physical well-being, contribute to forming first impressions.

The posture and gait of an individual may be indications of their emotions, self-concept, and quality of health. While observing an individual's posture and gait should not be considered as the sole basis for assessing their overall health, they may provide a clue to the individual's well-being.

Facial expressions can reflect many emotions, ranging from sadness to happiness. Additional expressions that may be noticed include fear, pain, and anger. Paying attention to an individual's facial expressions may provide information that can benefit the communication process. In addition, technologists should be aware of their own facial expressions and the message they are sending to the patient or family members. What patient would want their technologist to have a sad or unhappy expression on their face? Think about what your facial expression communicates to your patient and others around you.

In addition to being an important part of facial expressions, eye contact can indicate a willingness to communicate. Establishing eye contact during a conversation demonstrates respect for and a desire to listen to the other person. Likewise, a lack of eye contact may communicate a lack of interest, lack of confidence, anxiety, or disrespect for the other person. It is important to note that eye contact may be seen differently by various cultures. The technologist should be aware of the cultural differences and act accordingly.

Body gestures, such as pointing a finger, having arms folded across the chest, hand and arm movements, tapping a leg, and rolling the eyes, may have specific meanings in the communication process. Facial expressions along with a person's posture and gait work together to create a specific message.

Touch is a more personal form of communication. In medical imaging, touching a patient is necessary in positioning the patient. Touching can send a variety of messages to the patient or family member, such as emotional support and encouragement. Holding the hand of a grieving patient can often show understanding better than words. Touching that occurs when shaking hands during a greeting or putting an arm around a patient to assist them with getting up on the patient table for an examination is usually acceptable. Although some individuals and cultures may be unfamiliar to the technologist, it is important for the technologist to be aware of and sense the comfort level of the individual. Prior to touching a patient to help in positioning, the technologist should always ask permission and explain where they need to touch the patient and the reason. This demonstrates respect for the individual and improves the communication between the technologist and the patient. If family members, such as parents, are nearby, they will appreciate the thoughtfulness in asking permission.

In many situations, feelings and thoughts may be communicated through various types of sounds. These sounds include sighing, moaning, exhaling heavily, and crying. For example, a sigh may indicate relief or weariness. The technologist should observe all forms of nonverbal communication to facilitate better communication with individuals. Likewise, the sounds the technologist makes affect the communication with patients. Consider what the patient might feel or think if they ask a question and the technologist gives a sigh. Is it a sigh of boredom, frustration, or indifference? What will the patient think about the technologist and their facility? What if the patient fills out an evaluation form following their experiences in your care during their examination?

The space or distance between the technologist and an individual may be referred to as "personal space." If the personal space between individuals is invaded by decreasing this space, the patient may feel uncomfortable and threatened. Technologists are often used to being very close to patients when positioning them; however, patients may not be as comfortable with this proximity. Again, it is advised that the technologist always respect the patient and clearly communicate in a manner that will reduce a patient's discomfort.

In medical imaging, communicating with the patient and possibly the patient's family members, such as parents or legal guardians, is a process of social interaction where the technologist endeavors to gain the trust and cooperation of the patient. The technologist should understand that, for many people, being a patient can be a stressful experience that may not allow the patient to be seen at their best. Using verbal and nonverbal communication, the technologist begins the patient encounter by introducing themselves to the patient and explaining the examination in a step-by-step process, pausing at times to allow the patient to better understand and retain the information. Time and encouragement should also be provided for the patient to ask questions.

PHYSICAL SCREENING AND ASSESSMENT OF THE PATIENT

Following the initial introduction and verifying the patient and the exam that is to be performed, the technologist will review the MRI Safety Screening form with the patient or legal guardian.[1] This step is conducted to assess the patient for any information that might signal a contraindication to performing the exam. During this process, the technologist will verify that the information provided on the MRI Safety Screening form is correct and current by asking the patient specific questions. For patients who are hearing impaired, a note pad and pen can be used to assist the communication process.

Following the screening process, if there are no contraindications to performing the examination as ordered, the patient will need to change their clothes and put on a gown. If the exam is ordered with contrast media, lab work may need to be ordered and reviewed to verify that the patient's kidneys are functioning within acceptable limits. Accommodations for patients who arrive in wheelchairs, use a walker, or require oxygen or other items will need to be arranged to assure that no ferromagnetic device or component enters zone IV of the MRI environment. Portable devices that are metallic or partially metallic are to be categorized as MR Safe, MR Conditional, or MR Unsafe before being allowed to enter into zone III.

MRI Zones

Since most, if not all, MRI units are superconductive, site access should be restricted and limited to only individuals that have been approved to enter. This is accomplished by dividing the MRI department into four zones.[2]

Zone I: This zone includes all areas that are freely accessible to the public. This area is usually considered to be outside the MRI environment. It is the area where patients, health care personal, and other employees of the MR site access the MR environment.

Zone II: This zone is an interface between the public accessible zone (zone I) and the more restricted zones (zones III and IV). In zone II, the technologist screens the patient and obtains the patient history in a Health Insurance Portability and Accountability Act (HIPAA)–compliant environment.

Zone III: In zone III, all access to the general public and unscreened non–MR facility personnel is restricted.

Zone IV: Zone IV is the area where the MRI scanner magnet is located.

PATIENT SAFETY SCREENING FORM

Every MR facility has developed and tailored an MRI Safety Screening form to meet its specific needs. As a safety guideline for patients and other (nonpatient) individuals who may be entering into the strong magnetic field, it is required that they fill out the facility's MRI Safety Screening form and submit it for review prior to being scanned. Before entering into zone III, the MRI Safety Screening form is provided to the patient or individual requesting to enter the area where the main magnet is located. Once the form is completed, it must be reviewed by a qualified MR-trained health care worker employed at the imaging facility. The MRI Safety Screening form is made up of a few sections that focus on specific questions. Usually, in the first section, basic demographics about the patient are requested. The next section asks questions about the patient's medical history, such as prior imaging procedures or surgeries, possible metal or metallic object injuries, current medications, possible reactions to contrast media, any problems with their blood (eg, anemia) or kidneys (eg, failure, transplant, hypertension, diabetes), or history of seizures. A specific set of questions is provided for female patients to complete. In the next section, a list of possible implants or devices that may be contraindications or require special attention is provided for the patient's response. In addition, a figure representing a human body is provided so the patient can indicate any implants or devices located inside or on their body. At the end of the MRI Safety Screening form, is a signature area for the patient or legal guardian and the MRI technologist that reviewed the screening form with the patient to sign and date.

After completion of the MRI Safety Screening form, the designated qualified MR-trained health care worker should review the form and go over the questions and answers with the patient or individual to verify the information is accurate and current. By going over the form with the patient, any information that the patient may have forgotten to include will hopefully be recalled. This process may also be performed by two different employees to better ascertain the information and provide a safe experience. During the review process, the technologist should ask age-specific questions, encourage the patient to ask questions, observe nonverbal communication of the patient during the review process, and use the power of encouragement (eg, "You can do it" or "You are doing a good job holding still") to help the patient complete their examination.

An example of an MRI Safety Screening form is available at www.MRISafety.com.

Examination Overview

Performing an MRI examination on a patient includes several tasks. In addition to reviewing and verifying the accuracy of the patient's MRI Safety Screening form, reviewing the practical points or steps of the exam is helpful in better preparing the patient for their examination procedure. Discussing the key points of the procedure is time well spent in reducing patient anxiety and increasing patient cooperation and satisfaction. Points to consider in explaining the MRI procedure to be performed include the following:

- How the patient is to be positioned
- How the specific anatomic structure to be imaged will be positioned

- Approximate length of time for exam
- Ask the patient if they need to use the bathroom before beginning the exam
- Knocking noises
- Intravenous (IV) line if used for contrast media
- Use of professional terms to foster a professional environment (avoid using terms such as *dye* in place of contrast media or contrast agent)
- Where the technologist will be during the examination

In addition, before the exam, show the patient the MRI room and magnet. Patients who are claustrophobic or who deal with anxiety may benefit from a brief tour around the magnet to see that the magnet bore (opening) is open on both ends and that there is no such thing as a "closed" MRI unit.

After the Examination

At the conclusion of the examination, ask the patient how they are doing. Compliment and congratulate the patient regarding their participation in completing the examination and obtaining good-quality images for the doctor to see. Because they have been lying down for some time, helping the patient to sit up on the edge of the patient table will be appreciated and will allow the technologist to assure the patient's stability before they get off the table.

Patients may inquire as to the results of the examination and where to go next. The technologist should be familiar with instructions that answer these types of questions. Usually, the patient is scheduled to see the ordering physician, at which time the results of the examination (ie, report) will be discussed. If the technologist sees something on the images during the examination that needs to be reviewed by the radiologist before the patient leaves the MRI facility, the technologist may ask the patient to have a seat in the waiting room until further instructions are provided.

Documenting specific information in the patient's report regarding the examination should be performed by the technologist primarily involved with imaging the patient. This process should only focus on key components of the examination and may be as short and simple as stating the patient tolerated the procedure well without complications. If a contrast agent is used, that must be documented. Because contrast agents are drugs, they should be documented by the individual who started the IV and injected the contrast agent. Information to be documented includes the type and name of the contrast agent injected, the weight of the patient, the volume given, the gauge of the needle, the anatomical site or vein used, and any complications associated with the injection of the contrast agent. In most cases, the patient will tolerate the injection of the contrast agent with no complications.

References

1. Saraswat AK, Smith MA. MRI screening for patients and individuals. In: Shellock FB, Karacozoff AM, eds. *MRI Bioeffects, Safety, and Patient Management*. Biomedical Research Publishing Group; 2014:282-298.

2. Kanal E, Barkovich AJ, Bell C, et al. ACR guidance document on MR safe practices: 2013. *J Magn Reson Imaging*. 2013;37:501-530.

2

CT and MRI Contrast Agents

Technologists working in computed tomography (CT) or magnetic resonance imaging (MRI) are responsible for performing a wide variety of examinations on a diverse population of patients. Many of these examinations require the use of a contrast agent. It is very important, therefore, that the technologist has a working knowledge of how to perform venipuncture and how to safely administer the specific contrast agent required. To safely administer a contrast agent, the technologist must be able to determine five things:

- The specific contrast agent to be used
- The correct amount to be used
- The appropriate injection site
- The correct injection rate
- The appropriate gauge of the intravenous (IV) needle to be used

Upon completion of the examination, all pertinent details of the venipuncture and administration of the contrast agent should be documented in the patient chart by the technologist, along with the overall patient outcome. To ensure the safety of the patient, it would be beneficial for the technologist to have an overview of the main points to consider prior to using either a CT or an MRI contrast agent.

CT CONTRAST AGENTS

Water-soluble contrast agents, which consist of molecules containing atoms of iodine, are used extensively in CT. Although risk of adverse reaction is low, there is a real risk inherent in their use that can range from mild to life threatening. Due to these safety risks, newer but more expensive, low-osmolar contrast agents have replaced the older, cheaper, high-osmolar ionic contrast agents. Adverse side effects are uncommon for these agents, ranging from 5% to 12% with ionic to 1% to 3% with nonionic, low-osmolality intravascular contrast agents.

Mild reactions are the most common type of reaction and usually do not require treatment. Patients experiencing any of the typical reactions should be observed for 30 minutes after the onset to ensure that the reaction does not become more severe. Common signs and symptoms include the following:

- Nausea and vomiting
- Urticaria and pruritis
- Sneezing
- Itchy or scratchy throat
- Feeling warm or chills
- Headache, dizziness, anxiety, and altered taste

Moderate reactions are not life threatening but commonly require treatment for symptoms. Some of these reactions may become severe if not treated. Common signs and symptoms of moderate reactions include the following:

- Diffuse urticaria or pruritis
- Diffuse erythema with stable vital signs
- Facial edema without dyspnea
- Throat tightness or hoarseness without dyspnea
- Wheezing or bronchospasm with mild or no hypoxia
- Protracted nausea or vomiting
- Isolated chest pain
- Vasovagal reaction that requires and is responsive to treatment

Patients should be monitored until symptoms resolve. Benadryl is effective for relief of symptomatic hives. Beta agonist inhalers help with bronchospasm (wheezing), and epinephrine is indicated for laryngeal spasm. Leg elevation (Trendelenburg position) is indicated for vasovagal reactions and hypotension.

Severe reactions, which are potentially life-threatening reactions, usually occur within the first 20 minutes following the intravascular injection of contrast. Severe reactions are rare but should be recognized and treated immediately. Common signs and symptoms of severe reactions include the following:

- Diffuse edema or facial edema with dyspnea
- Diffuse erythema with hypotension
- Laryngeal edema with stridor and/or hypoxia
- Anaphylactic shock (hypotension with tachycardia)
- Vasovagal reaction resistant to treatment
- Arrhythmia
- Convulsions or seizures
- Hypertensive emergency

Severe bronchospasm or severe laryngeal edema may progress to unconsciousness, seizures, hypotension, dysrhythmias, or cardiac arrest and need for immediate cardiopulmonary resuscitation.

Local side effects, such as extravasation of the contrast agent at the injection site, may cause pain, swelling, skin slough, and deeper tissue necrosis. The affected limb should be elevated. A warm compress may help with absorption of the contrast agent, whereas a cold compress is more effective in reducing pain at the injection site. With the current use of power injectors, extra care should be taken in observing the injection site during the administration phase of the contrast agent.

Although the terms *extravasation* and *infiltration* have been used interchangeably, a difference should be noted. Infiltration is the inadvertent administration of a nonvesicant fluid (eg, normal saline) into the surrounding tissues. Extravasation is the inadvertent administration of a vesicant fluid (eg, contrast agent, chemotherapy) into the surrounding tissue. A vesicant fluid can cause necrosis or tissue damage when it escapes from the vein.

Contrast-Induced Nephropathy

Contrast-induced nephropathy (CIN) is defined as acute renal failure (sudden deterioration in renal function) occurring within 48 hours of contrast injection and is a significant source of morbidity. CIN is a subgroup of postcontrast acute kidney injury. The most prominent risk factors are diabetes and chronic renal insufficiency. Adequate hydration is essential in the prevention of CIN. Patients should be encouraged to drink several liters of water or fluid 12 to 24 hours before and after intravascular administration of contrast. As a prophylactic treatment, an IV bolus of *N*-acetylcysteine (Mucovit) may also be recommended at a dose given orally (600 mg twice daily) on the day before and on the day of contrast administration. Another option is to give 500 mL of normal saline over 30 minutes prior to the exam and 500 mL of normal saline over 4 hours after the examination.

Metformin (Glucophage)

Metformin (Glucophage) is an oral antihyperglycemic agent used to treat type 2 diabetes mellitus. It may potentially cause fatal lactic acidosis. Metformin should be discontinued for 48 hours following iodinated contrast administration and reinstated only after renal function is reevaluated and found to be normal.

Patients at high risk for adverse contrast reactions should be identified and consideration given as to whether a contrast agent should be given. In cases where administrating a contrast agent may not be in the best interest of the patient, alternative imaging such as ultrasound may be helpful. Further, it may be possible for the radiologist to monitor the noncontrast CT exam to assess the images as they are acquired. If contrast is needed, the patient should be adequately hydrated. Premedication should be considered.

Risk factors for adverse reactions to contrast agents include the following:

- Previous history of adverse reaction to IV contrast
- Clear history of asthma or allergies (a history of an allergy to shellfish or iodine is not a reliable indicator of a possible contrast reaction)
- Known cardiac dysfunction including severe congestive heart failure, severe arrhythmias, unstable angina, recent myocardial infarction, or pulmonary hypertension
- Renal insufficiency, especially in patients with diabetes mellitus
- Sickle cell disease
- Multiple myeloma
- Age over 65

All patients receiving CT contrast should be screened appropriately. For patients at risk for reduced renal function, serum creatinine and estimated glomerular filtration rate (GFR) should be obtained. Technologists need the patient's age, gender, weight, and serum creatinine to use the GFR calculator (which can be found online). Patients who have a GFR of less than 30 mL/min should not be given contrast.

Premedication has been proven to decrease but not eliminate the frequency of contrast reactions. Two regimens listed by American College of Radiology include either (1) prednisone 50 mg taken orally at 13 hours, 7 hours, and 1 hour before contrast administration or (2) methylprednisolone 32 mg taken orally at 12 hours and 2 hours before contrast administration. Benadryl 50 mg orally, intramuscularly, or IV should be administered 1 hour before contrast for either of the regimens. In addition, nonionic low-osmolality contrast should be used with either regimen.

MRI CONTRAST AGENTS

Gadolinium chelates are the most commonly used magnetic resonance (MR) contrast agents. These agents differ based on being either ionic or nonionic and based on their osmolality and viscosity. Their distribution and elimination are very similar to water-soluble, iodine-based contrast agents used in CT. Injected IV gadolinium chelates diffuse rapidly into extracellular fluid and blood pool spaces and are excreted by glomerular filtration. About 80% of an injected dose is excreted within 3 hours. MR imaging is usually done immediately after injection.

Adverse reactions to gadolinium contrast agents are quite uncommon. Common signs and symptoms for mild reactions include the following:

- Nausea and vomiting
- Headache
- Warmth or coldness at the injection site
- Paresthesia
- Dizziness
- Itching

Life-threatening reactions are rare. Gadolinium has no nephron toxicity at doses used for MRI. Since gadolinium agents are radiopaque, they have been used in conventional angiography in patients with renal impairment or severe reaction to iodinated contrast.

Nephrogenic Systemic Fibrosis

Nephrogenic systemic fibrosis (NSF), originally described in 2000, is a systemic disorder characterized by widespread tissue fibrosis following the administration of a gadolinium-based contrast agent in individuals with noticeable advanced renal failure. This disease causes fibrosis of the skin and connective tissues throughout the body. Patients with NSF develop skin thickening that may prevent bending and extending of joints, resulting in their decreased mobility. Affected patients also experience fibrosis that has spread to other parts of the body such as the diaphragm, muscles of the thigh and lower abdomen, and interior areas of the lung vessels. The clinical course is progressive and fatal.

Patients at high risk for reduced renal function include those with the following risk factors:

- Age 65 or over
- Diabetes mellitus
- History of renal disease or renal transplants
- History of liver transplantation or hepatorenal syndrome

As a safety precaution, serum creatinine and estimated GFR should be obtained in all patients with reduced renal function. Patients, who have a GFR of less than 30 mL/min should not be given contrast.

IV Contrast and the Pregnant Patient

The safety of fetal exposure to CT and MR contrast agents is not well described in the literature. The current recommendation is to avoid routine administration of contrast agents in pregnant patients unless the information is critical to the management of the patient (risk vs benefit). Alternate imaging studies like ultrasound also must be considered.

Reference

Reproduced with permission from Grey ML., Alinani JM. CT & MRI Pathology: A Pocket Atlas, 3rd ed. New York: McGraw-Hill; 2018.

3

Overview of Medical-Legal Issues in Magnetic Resonance Imaging for Technologists

The frequency of medical-legal issues continues to increase, including in the area of medical imaging. This chapter aims to better prepare medical imaging students and entry-level employees for the workforce and to help employers avoid ligation. The legal cases in this chapter are only examples of legal principles. It is important to note that health law is constantly changing and evolving over time. This chapter is not a substitute for legal advice.

RATE OF MRI ACCIDENTS

From 1995 through 2005, a total of 389 reported MRI safety incidents were reported by the Food and Drug Administration's (FDA's) Manufacturer and User Facility Device Experience (MAUDE) database.[1] At first glance, MRI appears to have a low rate of incidents; however, of the 389 reported incidents, "nine were deaths, 302 were incidents attributable to MR technology, and 87 were 'other' and not specific to MR technology."[2] Most deaths were caused by implantable device failures, "such as pacemakers and insulin pumps."[3] Other deaths included that of Michael Colombini (see The Michael Colombini Tragedy section later in this chapter) and the asphyxiation of an engineer.[4] Of the reported MRI injuries, "71% were burns, 10% were implant-related, and 10% resulted from projectiles."[5] Nevertheless, the actual number of MRI accidents may be much higher because of confusion about what is reported and what should be reported to the FDA.[6] It was estimated that the FDA MAUDE database "captures less than 10% of MR incidents and less than half of all deaths."[7]

Beginning June 2004, during a 16-month period, Pennsylvania reported 88 MRI incidents after it required all MRI incidents to be reported.[8] The mandatory reporting system included "near misses," which were frequently not reported to the FDA's MAUDE database.[9] Fortunately, all 88 reported incidents did not result in patient injuries but resulted from screening errors; contraindications discovered during or after imaging; incompatible equipment, which could become projectiles; and potential burns.[10]

The number of MAUDE-reported, MRI-related incidents fluctuated from 2009 to 2012.[11] A total of 194 incidents were reported in 2009, 169 in 2010, 186 in 2011, and 164 in 2012.[12] Further, the increase in MRI-related incidents is ever more worrisome because the number of MRI installations doubled between 2004 and 2009.[13]

RADIOLOGIC TECHNOLOGIST MALPRACTICE PAYMENTS

The National Practitioner Data Bank (NPDB) was established by the Health Care Quality Improvement Act of 1986.[14] The NPDB lists "adverse hospital privileging actions, professional society reports, and malpractice payments made on behalf of licensed health care practitioners."[15] Any entity, insurance company, or organization making a payment on behalf of a health care practitioner due to a malpractice settlement or judgment is required to report the payment to the NPDB.[16]

Between 1991 and 2008, a total of 155 radiologic technologist malpractice cases were reported to the NPDB.[17] Nationally, malpractice payments ranged from 2 to 16 per year.[18] Of the 155 radiologic technologist malpractice cases, 135 provided litigation information.[19] Ninety-four percent (ie, 127 cases) of the 135 cases resulted in negotiated settlements, and the remaining 6% (ie, 8 cases) resulted in court judgments.[20] Eighty-eight percent (ie, 137 cases) were paid by insurance companies or insurance guarantee funds, 8% (ie, 13 cases) were paid by self-insurance, and 3% (ie, 5 cases) were paid by state medical malpractice funds.[21]

Radiologic technologist malpractice payments ranged from $750 to $11.5 million, with a median payment of $57,500 and only 2 payments exceeding $1 million.[22] Extracting the 2 outlier payments of over $1 million, the mean payment was $177,598.[23] By comparison, during the same period, 325,104 malpractice cases were recorded in the NPDB for all health care providers, with a range of $50 to $27.5 million.[24] It is difficult to explain the infrequency of medical malpractice cases against radiologic technologists when the number of technologists and the nation's population have increased between 1991 and 2008.[25]

The most probable cause for the stability and low frequency of medical malpractice cases against radiologic technologists may be from the "shielding technologists receive from the hospitals and physicians with whom they are affiliated."[26] The injured plaintiff will often look to other codefendants for the capital to meet a settlement or jury verdict, even though the technologist was the party against whom negligent conduct was alleged.[27] Hospitals and radiologists take on a large amount of vicarious liability for the actions of technologists.[28]

A technologist is typically an "employee of a hospital, outpatient imaging facility, or radiology group."[29] Therefore, in these cases, the technologist's employer is named as a codefendant or sole defendant, rather than the technologist himself or herself.[30] The employer "becomes the deep pocket for the monies assessed by a jury or agreed on in a settlement."[31] Plaintiff's attorneys often formulate an allegation of wrongdoing to make the employer the sole or primary defendant because the technologist is less likely to have adequate assets or liability insurance to compensate the patient.[32]

Radiologists or supervising physicians are often included as codefendants or sole defendants.[33] Plaintiff's attorneys draw the physicians into the lawsuit under the legal theory of the borrowed servant doctrine, where the technologist is the "borrowed servant of the supervising physician."[34] For example, a supervising radiologist may be negligent for interpreting inadequate images acquired by a technologist.[35]

QUICK REFERENCE GUIDE TO AVOID LEGAL ISSUES

The reference guide below is a summary of the concepts that will be discussed in detail throughout this chapter and should help you avoid legal issues. If you have any questions, please review the relevant sections of this chapter. The list below is not exhaustive. After reading this chapter and spending time in the workplace, you may think of additional items to add to this list.

- Introduce yourself (name and position).
- Confirm that you have the correct patient, order, and imaging protocol.
- Explain the exam and answer the patient's questions. If you do not know the answer to a question, look it up or ask a colleague. Use correct terminology (eg, contrast media, not dye).
- Go over the screening form with the patient and individual(s) going back with the patient. Research any implants and determine whether it is safe to proceed.
- Obtain patient consent to proceed with the exam. If informed consent is required, verify that it has been obtained by a physician.
- If the exam requires contrast and the patient is female, a negative pregnancy test or a refusal of pregnancy testing waiver is required. Follow the policy at your facility.
- Position the patient correctly and use the correct coil.
- Immobilize the patient with straps, sandbags, and sponges, but be sure the patient is comfortable.
- Explain that you will need to touch the patient and explain why. Be respectful of the patient and respect their wishes. Do not just begin touching the patient without an explanation and consent.
- If the patient refuses to continue with the exam at any point, bring the patient out of the bore of the scanner and talk to the patient. Often, the patient just needs a short break and may decide to continue. If the patient refuses to continue, end the exam (within reason).
- When starting an intravenous (IV) line, explain what you are doing. Do not start an IV without notifying the patient. If a patient refuses the IV, discuss with the patient. Often, the patient just needs an explanation. If the patient continues to refuse, document this in the patient's chart and follow the protocol at your facility. Often, the radiologist and/or requesting physician may wish to be notified.
- Use the correct contrast media and the correct dosage.
- Document the following in the patient's chart:
  - Document pertinent exam details.
  - Document whether contrast media was administered and information about the IV.
  - Document using correct terminology (eg, contrast media, not dye; computed tomography [CT], not computerized axial tomography [CAT] scan).
- Do not make disparaging comments about the patient to anyone.
- When using social media, refrain from posting anything about the patient or exam.

AMERICAN SOCIETY OF RADIOLOGIC TECHNOLOGISTS PRACTICE STANDARDS

The American Society of Radiologic Technologists (ASRT), the premier professional association for medical imaging technologists, has established practice standards to serve as a guide for appropriate practice.[36] These practice standards are created by the profession to govern the quality of practice, education, and service provided by those in the medical imaging profession as technologists.[37] The practice standards may be utilized by facilities to create practice parameters or as an "overview of the role and responsibilities of the individual as defined by the profession."[38] The ASRT requires that a technologist be "educationally prepared and clinically competent as a prerequisite to professional practice."[39] The practice standards may be superseded by state and federal laws, lawful institutional policies and procedures, and governmental accreditation standards.[40] It is important for technologists to understand the practice standards and keep current. Adhering to the practice standards reduces the potential for litigation and helps the technologist provide excellent patient care. The practice standards will be used throughout this chapter.

THE US LEGAL SYSTEM

The US Constitution (federal) and state constitutions divide power among the legislative, executive, and judicial branches. The federal legislative branch makes or enacts laws and has authority to confirm or reject presidential appointments and declare war. This branch includes Congress, which is divided into the Senate and House of Representatives. The federal executive branch carries out and enforces laws. This branch includes the president, vice president, cabinet, executive departments, independent agencies, and other committees and commissions. The federal judicial branch evaluates and applies laws; in other words, the judicial branch interprets and applies laws to individual cases. It also decides if laws violate the Constitution. This branch includes the Supreme Court and other federal courts.

Each state has its own state constitution that is similar, if not identical, in structure to the US Constitution (ie, three branches of government). In addition, the specific duties of each branch (ie, legislative, executive, and judicial) of state government are similar to those of the federal government but pertain only to the state and not the federal government. For example, a state senate does not have authority to confirm or reject nominees to the US Supreme Court made by the President of the United States.

Federal law consists of the Constitution, statutes, regulations, treaties, and common law. State law consists of the state constitution, statutes, regulations, and common law. The federal government and all states, except Louisiana (which practices civil law), practice common law. The American common law system dates back to England. Common law is derived from court decisions and allows the law to adapt and grow as courts make rulings. Tort law is a function of common law that may have statutory restrictions and is largely a creature of state common law at that.

Judicial proceedings may be categorized as either a civil or criminal action. Civil actions are brought to enforce, compensate, or protect a civil right. Civil actions involve noncriminal matters, including torts (or civil wrongs). On the other hand, a criminal action is brought by the government against a party so the defendant may be punished for offenses made against the public. This chapter will focus on civil actions. In a civil suit, the plaintiff is the party that brings a lawsuit in a court of law against an opposing party, the defendant. The defendant is the party being sued.

Multiple people may be joined in a lawsuit (uniting parties or claims into a single lawsuit). For example, the defendants in a radiology department lawsuit could include the hospital, radiologist, and technologist. Conversely, if multiple people are harmed by the same physician, then their lawsuits can be joined into one suit, where multiple persons would be plaintiffs. Litigation is the process of bringing a lawsuit. A lawsuit, also known as a suit, is any legal action by a party against another party in a court of law.

THEORIES OF LIABILITY

This section focuses on several important theories of legal liability that apply to technologists. Generally, liability refers to a legal responsibility, obligation, or accountability to another person. The doctrine of professional liability is important for technologists to understand. Professional liability is accountability for an injured party, so that the injured person may seek damages. Technologists are accountable to patients, physicians, and all other health care professionals and may be liable for their misconduct. Technologists should understand the following doctrines and terminology and consult employer policies regarding specific procedures and protocols.

Agency

Agency is a fiduciary relationship, which means that one party—the agent—acts on behalf of another party—the principal. In this capacity, the agent's actions or words are binding upon the principal. For example, a supervising party is held vicariously (ie, indirectly) liable for the conduct of a subordinate or associate. In other words, a hospital may be held responsible for the actions of its employees, including technologists.

Respondeat Superior

Respondeat superior (ri-**spond**-dee-at soo-**peer**-ee-ər) is a Latin phrase that means "let the superior make answer." The doctrine of respondeat superior holds an employer (ie, the principal) liable for an employee's (ie, agent's) wrongful acts, when committed in the scope of employment. The elements of a cause of action for hospital liability under respondeat superior are:

1. An *employment relationship* existed between the defendant, as employer, and the employee whose negligence caused the plaintiffs injury;
2. The defendant employee was *acting within the scope of his or her employment* when negligently causing the plaintiffs injury; and
3. Proof of all of the elements necessary to establish the employee's liability as a defendant in a negligence action.[41]

Additionally, the plaintiff will most likely want to add the employer (eg, hospital, medical center, imaging facility) to a lawsuit because the employer has deeper pockets to pay damages. Insurance companies representing hospitals or imaging facilities are poised to pay large sums of money on behalf of the defendant. It is important to think about the job security of a technologist found to be at fault, even if the lawsuit bypasses the employee and focuses on the employer. The technologist employee could be looking for a new job, which may be difficult because the former employer would probably not give a favorable employee recommendation.

Borrowed Servant

The doctrine of borrowed servant uses the doctrine of respondeat superior to hold employers (ie, the principals) liable for the negligence of their employees (ie, agents). For example, a patient is injured because of the negligence of an MRI technologist. The patient brings a lawsuit against the technologist (ie, employee) and hospital (ie, employer). Often, the charge against the employer is negligent hiring practices or negligent supervision. Physicians may also be held liable for the negligence of employees under their control.

Temporary agency is common in health care, and the lines of who is in charge may be blurry. Technologists should be mindful of who is in charge during an exam and whose orders they are following. Technologists are generally under the direction and guidance of a radiologist; however, this is often disputed. Radiologists are typically not in the control room when the exam is performed but may be liable for the negligence of a technologist. Depending on the situation, technologists may be under the direction and guidance of other physicians, such as an anesthesiologist or emergency department physician.

MEDICAL-LEGAL ISSUES

The following subsections dive deeper into the Theories of Liability and discuss medical malpractice, intentional torts, defenses to the intentional torts, res ipsa loquitor, dam ages, defenses to negligence, agency, and ethics.

Medical Malpractice

Negligence is the failure of someone to practice to the standard of care that a reasonable, minimally competent professional in that field would have provided in the same or similar circumstances. The reasonable, minimally competent professional is a hypothetical person who practices with a level of knowledge, intelligence, attention, and judgment that society requires.

Medical malpractice is a specific kind of negligence claim, also known as professional negligence. Medical malpractice is the failure of a member of the medical profession to perform a duty of skill, care, and diligence exercised by members of the same profession. The elements of medical malpractice are the same as negligence (ie, duty, breach, causation, and damages), but the conduct occurs within a professional relationship and involves questions of medical judgment. However, some state legislatures have special rules in medical malpractice cases, such as limits on damages. The following five elements are required to satisfy a claim of medical malpractice:

1. Professional relationship (in this case, between the technologist and patient);
2. A duty of care to the patient;
3. The duty of care has been breached;
4. Causation; and
5. Damages

All of the elements must be met and are discussed further below.

Professional Relationship

Negligence and medical malpractice are similar but have several differences. Medical malpractice claims occur "within the course of a professional relationship" and "raise questions involving medical judgment."[42] Courts ask 2 questions when assessing whether a claim is ordinary negligence or medical malpractice: (1) whether the claim occurred within the course of a professional relationship and (2) whether the claim raises questions of medical judgment beyond common knowledge and experience.[43] If the answers to both questions are yes, then the action is considered within the realm of medical malpractice; if not, then it is ordinary negligence.[44] A professional relationship encompasses licensed health care professionals, licensed health care facilities, and agents or employees of a licensed health care facility, who owe a contractual duty to provide professional health care services.[45]

The following case example will help in differentiating medical malpractice and negligence.[46] A plaintiff (ie, a patient) filed suit against a medical center for injuries sustained during an MRI exam. The patient was involved in an all-terrain vehicle accident and sustained injury to her knee. The patient underwent successful surgery, and her leg was placed in a full brace. Ten days later, the patient underwent an MRI exam on the same leg. The technologists inspected, tested, and approved the leg brace to proceed with the MRI exam. As the exam began, the leg brace became attracted to the MRI unit and stuck to the bore of the unit. Movement of the leg brace caused the patient to suffer additional injuries.

The patient (ie, the plaintiff) filed suit against the medical center for ordinary negligence and breach of contract. The plaintiff argued that it was common knowledge of the general public that metallic objects, which are subject to magnetism, are not to be placed near or in the vicinity of an MRI unit. The plaintiff filed a second suit alleging medical malpractice, in conjunction with the ordinary negligence and breach of contract claims. Plaintiff argued that the defendant is liable for medical malpractice because the defendants failed to "conform and adhere to the recognized standard of acceptable professional practice and failed to give proper medical treatment to the plaintiff." The lawsuits were consolidated, and the defendant moved to have the suit dismissed. The trial court dismissed the plaintiff's claim because it did not comply with state law.

On appeal, the issue became whether the plaintiff's claims constituted ordinary negligence, medical malpractice, or both. The court determined that the distinction between ordinary negligence and medical malpractice depends on whether the acts or omissions in the complaint "involve a matter of medical science or art requiring specialized skills not ordinarily possessed by lay persons" or whether the acts or omissions may be "assessed on the basis of common everyday experience."

The court determined that the MRI technologist's evaluation of the patient prior to entering the MRI unit "required specialized expertise substantially related to the rendition of medical treatment." The technologist made a judgment regarding the amount and type of metal. These judgments are not matters that may be assessed on the "basis of common everyday experience" and require specialized training. Patient evaluation and preparation for the exam was a "substantial relationship to the rendition of medical treatment by a medical professional" and constitutes medical malpractice if it deviates from the standard of care.

The key takeaway from this example is that technologists may be liable for medical malpractice because technologists have a professional relationship with the patient and utilize special expertise when evaluating and preparing patients for exams.

Duty of Care

The next element of malpractice (ie, professional negligence) is duty of care, which is the legal responsibility one has toward the well-being of another. The duty of care is a legal obligation set to the level of the standard of care in professional situations. The standard of care may be divided into 4 parts: (1) care in the sense of attention, caution, alertness, and diligence; (2) care through education, training, skill, or experience; (3) sound professional judgment; and (4) use of personal superior abilities.[47] Sometimes, the standard of care varies by location and region, and courts may consider staffing, resources, and training opportunities, for example; however, this does not extend to professional judgments. The standard of care is established through expert testimony.

Author Daniel Penofsky published an article entitled "Diagnostic Radiology Litigation," in which he analyzed diagnostic radiology litigation. The article includes a list of the duties of a technologist. Generally, a technologist will most likely meet the standard of care if he or she satisfies the typical duties of a technologist. For example, the following are specific duties of care owed by a technologist to a patient:

- Duty to test radiologic imaging equipment before its use to make certain it is functioning properly
- Duty to document the proper functioning of radiologic imaging equipment
- Duty to initiate the repair of radiologic imaging equipment found to be defective or not functioning properly
- Duty to document the repair of defective radiologic equipment
- Duty to correlate the primary or referring physician's radiologic imaging order or requisition slip with the patient, to assure that the proper patient is about to undergo the radiologic imaging study
- Duty to inquire whether the patient has suffered any allergic reactions to contrast agents or media
- Duty to follow the primary or referring physician's orders or instructions pertaining to the radiologic imaging studies to be performed
- Duty to adhere to the hospital's or private facility's policies and procedures manual or similarly titled directives governing the use and operation of radiologic equipment
- Duty to comply with applicable state and federal requirements governing the use and operation of radiologic equipment
- Duty to exercise due care, skill, and diligence in the positioning of the patient, aiming and focusing the radiologic camera, taking diagnostic images, and taking all necessary steps and precautions to obtain radiologic films that are readable and capable of interpretation by the radiologist
- Duty to exercise due care, skill, and diligence so as not to injure the patient during the performance of the radiologic imaging study
- Duty to timely transmit the radiologic films of the correct patient to the radiologist for interpretation[48]

While this list is not exclusive, these duties are applicable to all technologists, no matter the modality. The duties closely align with the ASRT practice standards (see the ASRT Practice Standards for Medical Imaging and Radiation Therapy at https://www.asrt.org/main/standards-and-regulations/professional-practice/practice-standards-online). Following these duties will protect the patient and technologist and also may avoid legal issues.

Breach of Duty

The next element of professional negligence is a breach of duty. The defendant breaches their duty when, under the circumstances, their conduct falls short of the standard of care owed to the plaintiff. In other words, a breach of duty is a violation of the duty of care technologists owe to patients, physicians, and all other health care workers. The standard of care asks, "What would a reasonable health care professional who is minimally competent and reasonably situated do in a similar circumstance?" The plaintiff (ie, the patient) must use the testimony from an expert witness to establish the standard of care and the defendant's failure to meet that standard. Generally, expert witnesses are individuals who have the required education and experiences to testify as to the subject of the lawsuit.

Causation

The next element of malpractice (ie, professional negligence) is causation. Causation is shown by evidence that the injury to the plaintiff is a natural and probable consequence of the defendant's negligence. Causation is established by showing (1) a causal connection between the defendant's breach of the duty and the resulting injury[49] and (2) that it is fair to hold the defendant responsible for the plaintiff's injuries under the law.[50]

Damages

The final element of professional negligence is damages, which is the term for the monetary award after winning a lawsuit. Damages are awarded only if a physical or emotional injury is proven and was caused by the defendant's breach of duty. Damages that the plaintiff suffered must be a direct result of the injury. In tort cases, including negligence, the purpose of damages is to restore the plaintiff (ie, the patient) to *status quo ante* (Latin for "the way things were before"). In other words, the monetary award is to restore the plaintiff to the way they were before the injury. The plaintiff is potentially eligible for two forms of monetary damages: compensatory and punitive.

Compensatory Damages Compensatory damages are awarded to compensate the plaintiff for the harm they suffered. In personal injury cases, compensatory damages are based on economic and noneconomic losses. The plaintiff is compensated for economic losses, such as past and future medical expenses, permanent disability and disfigurement, and loss of earning capacity or reduced earning capacity. The plaintiff may also be compensated for past and future pain and suffering and loss of enjoyment.

Punitive Damages In addition to compensatory damages, punitive damages are awarded to the plaintiff and aimed at punishing the defendant for willfully or recklessly causing the plaintiff harm. The policy behind punitive damages is to penalize the defendant or to make them an example. It is intended to deter undesirable conduct. Punitive damages are only awarded in extreme cases.

Res Ipsa Loquitor: A Presumption of Negligence Based on the Injury

Res ipsa loquitor (rays **ip**-sə **loh**-kwə-tər) is a Latin phrase that means "the thing speaks for itself." Under this doctrine, the fact that an accident occurred raises enough of an inference of negligence to establish a case. It occurs when (1) an accident would not normally occur unless the defendant's (ie, hospital's) conduct was negligent; (2) the accident was caused by an agent or instrumentality under the exclusive control of the defendant; and (3) the accident was not attributable to the plaintiff (ie, the patient).[51]

The first use of the res ipsa loquitur doctrine was in *Byrne v. Boadle*.[52] In this case, the plaintiff was passing by the defendant's warehouse. A barrel of flour rolled from the defendant's shop window, fell on the plaintiff's head, and injured him. At trial, the plaintiff did not show how the barrel of flour fell from the window. The trial judge sided with the plaintiff. On appeal, the judge stated: "There are certain cases of which it may be said *res ipsa loquitur* and this seems one of them. In some cases, the Court has held that the mere fact of the accident having occurred is evidence of negligence."[53] Two years later, in the case *Scott v. London & St. Katherine Docs Co.*, Chief Justice Erle offered the first clear statement of the res ipsa loquitur doctrine:

> There must be reasonable evidence of negligence. But where the thing is shown to be under the management of the defendant or his servants, and the accident is such as in the ordinary course of things does not happen if those who have the management use proper care, it affords reasonable evidence, in the absence of explanation by the defendant that the accident arose from want of care.[54]

Res ipsa loquitur has been applied in negligence and malpractice actions.[55] Res ipsa allows plaintiffs without evidence of the elements of negligence to present their case on a suggestion of negligence. The plaintiff shows the facts and circumstances regarding the injury and makes the argument that the defendant's negligence is the reasonable cause. "It is not enough that plaintiff's counsel can suggest a possibility of negligence."[56]

The case of *Ybarra v. Spangard* is a good example of the res ipsa loquitur doctrine as applied to the medical arena.[57] In the case, the plaintiff brought an action for damages for personal injuries alleged to have been caused by defendants (Dr. Spangard and others) during a surgical operation.[58]

Plaintiff consulted defendant Dr. Tilley, who diagnosed his ailment as appendicitis and made arrangements for an appendectomy to be performed by defendant Dr. Spangard at a hospital owned and managed by defendant Dr. Swift. Plaintiff entered the hospital, was given a hypodermic injection, slept, and later was awakened by Drs. Tilley and Spangard and wheeled into the operating room by a nurse whom he believed to be defendant Gisler, an employee of Dr. Swift. Defendant Dr. Reser, the anesthetist, also an employee of Dr. Swift, adjusted plaintiff for the operation, pulling his body to the head of the operating table and, according to plaintiff's testimony, laying him back against two hard objects at the top of his shoulders, about an inch below his neck. Dr. Reser then administered the anesthetic, and plaintiff lost consciousness. When he awoke early the following morning, he was in his hospital room attended by defendant Thompson, the special nurse, and another nurse who was not made a defendant.

Plaintiff testified that, prior to the operation, he had never had any pain in, or injury to, his right arm or shoulder, but that when he awakened, he felt a sharp pain about halfway between the neck and the point of the right shoulder. He complained to the nurse and then to Dr. Tilley, who gave him diathermy treatments while he remained in the hospital. The pain did not cease but spread down to the lower part of his arm, and after his release from the hospital, the condition grew worse. He was unable to rotate or lift his arm and developed paralysis and atrophy of the muscles around the shoulder. He received further treatments from Dr. Tilley until March of 1940 and then returned to work, wearing his arm in a splint on the advice of Dr. Spangard.

Plaintiff also consulted Dr. Wilfred Sterling Clark, who had x-rays taken that showed an area of diminished sensation below the shoulder and atrophy and wasting away of the muscles around the shoulder. In the opinion of Dr. Clark, plaintiff's condition was due to trauma or injury by pressure or strain applied between his right shoulder and neck. Plaintiff was also examined by Dr. Fernando Garduno, who expressed the opinion that plaintiff's injury was a paralysis of traumatic origin, not arising from pathologic causes, and not systemic, and that the injury resulted in atrophy, loss of use, and restriction of motion of the right arm and shoulder.

The Supreme Court of California found for the plaintiff. The court found that every defendant in whose custody the plaintiff was placed for any period was bound to exercise ordinary care to see that no unnecessary harm came to him and each would be liable for failure in this regard. Any defendant who negligently injured him, and any defendant charged with his care who so neglected him as to allow injury to occur, would be liable. The defendant employers would be liable for the neglect of their employees, and the doctor in charge of the operation would be liable for the negligence of those who became his temporary servants for the purpose of assisting in the operation.

Defenses to Medical Malpractice and Negligence

Comparative Negligence

Comparative negligence is when the plaintiff's (ie, the patient's) own negligence comparably reduces recoverable damages. The negligence of the plaintiff is compared to the negligence of the defendant. The reduction in damages is comparable to the plaintiff's level of fault in causing the injury. Most states have adopted a form of the comparative negligence doctrine.[59] Some states only allow recovery of damages if the plaintiff's negligence is less than 50% or 51%.

For example, a patient (ie, the plaintiff) fails to disclose their full medical history to the technologist and suffers an injury as a result. The technologist may claim that the patient was comparatively negligent by not disclosing their full medical history. The court may reduce the amount the plaintiff recovers by the level of fault. Alternatively, the court could find the patient was 60% negligent because their own negligence was a part in causing the injury, and in some states, the patient may not be able to recover damages.

Assumption of the Risk

Assumption of the risk is the principle that some activities have inherent risks. A plaintiff assumes the risk and is unable to recover for the negligent conduct that causes the harm. In other words, a plaintiff may be barred from recovering damages due to an injury because they knew the risk involved. Many states have incorporated assumption of risk into comparative and contributory negligence.[59]

Informed Consent

Certain exams and procedures require the patient's informed consent prior to entering the MRI suite. The technologist must know which exams require informed consent. A majority of states have adopted the professional disclosure standard, where the duty to inform the patient is by the standard of what a reasonable medical practitioner similar situated would disclose to the patient.[60] Testimony by an expert witness is required to establish what information should be disclosed to the patient.[61] A minority of states use a reasonable patient standard, where the standard is what a reasonable patient in the same or similar circumstance would like to know when deciding whether to undergo a proposed medical action (eg, therapy or surgery).

Informed consent must be obtained by a physician and requires the physician to discuss (1) the nature of the treatment, (2) risks and benefits of the treatment, and (3) alternative procedures and associated risks.[62] The patient must have the appropriate mental capacity to make the decision voluntarily and without coercion.[63] Many cases of battery involve physicians who perform treatments that exceed the informed consent they gave, where the patient did not consent to the new treatment.[64]

Physicians obtain informed consent because it involves the practice of medicine and only physicians are licensed to practice medicine. The ASRT practice standards require technologists to verify that informed consent has been obtained.[65] Policies and procedures for obtaining informed consent may differ among imaging facilities, but a radiologist will most likely obtain informed consent. Informed consent must be reduced to writing, and technologists must have this documentation before escorting the patient to the MRI suite. Performing additional unconsented procedures makes the technologist liable if something goes wrong. It is important to note that the practice standards require technologists to educate and inform the patient regarding the exam; however, only physicians are qualified to discuss treatment risks, benefits, and alternative procedures. Further, it is important for the technologist to read their employer's policies regarding informed consent.

Statutes of Limitations and Repose

Statutes of limitation and repose establish a time limit on when a plaintiff (ie, the patient) may bring a suit against a defendant. The statutes allow a plaintiff a reasonable amount of time to bring a suit. Without the time limit, a defendant could face the threat of litigation for an indefinite period of time.

Malpractice Examples

Example 1[66]

Plaintiff (ie, a patient) presented to defendant's MRI facility for imaging. Following the MRI, plaintiff, who was lying on a table, attempted to stand. Plaintiff became lightheaded, lost his balance, and fell. Plaintiff alleged that defendant's employee failed to properly assist plaintiff in standing, in violation of the duty of care. Defendant (employer) contended that its technologist was making his way toward plaintiff to assist plaintiff in standing when the accident occurred and that plaintiff failed to exercise due care for his own safety by getting up too fast from a prone (lying flat and face down) position. Per plaintiff's counsel, the fact that plaintiff had preexisting back problems and that there was no permanency to plaintiff's injuries had an impact on the outcome. The jury awarded plaintiff damages.

The important takeaways from this case are that technologists need to guard against patient falls and technologists should follow the policies and procedures of their employer. The ASRT practice standards allow the technologist to immobilize the patient for the exam. Straps and sandbags will restrict patient movement and could prevent a patient from falling off the scanner table.

Example 2[67]

Plaintiff went to defendant's MRI and CT center for an MRI examination of his lumbar spine. While being introduced into the MRI, he felt a pressure on his head, and the machine continued to move, bending his head forward and to the left and injuring his neck. Plaintiff alleged that the MRI technologist did not stop when plaintiff first indicated that he was in trouble and that he was improperly positioned in the unit. Defendants contended that plaintiff's description of the occurrence was not possible, that plaintiff simply raised his head and bumped it slightly against the side of the unit, and that plaintiff did not complain of any injuries at the time of the incident. Defendants also contended that plaintiff had contacted the manager of the facility within two or three days and had only complained about being treated rudely and that he had not alleged that he had twisted his neck in the unit or alleged any problems with his neck. Defendants further contended that plaintiff had a preexisting condition, that the bump the plaintiff incurred had at most aggravated his condition for a short time, and that plaintiff's condition was caused by degenerative changes.

At trial, plaintiff introduced evidence to prove that the incident could have occurred as plaintiff stated and that defendant's account of what occurred was inconsistent with their actions subsequent to the incident, including the calling of a technologist to look at the unit, and plaintiff provided the testimony of an independent doctor who stated that she had contacted the facility to question them about plaintiff's incident and had informed them of the details of that incident. The case was one of credibility, and the jury evidently accepted plaintiff's statement of what had occurred even though plaintiff stated that he did not know what he had hit and could not explain how it had happened. The jury awarded plaintiff $25,000 in damages and $7,000 for costs.

An important takeaway from this case is that the ASRT practice standards require technologists to provide optimal patient care and to assume responsibility for patient needs during exams. Further, technologists are to explain each step of the exam and obtain patient cooperation. When positioning the patient, it is important to respect patient comfort. A comfortable and content patient will provide for a quality exam. Remember, patients may retract consent at any time, and the technologist must respect the wishes of the patient or legal guardian.

Example 3[68]

Plaintiff was admitted to a hospital with a possible stroke. During her visit to the emergency department, a neurologist was reportedly consulted and recommended an MRI. According to the plaintiff, the technologist who performed her MRI failed to question her concerning her implanted transcutaneous electrical nerve stimulation (TENS) unit for her neurogenic bladder. As a result of the MRI, plaintiff said her TENS unit became dysfunctional and had to be surgically replaced. She said she continued to have bladder dysfunction due to the incident. Plaintiff filed suit alleging the defendant was liable via the doctrine of respondeat superior as the employer of the alleged negligent party.

The plaintiff sought compensation for her mental anguish, physical pain and suffering, loss of enjoyment of life, lost wages, and unnecessary medical expenses. The jury found in favor of the plaintiff, awarding $100,000 in damages for permanent disability, physical and mental pain and suffering, inconvenience, and anxiety; $150,000 for loss of enjoyment of life; $334,412.25 for past medical expenses; and $15,587.75 for future medical expenses.

An important takeaway from this case is that technologists must properly screen the patient and review the patient's medical record for potential contraindications, such as implanted hardware. Once again, it is important to follow the employer's policies and procedures. The *Reference Manual for Magnetic Resonance Safety, Implants, and Devices* and the website MRIsafety.com (http://www.mrisafety.com) by Frank Shellock provide information about MRI screening forms and whether hardware is safe, conditional, or unsafe. It is important to document your findings in the patient's chart.

Example 4[69]

Plaintiff underwent a breast MRI exam. Plaintiff was face down on the table when a technologist attempted to place an earplug into her ear. Plaintiff said she was frightened and somewhat startled and she asked the technologist if an earplug was really necessary. Plaintiff claimed the technologist said it was not and proceeded with the MRI. During the exam, plaintiff experienced ear pain, which she claimed caused permanent damage, including tinnitus (ringing in the ears) and hyperacusis (oversensitivity to frequency and sound volume ranges). Plaintiff alleged the American College of Radiology's guidelines and the policies and procedures of defendant MRI center mandated ear protection. Defendant contended plaintiff knowingly and voluntarily declined ear protection. The parties resolved the matter during mediation for the sum of $132,500 plus payment of the mediator's fees by defendant.

An important takeaway from this case is that the technologist should not have said that the earplugs were not necessary. The technologist should educate the patient about the loud noises the MRI unit will produce and the length of exam. Further, the patient and anyone else in the MRI suite during the exam should be provided with hearing protection.

Example 5[70]

Plaintiff took her mother to the MRI center for an MRI of her spine. In the MRI center reception area, the technologist had plaintiff's mother fill out some screening forms and then took her into the MRI room. After a few minutes, the technologist reappeared and told plaintiff to come into the MRI room and sit with her nervous mother. The technologist then placed plaintiff at the head of the MRI unit and told her to lean over into the MRI unit and talk to her mother during the exam to calm her. The technologist left the room and started the exam.

After a few minutes, plaintiff became dizzy and nauseous. She pulled her head away from the MRI unit and began screaming for help. The technologist stopped the exam, ran into the MRI room, and asked plaintiff what was wrong. Plaintiff explained that she felt like her head was going to explode. Then, for the first time, the technologist asked the plaintiff if she had any metal in her body. Plaintiff informed the technologist that she had undergone prior brain surgery in 1972 during which a metal aneurysm clip had been placed.

Plaintiff suffered a recurring aneurysm, left cerebral ischemia, and permanent right-side deficits and memory loss. Plaintiff later underwent brain surgery to repair a recurring aneurysm at the site of the aneurysm clip. She spent several months undergoing therapy to regain minimal function in her right arm. She has since learned to write with her left hand. Plaintiff alleged that the MRI technologist failed to screen her before she entered the MRI room and that the magnetic forces emitted by the MRI unit caused the aneurysm clip to move, causing plaintiff's subsequent brain injury. After the incident, defendant adopted a policy that all persons (not just patients) were to be screened before entering the MRI room. Defendants contended that the MRI did not cause the aneurysm clip to move and that the MRI technologist adequately screened plaintiff before she entered the room. Plaintiff was awarded $1,250,000 and $74,839.23 for attorneys' fees and expenses.

An important takeaway from this case, as stated earlier for Example 3, is that technologists must properly screen anyone who enters the MRI suite and review the patient's medical record for potential contraindications, such as implanted hardware. Once again, it is important to follow the employer's policies and procedures. The *Reference Manual for Magnetic Resonance Safety, Implants, and Devices* and the website MRIsafety.com (http://www.mrisafety.com) by Frank Shellock provide information about MRI screening forms and whether hardware is safe, conditional, or unsafe. It is important to document your findings in the patient's chart.

Example 6[71]

Plaintiff sustained a right hip fracture that required surgical repair when she fell off a radiography table after undergoing a radiology exam under the care of defendants. The plaintiff claimed the defendants were vicariously liable for the radiology technologist's violation of the standard of care. She claimed the technologist failed to assist her off the radiography table. Plaintiff was legally blind. The defendants denied liability and denied that the technologist violated the standard of care. Defendants claimed that the technologist instructed the plaintiff to stay on the table until she could assist her. The jury determined the plaintiff and the defendants were comparatively negligent (see below) and allocated 40% of the negligence to the defendants and 60% to the plaintiff. The plaintiff was awarded $72,000.

An important takeaway from this case, as stated earlier in Example 1, is that technologists need to guard against patient falls.

Technologists should follow the policies and procedures of their employer. The ASRT practice standards allow the technologist to immobilize the patient for the exam. Straps and sandbags will restrict patient movement and could prevent a patient from falling off the scanner table.

Negligent Infliction of Emotional Distress

Negligent infliction of emotional distress is another specific form of negligence and occurs when the plaintiff suffers severe emotional distress resulting from the defendant's negligence. Most courts will allow the recovery of damages when physical contact occurs or if the plaintiff is in the "zone of danger." The zone of danger refers to the dangerous area created by the negligence of the defendant. The plaintiff must be in the zone of danger, which unreasonably threatens the physical safety of the plaintiff. For example, a plaintiff's distress is from a physical injury caused by the defendant, or the plaintiff witnessed a severe injury or death of a close family member caused by the defendant.

Liability may relate to the delivery of medical services because medical services can involve life-and-death situations that may induce mental pain, suffering, and anguish. An example seen in many cases is when a parent witnesses the horrific death of a child caused by the defendant. Case law varies on whether the parent must fear for their own safety as a result of the negligence of the medical professional.

Intentional Torts

A tort is a breach or violation of a duty (responsibility) that is imposed on one person in relation to another. Similar to the legal doctrine of liability, technologists owe a duty to patients, physicians, and all other health care professionals. Of the many established torts, technologists need to be familiar with the intentional torts. *Intentional torts require the defendant to have an intent to cause harm and may be either specific or general intent.* Specific intent is when the defendant intends their actions to bring about a specific harm. In contrast, general intent is when the defendant knew to a substantial certainty that their actions would cause harm to another. Intent may also be inferred from a person's conduct or speech. The intentional torts discussed in this section are battery, assault, false imprisonment, intentional infliction of emotional distress, misrepresentation, and defamation.

Battery

Battery is an *intentional harmful or offensive contact to the plaintiff's person.* Harmful or offensive contact may be as simple as nonconsented touching of another person. The plaintiff's person encompasses anything connected or attached to plaintiff's body (eg, a hat or purse). In *Fisher v. Carrousel Motor Hotel,* the issue in the case was whether a plaintiff may recover for battery even though he was not physically touched by the defendant.[72] The case arose when the defendant's employee seized a plate

from the hand of an African American and shouted "a Negro could not be served in the club."[73] The plaintiff sought damages for assault and battery.[74] The court held that the "intentional grabbing of plaintiff's plate constituted a battery. The intentional snatching of an object from one's hand is as clearly an offensive invasion of his person as would be an actual contact with the body."[75] The court further stated that "it is not necessary to touch the plaintiff's body or even his clothing; knocking or snatching anything from plaintiff's hand or touching anything connected with his person, when done in an offensive manner, is sufficient."[76]

Applying the concept of battery to health care leads to one of the most quoted statements regarding medical battery.[77] Justice Cardozo said: "Every human being of adult years and sound mind has a right to determine what shall be done with his own body; and a surgeon who performs an operation without his patient's consent commits . . . [battery], for which he is liable in damages."[78] Lack of consent (see Consent section) is an essential element of battery.[79] A diagnostic exam performed without the patient's consent may be considered battery.[80]

Some courts have applied a 2 element standard test to determine medical battery: (1) Was the *patient aware* of the procedure or diagnostic operation? And if so, (2) did the *patient consent*?[81] Generally, this means that the patient knew and understood they were undergoing an MRI exam and the general details of the exam prior to signing the consent from. Further, the administration or injection of drugs (eg, contrast media) against the patient's will may be battery.[82] It is important to note that the ASRT practice standards consider the use of peripherally inserted central catheter (PICC) lines or implanted ports as being within the scope of practice for technologists.[83] A technologist could use a PICC line to inject contrast media.

Another situation in which a battery could arise is if a patient retracts consent for an exam. In *Coulter v. Thomas,* an automatic blood pressure cuff was placed on the patient's arm before surgery.[84] The first time the blood pressure cuff inflated, the patient felt "extreme pain, began to sweat and tremble, and demanded the cuff to be removed."[85] The cuff inflated a second time, and she demanded that the cuff be removed.[86] The cuff was finally removed after it inflated again.[87] The blood pressure cuff was removed prior to surgery.[88] It was discovered that the blood vessels in the arm on which the blood pressure cuff was placed had hemorrhaged and blood had collected around the patient's median nerve, causing her severe and permanent injury.[89] The hemorrhage occurred below the elbow, but the cuff was placed above the elbow.[90] The patient brought a claim of battery, arguing that she expressly revoked consent to use the cuff and demanded that it be removed.[91] The court determined that in order to constitute a withdrawal of consent after the exam has begun, two elements are required:

1) The patient must act or use language which can be subject to no other inference and which must be unquestioned responses from

a clear and rational mind. These actions and utterances of the patient must be such as to leave no room for doubt in the minds of reasonable men that in view of all the circumstances consent was actually withdrawn.

2) When medical treatments or examinations occurring with the patient's consent are proceeding in a manner requiring bodily contact by the physician with the patient and consent to the contact is revoked, it must be medically feasible for the doctor to desist in the treatment or examination at that point without the cessation being detrimental to the patient's health or life from a medical viewpoint.[92]

The court determined that the patient satisfied both elements because she used very clear and specific language in demanding that the blood pressure cuff be removed.[93] The patient testified that she said, "Take it [the blood pressure cuff] off. I can't stand it," after the first inflation.[94]

It is important that MRI technologists pay attention to the patient's wishes. As the court in *Coulter v. Thomas* determined, the patient must make a clear statement that they wish to stop the exam and it must be feasible to stop without harm to the patient. If a patient uses clear and specific language that they refuse to continue with an exam, the technologist should obey the wishes of the patient and stop the exam as soon as possible. Further, a patient may terminate consent at any time. As stated in the ASRT practice standards, the technologist should inform the patient of the consequences of not completing the exam. If the patient decides to continue with the exam, they have given consent to continue and the elements of battery are not satisfied.

Assault

Assault is an intentional act by the defendant that creates a reasonable apprehension of immediate harmful or offensive contact to the plaintiff's person. It may also be considered an attempted battery. The plaintiff must have knowledge of defendant's act and a reasonable expectation that it will result in harmful or offensive contact. Also, words or threats alone are usually not enough, unless in coordination with an overt act (eg, clenching fists).

Assault and Battery Example Examples of circumstances where assault and battery could occur in the medical provider-patient setting are as follows: "1) when a physician *performs a procedure other than that for which consent was granted*; 2) when a physician performs a procedure *without obtaining any consent* from the patient; and 3) when the physician *realizes that the patient does not understand* what the procedure entails."[95] The court in *Pallacovitch v. Waterbury Hospital*, applied this physician standard to a technician (phlebotomist) who performed a routine blood draw. This standard may further be applied to MRI technologists. Proper patient education and consent to the exam are important to avoid an allegation of battery.

The ASRT practice standards require the technologist to verify that the patient consented (see Consent and Informed Consent sections) to the exam and "fully understands its risks, benefits, alternatives, and follow-up."[96] The requested exam is to be verified for appropriateness before the exam begins. The technologist is to further verify that "written or informed consent has been obtained." The technologist is to explain each step of the exam to the patient and ask for cooperation of the patient.

All patients must be positioned for MRI exams. The technologist must obtain consent before touching the patient. It is good practice to ask the patient if you may position them by touching them and to explain why. Patients need to be informed and consent to each step of the exam. As stated in the ASRT practice standards, patients need to be immobilized for the exam. Immobilization is necessary to restrict patient movement and provide good-quality diagnostic images. Just as when positioning the patient, the technologist must obtain consent before touching the patient. Technologists may use straps, sandbags, and sponges to immobilize the patient, especially the anatomic area of interest. It is important that the patient is comfortable because of the long duration of the exam and the need for the patient not to move. If the patient becomes upset and refuses to continue the exam, the technologist must stop the exam. It is good practice to remove the patient from the bore of the MRI unit and discuss why the patient wishes to stop before removing the immobilizing items, unless it is an emergency.

False Imprisonment

False imprisonment is an act or omission to act by the defendant that restrains or confines the plaintiff to a bounded area. The restraint or confinement need not be physical; threats of force may be enough. Also, the duration of restraint or confinement need not be long; a brief confinement may suffice. The plaintiff must be aware of the confinement or harmed by it. The plaintiff must not have a reasonable means of escape from the bounded area.

A patient is restrained once they are positioned, immobilized, and placed in the bore of the MRI unit. The restraint of the patient must be performed with patient consent and justification. Consent applies to false imprisonment just as it did with battery. The technologist must respect the wishes of the patient. Immobilization of the patient is justified, so that good diagnostic images may be obtained; however, the patient should be comfortable.

Once positioned, immobilized, and placed in the bore of the MRI unit, patients know that they are confined. Prior to entering the bore of the MRI unit, the technologist should inform the patient, in a professional manner, about the confining nature of the exam and how to communicate with the technologist during the exam. Also, the technologist should inform the patient that, they will be continuously monitoring the exam. After placing the patient in the bore of the MRI unit, the technologist should assess the patient and talk to the patient. This will reduce anxiety and lead to a better exam. It is important to note that the patient has consented to this confinement but may withdraw consent and refuse the exam at any time.

Positioned and immobilized patients who are in the bore of the MRI unit cannot easily remove themselves. Patients rely on the technologist to remove them from the bore of the MRI unit and to remove immobilizing devices. Ignoring patients may lead to patients attempting to extract themselves from the bore, which could lead to injury and may constitute false imprisonment. Once again, the technologist should respect the wishes of patients. Further, the technologist should assess and monitor patients' physical, mental, and emotional status throughout the exam.

Intentional Infliction of Emotional Distress

Intentional infliction of emotional distress is intentional or reckless, extreme and outrageous conduct by the defendant that causes the plaintiff to suffer severe emotional distress. Courts require the defendant's conduct to meet the high threshold of outrageous conduct. Outrageous conduct is conduct that exceeds all bounds of decency in society, and the plaintiff must suffer severe emotional distress as a result of the conduct.

Bystander Claim of Emotional Distress

A bystander may claim emotional distress if the bystander is closely related to the person physically injured or killed by the defendant's conduct. The defendant's actions may be negligent (see Negligent Infliction of Emotional Distress section) or intentional (see Intentional Infliction of Emotional Distress section). Also, the plaintiff must witness the injury-causing event. For example, a father may bring a bystander claim of emotional distress after witnessing the death of a child if the child was struck and killed by a car in the father's presence.

Misrepresentation

Misrepresentation is the intent to deceive someone by making false statements or concealment of important facts. Technologists could misrepresent themselves as medical doctors. For example, after completing an exam, a technologist tells a patient that the patient has cancer. The technologist may be liable for misrepresentation because they concealed that they were a technologist, not a physician, and acted outside the scope of practice for a technologist.

Defamation

Defamation is harm to the plaintiff's reputation caused by a statement made by the defendant to a third person that concerns the plaintiff. If the statement is a matter of public concern or involves a public figure or official, then the plaintiff must prove that the statement was false and the defendant was at fault. Technologists must not make false statements about

patients or coworkers. Statements may quickly spread and harm the reputation of the plaintiff. Also, social media allows for the quick dissemination of information, regardless of whether the information is true or false.

Defenses to Intentional Torts

The first defense is that the plaintiff did not meet the elements, but if the plaintiff did meet the elements, then the defendant may offer several defenses. In addition to consent, discussed in the next section, the defendant can argue that the plaintiff gave informed consent to perform the exam or procedure (see Informed Consent section).

Consent

Consent is a defense to all intentional torts. Consent is approval or permission voluntarily given by a competent person to the defendant's otherwise tortious conduct. Patients or patient representatives must consent to the MRI exam, venipuncture, and administration of contrast agents after being informed. The ASRT practice standards require technologists to verify and document that the patient consents to the exam prior to entering the MRI suite. Technologists may be liable for an intentional tort if the patient retracts consent and the exam continues or if the patient has not given consent in the first instance. If a patient refuses the exam or retracts consent, it is good practice for a technologist to inform his or her supervisor and document the incident.

Consent may not be necessary in emergency situations, where consent may not be obtained and medical treatment is crucial. In emergency situations where consent has not been obtained, technologists should follow the written policy of their employer and direction of the attending physician and/or attending radiologist. Hospitals may have internal emergency policies regarding consent. Also, surrogates (eg, family members) may consent for the patient to undergo the exam. Once again, technologists should follow the written policy of their employer and the direction of the attending physician and/or attending radiologist.

DOCUMENTATION

Technologists need to document "information about patient care, the procedure, and the final outcome" because "clear and precise documentation is essential for continuity of care, accuracy of care and quality of assurance."[97] Generally, the technologist should document all pertinent information. For example, the technologist should:

- Verify the patient's medical history
- Note important facts in the patient's medical history (eg, implant records, labs)
- Verify and record pertinent information on the MRI screening form and then sign the form

- Document pertinent exam details in the patient's medical record (following the employer's policies and procedures)
- Document whether contrast media was administered and, if so, specifically document:
  - Injection site
  - Type of needle
  - Gauge of needle
  - Type of contrast administered
  - Amount administered
  - Whether it was hand injected or power injected
  - Flow rate
  - Any complications
- Sign and date documentation

This list is not exhaustive, and the technologist should follow their employer's policies and procedures. Generally, it is good to document all information that the technologist believes is important because if a supervisor, an attorney, or anyone else has a question about an exam, then they may review the technologist's notes.

HEALTH INSURANCE PORTABILITY AND ACCOUNTABILITY ACT AND HEALTH INFORMATION TECHNOLOGY FOR ECONOMIC AND CLINICAL HEALTH ACT

The Health Insurance Portability and Accountability Act (HIPAA) is a federal law that all technologists need to understand, particularly the HIPAA Privacy Rule. It is important to note that HIPAA is only one of many complex confidentiality laws.

The Health Information Technology for Economic and Clinical Health (HITECH) Act revised HIPAA and amended enforcement regulations. The Privacy Rule applies to most health care plans and providers that use electronic transmission of protected patient health information. The Privacy Rule limited the disclosure or use of someone's protected health information by a covered entity. The protected health information must be disclosed to (1) individuals or authorized representatives, if they specifically requested access or an accounting of their health information; and (2) the Department of Health and Human Services when completing a compliance review, enforcement action, or investigation. Disclosure or use of protected health information without the person's authorization is permitted for payment, treatment, or health care operations. Any other purposes require the covered entity to obtain the person's written authorization.

The covered entity must make an effort to only allow the minimum disclosure and use of protected health information. Health care employees should be provided only the necessary information to complete their job. Covered entities, such as hospitals and clinics, also limit employee access to patient information, where they only have sufficient information to perform their job functions and roles. A common example of unlawful disclosure and use is when a third party overhears employees discussing a patient. The third party would have received access to patient information that they did not have authorization to receive.

The covered entity may disclose protected health information without authorization when required by law (eg, victims of abuse, neglect, or domestic violence; law enforcement purposes; or judicial and administrative proceedings); to prevent or control disease, disability, or injury; for authorized health oversight activities; when decedents (eg, funeral directors, coroners, medical examiners) are involved; to facilitate organ or tissue donation; when research is involved; to prevent or reduce a serious and imminent threat to someone; for essential government functions; and for workers' compensation.

Limited data sets may also be released when direct identifiers of individuals, household members, relatives, and employers have been removed. Direct identifiers include the following:

1. Names
2. Postal address information, other than town or city, state, and zip code
3. Telephone numbers
4. Fax numbers
5. Email addresses
6. Social Security numbers
7. Medical record numbers
8. Health plan beneficiary numbers
9. Account numbers
10. Certificate/license numbers
11. Vehicle identifiers and serial numbers, including license plate numbers
12. Device identifiers and serial numbers
13. Web universal resource locators (URLs)
14. Internet protocol (IP) address numbers
15. Biometric identifiers, including finger and voice prints
16. Full face photographic images and any comparable images[98]

The limited data set information may be used in research, for public health purposes, or for health care operations. The covered entity should obtain satisfactory assurance, in the form of a data use agreement, that the limited data set recipient will only use or disclose the protected health information for limited purposes.[99] It is important for technologists to read their employers' HIPAA policies. For research and educational purposes, images with all direct identifiers removed should not be a problem.

AMERICAN REGISTRY OF RADIOLOGIC TECHNOLOGISTS STANDARD OF ETHICS

The first part of the American Registry of Radiologic Technologists (ARRT) Standard of Ethics is the Code of Ethics, which is a guide of "professional conduct as it relates to patients, healthcare consumers, employers, colleagues, and other members of the healthcare team."[100] The Code of Ethics is aspirational, with the intent of "maintaining a high level of ethical conduct and in providing for the protection, safety, and comfort of patients."[101]

1. The Registered Technologist *acts in a professional manner*, responds to patient needs, and supports colleagues and associates in providing quality patient care.
2. The Registered Technologist acts to advance the principal objective of the profession to *provide services to humanity* with full respect for the dignity of mankind.
3. The Registered Technologist delivers patient care and service unrestricted by the concerns of personal attributes or the nature of the disease or illness, and without discrimination on the basis of race, color, creed, religion, national origin, sex, marital status, status with regard to public assistance, familial status, disability, sexual orientation, gender identity, veteran status, age, or any other legally protected basis.
4. The Registered Technologist practices technology founded upon theoretical knowledge and concepts, *uses equipment and accessories consistent with the purposes for which they were designed*, and *employs procedures and techniques appropriately*.
5. The Registered Technologist assesses situations; exercises care, discretion, and judgment; assumes responsibility for professional decisions; and *acts in the best interest of the patient*.
6. The Registered Technologist acts as an agent through observation and communication to *obtain pertinent information for the physician* to aid in the diagnosis and treatment of the patient and recognizes that *interpretation and diagnosis are outside the scope of practice* for the profession.
7. The Registered Technologist uses equipment and accessories, employs techniques and procedures, *performs services in accordance with an accepted standard of practice*, and demonstrates expertise in *minimizing radiation exposure* to the patient, self, and other members of the healthcare team.
8. The Registered Technologist *practices ethical conduct* appropriate to the profession and protects the patient's right to quality radiologic technology care.
9. The Registered Technologist *respects confidences* entrusted in the course of professional practice, *respects the patient's right to privacy*, and reveals confidential information only as required by law or to protect the welfare of the individual or the community.
10. The Registered Technologist continually strives to improve knowledge and skills by *participating in continuing education and professional activities*, sharing knowledge with colleagues, and investigating new aspects of professional practice.
11. The Registered Technologist *refrains from the use of illegal drugs and/or legally controlled substances which result in impairment of professional judgment* and/or ability to practice radiologic technology with reasonable skill and safety to patients.[102]

The Rules of Ethics compose the second part of the Standard of Ethics.[103] The Rules of Ethics are mandatory standards of minimal professional conduct for registered technologists and applicants.[104] The rules are intended to promote safety, protection, and comfort of patients and are enforceable.[105] Registered technologists are required to notify the ARRT of any ethics violation within 30 days of the occurrence or during annual renewal and registration.[106] The rules cover (1) fraud or deceptive practices; (2) subversion; (3) unprofessional conduct and scope of practice; (4) fitness to practice; (5) improper management of patient records; (6) violation of state or federal law or regulatory rule; and (7) duty to report.[107] For a comprehensive explanation of each rule, please review the ARRT Standards of Ethics.

THE MICHAEL COLOMBINI TRAGEDY

One of the most publicized accidents in MRI history involved a 6-year-old child named Michael Colombini.[108] Soon after graduating from kindergarten, he suffered a nasty fall.[109] Physicians suspected his balance problems had an underlying cause and were not simply the result of being an active six-year-old child.[110] A CT exam revealed a benign brain tumor, and the tumor was removed in a routine operation.[111] Subsequent to the surgery, physicians placed an imaging request for a postoperative MRI brain exam.[112] Postoperative MRI exams are often used to determine whether a tumor was removed and if there were any complications.[113]

Michael was sedated inside the MRI suite, on the MRI table, by an anesthesiologist.[114] At the outset, the anesthesiologist told the MRI technologist in charge of the exam that Michael would need oxygen.[115] The MRI suite did not use the hospital's oxygen supply system; instead, oxygen had to be fed from an independent tank.[116]

The technologist assured the anesthesiologist that the oxygen was set, and she checked the oxygen flow meter before leaving the MRI suite and going to the MRI control room.[117] Approximately one minute later, the anesthesiologist noticed that Michael was not receiving oxygen and motioned to the technologist that he needed immediate assistance.[118] The technologist opened the MRI suite door, and the anesthesiologist told her that Michael needed oxygen.[119] The technologist asked her supervising technologist for help.[120] The technologist thought her supervisor checked the oxygen tank levels in the computer room earlier that morning.[121] However, the technologist did not check the oxygen levels, despite assuring the anesthesiologist that oxygen supply was ready.[122] The technologist asked the supervisor for assistance with the oxygen.[123] The supervisor suggested they change the oxygen tanks in the computer room.[124]

The technologist did not know how to change the tanks, so the supervisor made the change.[125] While attending to the oxygen supply, the MRI suite was left unattended.[126]

The anesthesiologist opened the MRI suite door and urgently called for oxygen.[127] A hospital nurse passing in the hallway outside the MRI suite heard the calls of the anesthesiologist.[128] She found a portable oxygen tank, which was about the size of a fire extinguisher, in the control room and brought it to the anesthesiologist inside the MRI suite.[129] The ferromagnetic oxygen tank was attracted by the static magnetic field of the MRI unit.[130] Like a missile, the oxygen tank flew across the room into the bore of the MRI unit where Michael was lying.[131] The oxygen tank hit Michael's face and head, causing serious injuries.[132] Michael clung to life for two days before passing away from injuries he sustained from the oxygen tank.[133] The medical examiner's office said Michael's cause of death was "blunt-force trauma, a fractured skull, and [a] bruised brain."[134]

The hospital launched an investigation into the accident and discovered many errors and lapses.[135] The hospital found six "critical factors" that led to the accident, including a "lack of training for staff members on the dangers of the [MRI] machine and the absence of written procedures for administering oxygen."[136] The MRI suite had a faulty intercom so communication between the anesthesiologist inside the MRI suite and the technologist in the MRI control room was impeded.[137] Further, the MRI suite did not "safely identify and safely secure the restricted magnetic field area."[138] As a result of the study, the hospital made 32 safety changes.[139] Hospital administrators invited Dr. Emanuel Kanal to visit the medical center and head a panel about the accident.[140] Dr. Kanal is a professor of radiology and neuroradiology at the University of Pittsburg.[141] Dr. Kanal is also a consultant to the FDA on MRI safety issues; he has chaired and/or served on many MRI safety committees, was the chairman of the first MR safety committee, and is the "Chair of the American College of Radiology's (ACR) Blue Ribbon Panel on MRI safety and is the lead author of the ACR's White Paper on MRI Safety."[142] Dr. Kanal said the accident awakened some to the issues of MRI safety, and he recommended that the MRI suite be "strictly limited to highly trained professionals," even barring the patient's doctor if not properly trained.[143]

Following Michael's death, his family filed a complaint seeking damages for negligence, medical malpractice, breach of warranty, strict products liability, lack of informed consent, infliction of emotional distress, loss of services, and wrongful death.[144] The complaint named the medical defendants, anesthesiologist, anesthesiologist firm, two MRI technologists, a nurse, the hospital, and the MRI unit manufacturer as defendants.

The Supreme Court of New York dismissed all claims against the defendants except the hospital. The supervising technologist was found to have, at best, only minimal safety training; however, the court found this did not indicate he was responsible. Further, the court determined he was not responsible for the area outside the MRI suite and was not "present in the immediate area at the time of the accident such that he could have prevented it." The court found that the supervisor was only secondarily involved in Michael Colombini's MRI exam and was not legally responsible for the tragedy.

The primary technologist in charge of Michael Colombini's MRI exam "received no training in MRI safe practices and procedures when she began working at the MRI facility." The technologist knew that no ferrous objects should be brought into the MRI suite but was never instructed as to any procedure for excluding ferrous objects. The court found that the technologist had a limited job to do and she had minimal safety training. Moreover, the technologist was not in a supervisory role and had no authority or responsibility outside the MRI suite, which was controlled by the physician at the time. The court's reasoning indicates that the physician was in control of the MRI suite at the time of the accident, not the technologist. Further, the technologist was not "'absolutely reckless,' with a 'conscious disregard for safety' to support an award of punitive damages." It was not the technologist's responsibility to oversee the MRI suite safety protocols, and there were no protocols in place for her to follow. The court also held that it is a matter for trial to determine if the technologist was negligent in leaving the MRI suite and control room to check the oxygen, but the technologist did not act with "malicious intent or a high degree of moral culpability, [and it] was not so flagrant as to transcend mere carelessness, and did not constitute willful or wanton negligence or recklessness."

It is important to note that since this tragedy, MRI safety has been a focus of the ARRT, ASRT, hospitals, and imaging facilities. Much has changed since this tragedy, but what happened to Michael was not unique. Please do not allow the holding of this court in regard to technologists lead you to believe that you are not subject to liability. As previously discussed throughout this chapter, the theories of liability may be applied to technologists.

Bibliography

American Hospital Association. Patient Bill of Rights. Accessed February 2022. https://www.americanpatient.org/aha-patients-bill-of-rights/

American Law Institute. Restatement of the Law Second, Torts. American Law Institute; 1979.

American Registry of Radiologic Technologists. ARRT Standards of Ethics. September 1, 2021. Accessed August 8, 2022. https://assets-us-01.kc-usercontent.com/406ac8c6-58e8-00b3-e3c1-0c312965deb2/eac1b19c-a45a-4e65-917b-922115ff2c15/arrt-standards-of-ethics.pdf

American Society of Radiologic Technologists. *The ASRT Practice Standards for Medical Imaging and Radiation Therapy*. June 20, 2021. Accessed August 8, 2022. https://www.asrt.org/docs/default-source/practice-standards/asrt-practice-standards-for-medical-imaging-and-radiation-therapy.pdf?sfvrsn=de532d0_24

Boumil MM, Elias CE, Moes DB. *Medical Liability: In a Nutshell*. 2nd ed. West; 2003.

Bryant v. Oakpointe Villa Nursing Ctr., 684 N.W.2d 864, 871 (Mich. 2004).

Byrne v. Boadle, 159 Eng. Rep. 299 (Ex. 1863).

Caldwell v. Vanderbilt U., M2012-00328-COA-R3CV, 2013 WL 655239, slip op. at 1 (Tenn. App. 2013); *Brief of Defendants/Appellee the Vanderbilt U. d/b/a Vanderbilt U. Medical Center*, 2011 WL 10549728 (Tenn. Cir. Ct.).

Colombini et al. v. Westchester County Healthcare Corporation et al., 2002 WL 34160371 (N.Y. Sup.).

Colombini v. Westchester County Health Care Corp., 899 N.Y.S.2d 58, 2009 NY Slip Op 51555(U).

Coulter v. Thomas, 33S.W.3d 522, 523 (Ky. 2000).

Defense Against a Prima Facie Case § 14:48, Intentional Infliction (Rev. ed., March 2014).

Defense Against a Prima Facie Case § 14:49, Negligent Infliction (Rev. ed., March 2014).

Furrow BR, Greaney TL, Johnson SH, Jost TS, Schwartz RL. *Law and Health Care Quality, Patient Safety, and Medical Liability*. West Academic Publishing; 2013.

Garner BA, ed. *Black's Law Dictionary*. 9th ed. West Group; 2009.

Harris DM. *Healthcare Law and Ethics: Issues for the Age of Managed Care*. Health Administration Press; 1999.

Pallacovitch v. Waterbury Hosp., No. CV126013332, 2012 WL 3667310 (Conn. Super. Ct. Aug. 3, 2012).

Restatement (Second) of Torts

Trinckes JJ Jr. *The Definitive Guide to Complying with the HIPPA/HITECH Privacy and Security Rules*. CRC Press; 2013.

Twerski AD, Henderson JA, Wendel WB. *Torts: Cases and Materials*. Wolters Kluwer Law & Business; 2012.

USA.gov. Branches of the U.S. Government. Accessed August 8, 2022. https://www.usa.gov/branches-of-government

US State Courts. *Federal Rules of Civil Procedure*. December 1, 2020. Accessed August 8, 2022. https://www.uscourts.gov/sites/default/files/federal_rules_of_civil_procedure_-_december_2020_0.pdf

Ybarra v. Spangard, 25 Cal. 2d 486, 487, 154 P.2d 687 (1944).

Yeazell SC. *Civil Procedure*. 8th ed. Wolters Kluwer Law & Business; 2012.

References

1. Mitka M. Safety improvements urged for MRI facilities. *J Am Med Assoc*. 2005;294:2145.
2. *Id.*
3. *Id.*
4. *Id.*
5. *Id.*
6. *Id.*
7. *Id.*
8. *Id.*
9. *Id.*
10. *Id.*
11. Forrest W. MRI safety remains a concern, as does need for more formal training. *Aunt Minnie*. July 14, 2014. http://www.auntminnie.com/index.aspx?sec=ser&sub=def&pag=dis&ItemID=107923
12. *Id.*
13. *Id.*
14. Duszak R Jr, Berlin L, Ellenbogen PH. Stability and infrequency of radiologic technologist malpractice payments: an analysis of the National Practitioner Data Bank. *J Am Coll Radiol*. 2010;7:705. The NPDB is maintained by the Department of Health and Human Services. *Id.*
15. *Id.*
16. *Id.*
17. *Id.* at 706. Health care providers are categorized according to their state license types. *Id.* Applicable categories included nuclear medicine technologists, radiologic technologists, and x-ray technicians or operators. *Id.* These 4 categories were grouped together for the study. *Id.*
18. *Id.*
19. *Id.* Thirty of the 155 cases listed in the NPDB were reported as a malpractice act or omission, and 24 cases were reported as allegation not otherwise specified. *Id.* at 707. A third of the 131 cases listed in a specific and identifiable category were reported as diagnostic errors, which included "failure to diagnose and wrong or misdiagnosis." *Id.* Another third of the 131 cases were reported as "improper technique; failure to monitor; failure to conform with regulation state, or rule; and improper conduct." *Id.*
20. *Id.* at 706.
21. *Id.*
22. *Id.* Payments were adjusted to 2008 dollars by using the Bureau of Labor Statistics Consumer Price Index. *Id.*
23. *Id.* at 706-707.
24. *Id.* at 707.
25. *Id.* at 708. The nation's population increased from 252,980,941 to 304,059,724, representing a 20% increase. *Id.* The government's labor statistics indicated that from 1988 to 2008, the number of radiologic technologists increased from 132,000 to 214,700, representing a 63% increase. *Id.* The American Registry of Radiologic Technologists estimated that the actual number of technologists in 2008 was 278,415. *Id.*
26. *Id.*
27. *Id.*
28. *Id.* at 709.
29. *Id.* at 708.
30. *Id.*
31. *Id.*
32. *Id.*
33. *Id.* at 709.
34. *Id.* Here, borrowed servant may be defined as "[a] physician . . . who borrows [temporarily] another's employee may be liable for the employee's negligent acts if he acquires the same right of control over the employee as originally possessed by a lending employer." *Id.*
35. *Id.* The Oregon Supreme Court held in a case involving a misdiagnosis that, while technologists are skilled in taking x-rays, they are not experts in determining whether the images are sufficient. *Id.* The radiologist is responsible for reading the images and determining whether the images are sufficient. *Id.*
36. See, generally, American Society of Radiologic Technologists. *The ASRT Practice Standards for Medical Imaging and*

Radiation Therapy. June 20, 2021. https://www.asrt.org/docs/default-source/practice-standards/asrt-practice-standards-for-medical-imaging-and-radiation-therapy.pdf?sfvrsn=de532d0_24

37. *Id.* at PS 3.

38. *Id.*

39. *Id.*

40. *Id.*

41. Leahy MCM. *Radiation Overexposure From CT Scans and Resulting Cancer Risk.* 127 Am. Jur. Trials 395 (originally published in 2012). *Emphasis added.*

42. *Bryant v. Oakpointe Villa Nursing Ctr.*, 684 N.W.2d 864, 871 (Mich. 2004).

43. *Id. Emphasis added.*

44. *Id.*

45. *Id.*

46. *Caldwell v. Vanderbilt U.*, M2012-00328-COA-R3CV, 2013 WL 655239 (Tenn. App. 2013); *Brief of Defendants/Appellee the Vanderbilt U. d/b/a Vanderbilt U. Medical Center*, 2011 WL 10549728 (Tenn. Cir. Ct.).

47. James AE Jr, ed. *Legal Medicine With Special Reference to Diagnostic Imaging.* Urban & Schwarzenberg; 1980.

48. Penofsky D. *Diagnostic Radiology Malpractice Litigation.* 75 Am Jur. Trials (2000) 55, at § 78 (May 2016 Update).

49. Actual causation.

50. Proximate causation.

51. Furrow BR, Greaney TL, Johnson SH, Jost TS, Schwartz RL. *Law and Health Care Quality, Patient Safety, and Medical Liability.* West Academic Publishing; 2013:305.

52. *Byrne v. Boadle*, 159 Eng. Rep. 299 (Ex. 1863).

53. Twerski AD, Henderson JA, Wendel WB. *Torts: Cases and Materials.* Wolters Kluwer Law & Business; 2012

54. *Scott v. London & St. Katherine Docs Co.*, 159 Eng. Rep. 665, 667 (Ex. 1865).

55. *Toogood v. Owen J. Rogul, D.D.S., P.C.*, 824 A.2d 1140 (Pa. 2003).

56. Prosser & Keeton. (5th ed. 1995). *The Law of Torts* § 39, p. 243.

57. *Ybarra v. Spangard*, 25 Cal. 2d 486, 154 P.2d 687 (1944).

58. *Id.* at 487, 154 P.2d at 688.

59. Contributory negligence is another defense to negligence, but most states have abolished contributory negligence doctrine in favor of comparative negligence doctrine. Contributory negligence is when the plaintiff's own negligence was a part in causing the injury. In some states, this is enough to prevent the plaintiff from recovering any damages, but other states reduce the plaintiff's recoverable damages by the percent fault attributed to their own misconduct. For example, a patient (plaintiff) fails to disclose their full medical history to the technologist and suffers an injury as a result. The technologist may claim that the patient was contributory negligent by not disclosing their full medical history. The court could find the patient was 40% contributory negligent because their own negligence was a part in causing the injury and could therefore reduce their total awards by 40%.

60. Furrow B., Greaney TL, Johnson SH, Jost TS, Schwartz RL. *Law and Health Care Quality, Patient Safety, and Medical Liability.* West Academic Publishing; 2013:195.

61. *Id.*

62. *Conte v. Girard Orthopaedic Surgeons Med. Group, Inc.*, 132 Cal. Rptr. 2d 855, 859 (Cal. App. 4th Dist. 2003); *Cobbs v. Grant*, 502 P.2d 1, 7-10 (Cal. 1972); *M.G. v. A. I. Dupont Hosp. for Children*, 393 Fed. Appx. 884, 889 (3d Cir. Pa. 2010).

63. *Conte v. Girard Orthopaedic Surgeons Med. Group, Inc.*, 132 Cal. Rptr. 2d 855, 859 (Cal. App. 4th Dist. 2003).

64. *Id.*

65. American Society of Radiologic Technologists. *The ASRT Practice Standards for Medical Imaging and Radiation Therapy.* PS 14. June 20, 2021. https://www.asrt.org/docs/default-source/practice-standards/asrt-practice-standards-for-medical-imaging-and-radiation-therapy.pdf?sfvrsn=de532d0_24

66. *Steve Herbst v. IMI Acquisition Arlington Corp.*

67. Reproduced with permission from *Gumm vs. North Valley MRI & CT Center.* 30 Trials Digest 63 (1993). Westlaw/Thomson Reuters Corporation.

68. Reproduced with permission from *Barras v. Univ. Healthcare Sys.*, 2010 WL 3840287. Westlaw/Thomson Reuters Corporation.

69. Reproduced with permission from *Confidential vs. Confidential*, 32 Trials Digest 15th 17. Westlaw/Thomson Reuters Corporation; 2012.

70. Reproduced with permission from *Thrallkill, et al vs. Chumptons MRI & Diagnostic Center and Mohammed Athari, MD v. Hartford Lloyd's Insurance Company*, 99 Tex. J.V.R.A. 9 (1999). Westlaw/Thomson Reuters Corporation.

71. Reproduced with permission from *Newton, Estate of v. Botsford General Hospital; Botsford Medical Imaging PC.* JVR No. 1306250010. Westlaw/Thomson Reuters Corporation.

72. *Fisher v. Carrousel Motor Hotel*, 424 S.W.2d 627, 628 (Tex. 1967).

73. *Fisher v. Carrousel Motor Hotel*, 424 S.W.2d 627, 628-629 (Tex. 1967).

74. *Fisher v. Carrousel Motor Hotel*, 424 S.W.2d 627, 628 (Tex. 1967).

75. *Fisher v. Carrousel Motor Hotel*, 424 S.W.2d 627, 629 (Tex. 1967).

76. *Id.*

77. James AE Jr, ed. *Legal Medicine With Special Reference to Diagnostic Imaging.* Urban & Schwarzenberg; 1980.

78. *Schloendorff v. Society of New York Hospital*, 105 N.E. 92, 129-130 (N.Y. App. 1914). Justice Cardozo misstated when he said the surgeon committed an assault; the surgeon actually committed a battery. James AE Jr, ed. *Legal Medicine With Special Reference to Diagnostic Imaging.* Urban & Schwarzenberg; 1980.

79. *Vitale v. Henchey*, 24 S.W.3d 651, 658 (Ky. 2000).

80. James AE Jr, ed. *Legal Medicine With Special Reference to Diagnostic Imaging.* Urban & Schwarzenberg; 1980.

81. *Shuler v. Garrett*, 743 F.3d 170, 173 (6th Cir. 2014). *Emphasis added.* This is a federal court case and is not applicable to all state medical malpractice cases.

82. *Shuler v. Garrett*, 743 F.3d 170, 174 (6th Cir. 2014).

83. American Society of Radiologic Technologists. *The Practice Standards for Medical Imaging and Radiation Therapy Advisory Opinion Statement: Injecting Medication in Peripherally Inserted Central Catheter Lines or Ports with a Power Injector.* American Society of Radiologic Technologists; June 2018.

84. *Coulter v. Thomas*, 33 S.W.3d 522, 523 (Ky. 2000).

85. *Id.*

86. *Id.*

87. *Id.*

88. *Id.*

89. *Id.*

90. *Id.*

91. *Id.*

92. *Id.* at 524.

93. *Id.*

94. *Id.*

95. *Pallacovitch v. Waterbury Hosp.*, No. CV126013332, 2012 WL 3667310 (Conn. Super. Ct. Aug. 3, 2012), quoting *Logan v. Greenwich Hospital Assn.*, 465 A.2d 294, 298 (Conn. 1983). *Emphasis added.*

96. American Society of Radiologic Technologists. *The ASRT Practice Standards for Medical Imaging and Radiation Therapy.* June 20, 2021. https://www.asrt.org/docs/default-source/practice-standards/asrt-practice-standards-for-medical-imaging-and-radiation-therapy.pdf?sfvrsn=de532d0_24

97. *Id.* at PS 40.

98. 45 CFR § 164.514(e)(2).

99. 45 CFR § 164.514(e)(4)(i).

100. American Registry of Radiologic Technologists. *ARRT Standards of Ethics.* September 1, 2021. https://assets-us-01.kc-usercontent.com/406ac8c6-58e8-00b3-e3c1-0c312965deb2/eac1b19c-a45a-4e65-917b-922115ff2c15/arrt-standards-of-ethics.pdf

101. *Id.*

102. *Id. Emphasis added.*

103. *Id.*

104. *Id.*

105. *Id.*

106. *Id.*

107. *Id.*

108. Chen D. Small town reels from boy's M.R.I. death. *New York Times.* August 1, 2001. http://www.nytimes.com/2001/08/01/nyregion/small-town-reels-from-boy-s-mri-death.html

109. *Id.*; Robin, *supra* note 1.

110. Beach M. "Mistake" killed MRI boy Michael. *The Daily Telegraph*, August 2, 2001, at 25.

111. *Id.*

112. *Id.*

113. Robin, *supra* note 1.

114. Martinez J, et al. Freak MRI accident kills Wichester Boy: magnet sends canister flying into him. *N.Y. Daily News*, July 31, 2001, at 3; *Colombini v. Westchester Cnty. Healthcare Corp.*, 808 N.Y.S.2d 705, 707 (N.Y. 2005) (an anesthesiologist is a physician who specializes in anesthesia and anesthetics. Anesthesiologist, Merriam-Webster Dictionary, http://www.merriam-webster.com/dictionary/anesthesiologist [last visited February 2022]).

115. *Colombini v. Westchester Cnty. Health Care Corp.*, 899 N.Y.S.2d 58, 2009 NY Slip Op 51555(U) at *11.

116. Gilk, *Did the MRI Community Learn From the Colombini Tragedy*, *supra* note 5.

117. *Colombini v. Westchester Cnty. Health Care Corp.*, 899 N.Y.S.2d 58, 2009 NY Slip Op 51555(U) at *11.

118. *Id.*

119. *Id.*

120. *Id.*

121. *Id.* at *10-11.

122. *Id.* The computer room is often referred to as the "cold room." The room was located next to the MRI suite but was separated by a wall. This room could only be accessed by leaving the MRI suite and walking through the control room. The equipment inside the room is very noisy, which makes it difficult to hear anything else.

123. *Id.* at *11.

124. *Id.*

125. *Id.*

126. *Id.*

127. *Id.*

128. *Colombini v. Westchester Cnty. Healthcare Corp.*, 808 N.Y.S.2d at 707.

129. Gilk, *Did the MRI Community Learn From the Colombini Tragedy* *supra* note 5.

130. *Id.*

131. Gilk, *Did the MRI Community Learn From the Colombini Tragedy*, *supra* note 5; Martinez et al, supra note 12.

132. *Colombini v. Westchester Cnty. Healthcare Corp.*, 808 N.Y.S.2d at 707.

133. Martinez et al, *supra* note 12.

134. *Id.*

135. Archibold R. Hospital details failures leading to M.R.I. fatality. *New York Times.* August 22, 2001. http://www.nytimes.com/2001/08/22/nyregion/hospital-details-failures-leading-to-mri-fatality.html; Associated Press. Training, communication cited in boy's MRI death: the report does not blame any one person. *Grand Rapids Press*, August 22, 2001.

136. Archibold, *supra* note 33.

137. *Id.*

138. *Id.*

139. *Id.*

140. *Id.*

141. *Id.*

142. About Dr. Kanal. University of Pittsburgh: Center for Magnetic Resonance Education. https://www.rad.pitt.edu/mredu-about.html (last visited February 2022).

143. Archibold, *supra* note 33.

144. *Colombini et al. v. Westchester County Healthcare Corporation et al.*, 2002 WL 34160371 (N.Y.Sup.).

4

Spin Echo Sequences: T1-Weighted Images

T1-weighted images are one of the most commonly used pulse sequences in MRI. They are used to image virtually any area of the body. T1-weighted images usually provide excellent anatomic detail. Another advantage of T1-weighted images is their ability to provide the best tissue contrast when using paramagnetic contrast agents such as gadolinium. However, detecting pathology usually requires additional sequences. The various manufacturers use different terminology to name the various sequences. Luckily, most use "SE" to signify spin echo sequences.

We can distinguish various soft tissues from one another on T1-weighted images based on each tissue's longitudinal relaxation time. Tissues with a short longitudinal relaxation time will have a higher signal intensity on T1-weighted images. Briefly, proton spins are aligned along an external magnetic field, either parallel or antiparallel to the main magnetic field (Bo) (along the bore of the magnet). A brief radiofrequency pulse then excites the protons and causes them to spin in the plane transverse to the magnetic field (Mxy). After the radiofrequency pulse ends, the protons return to their prior alignment along the magnetic field. Not all protons return to their equilibrium state at the same rate. Tissues such as fat, proteinaceous fluids, and tissues in very close approximation with gadolinium contrast have protons that recover to equilibrium faster than protons in water, for instance. T1-weighted images are obtained by using short TR (repetition time) and TE (echo time) times.

As mentioned before, in T1-weighted images, fat exhibits very intense signal (hyperintense). This can sometimes be problematic when attempting to characterize areas with a large amount of fat. There are various methods of decreasing the signal of fat, such as applying a homogeneity spoiling gradient pulse to diphase lipid signal. The final result is an image with much less fat signal, hopefully allowing a more detailed view of the adjacent soft tissues.

It is useful to know the signal characteristics of the various MRI pulse sequences. This will not only allow you to quickly determine the sequence used to obtain the image you are viewing but also let you pick up on potential problems that may arise in the course of an imaging exam. Table 4–1 briefly describes tissues based on their T1-weighted imaging characteristics.

Now let's apply this knowledge to some images (Figures 4–1 to 4–6).

TABLE 4–1 • T1-Weighted Imaging Characteristics	
Dark (Hypointense)	**Bright (Hyperintense)**
Water	Fat
Cerebrospinal fluid	Proteinaceous fluid
Arterial flow voids (quickly flowing blood)	Slowly flowing blood
Brain: gray matter	Gadolinium
	Brain: white matter

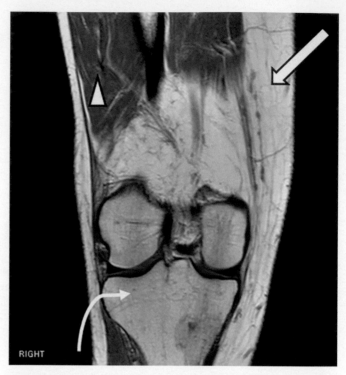

FIGURE 4–2. Coronal T1-weighted image of the right knee. Notice again how intense the signal is from not only the subcutaneous adipose tissue (*straight arrow*) but also the bone marrow of the tibia (*curved arrow*), which contains a large amount of fat. Muscle (*arrowhead*), which contains more water, is much less intense.

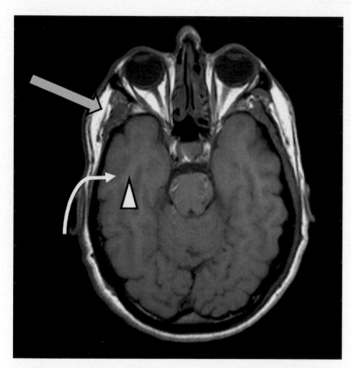

FIGURE 4–1. Axial T1-weighted image of the brain. Note that fat is hyperintense (bright) on T1. You can see the intense signal of the fat underlying the skin on this image (*straight arrow*). Also, notice that the gray matter (*curved arrow*) on the peripheral portion of the brain is darker than the white matter (arrowhead), which is found just deep to the gray matter. This is because of the increased amount of fat in white matter. Also notice that the eyes, which have a high water content, are dark on this T1-weighted image.

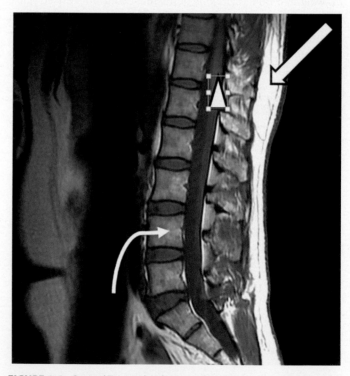

FIGURE 4–3. Sagittal T1-weighted image of the lumbar spine. Notice how intense the signal from the fat (*straight arrow*) is. The L4 vertebral body (*curved arrow*) and spinal cord (arrowhead) demonstrate moderate signal intensity. The cerebrospinal fluid (CSF) exhibits low-intensity signal. This will be important when distinguishing T1- from T2-weighted images. On T2-weighted images, CSF and water will be very bright.

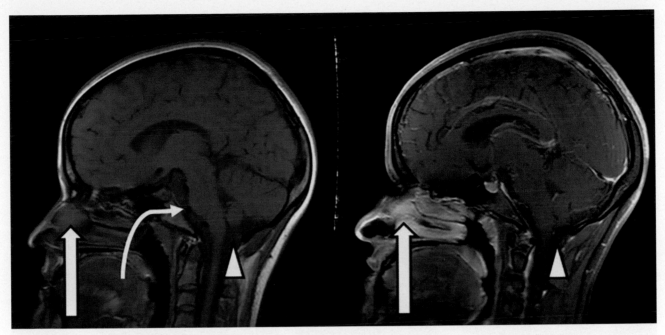

FIGURE 4–4. Two midline sagittal T1-weighted images of the brain. The left image is without contrast, and the image on the right is after contrast administration. A good quick way to distinguish pre- and postcontrast images is to look at the nasal mucosa (*straight arrows*), which avidly enhances. The signal intensity in the nasal sinuses is much greater on the postcontrast images than the precontrast images. This image also demonstrates a good example of a flow void within an artery (*curved arrow*) exhibiting little or no signal. Note also the low signal intensity of the cerebrospinal fluid (*arrowhead*).

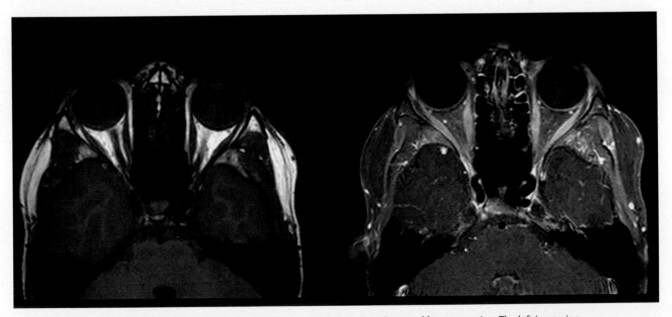

FIGURE 4–5. Two axial T1-weighted images of the orbits, demonstrating the use of fat suppression. The left image is a conventional T1-weighted sequence, whereas the right image was obtained using a spoiling gradient pulse to decrease the signal intensity of the fat after administration of gadolinium contrast. This may also be termed *T1 fat sat*. We will explore other sequences in other chapters of the Overview of Pulse Sequences Section that make use of other fat-suppression techniques. Notice that the subcutaneous fat as well as the fat within the orbits is much less intense on the right image.

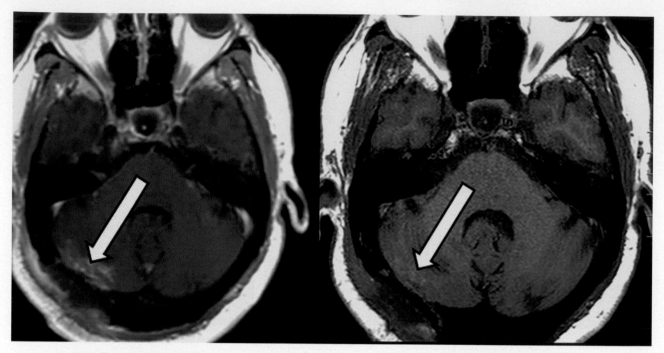

FIGURE 4–6. Two axial T1-weighted images of the brain demonstrating the benefit of contrast agents such as gadolinium with T1-weighted images. The right image is without contrast, whereas the left image is following contrast administration. There is a region of enhancement in the left cerebellum (*straight arrow*) representing metastatic disease. The metastasis is not nearly as apparent without the use of contrast.

5

Spin Echo Sequences: T2-Weighted Images

T2-weighted images are a common MRI sequence and are used on nearly every body part imaged. One of the great benefits of T2-weighted imaging is its property of showing water as hyperintense (bright). Much of MRI is detecting where water should not be. For example, most infections, fractures, tumors, and inflammatory conditions have edema (swelling) as a disease characteristic. Simply put edema results in more water in a particular body part than there should be. T2-weighted imaging will let us see these areas clearly.

Notice that T2-weighted images contrast nicely with T1-weighted images in this respect. T1-weighted images will display water as dark (hypointense), whereas T2-weighted images will display water as very bright (hyperintense). Let's use a fracture as an example of how these principles can help detect pathology. In a fracture, the surrounding bone will be inflamed and edematous. Sometimes fractures are nondisplaced and therefore unable to be seen on a conventional radiograph. On MRI, however, nearly every fracture will be apparent even if it is nondisplaced. This may seem counterintuitive considering the much higher spatial resolution of radiography. The key is the principle of detecting water in tissues where it should not be. On T2-weighted images, bones are normally dark because of their high fat content. In the case of a fracture with surrounding edema, the edematous marrow will be hyperintense to normal bone. A similar phenomenon is observed with T1-weighted imaging. Instead of the bone being hyperintense on T1, in the case of a fracture, water from edema will cause the bone to appear hypointense to normal bone.

Note that instead of the short TR and TE times used in T1-weighted images, T2-weighted images use long TR and TE times. Table 5–1 briefly describes tissues based on their T2-weighted image characteristics.

Let's take a look at some images to see how normal tissue and diseased tissue appear on T2-weighted images (Figures 5–1 to 5–3).

TABLE 5–1 • T2-Weighted Image Characteristics

Dark (Hypointense)	Bright (Hyperintense)
Bones	Water
Brain: white matter	Fat
	Cerebrospinal fluid
	Brain: gray matter

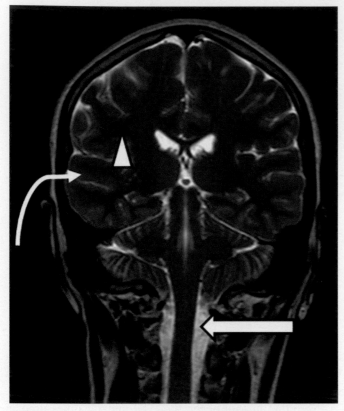

FIGURE 5–1. Coronal T2-weighted image of the brain and cervical spine. Note the intense signal from the cerebrospinal fluid (*straight arrow*). Another way to distinguish this sequence from T1-weighted images is the differences in gray and white matter signals. In T2-weighted images, gray matter (*curved arrow*) will appear more intense than the underlying white matter (*arrowhead*). This is opposite from T1-weighted images, which show gray matter as darker than the white matter.

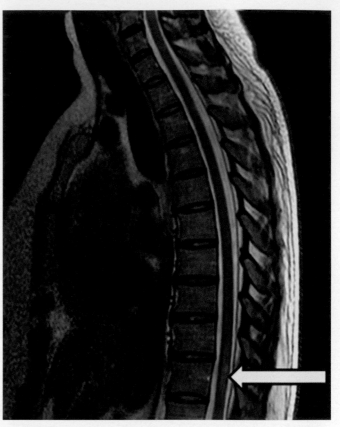

FIGURE 5–2. Sagittal T2-weighted image of the thoracic spine. Notice again the intense signal from the cerebrospinal fluid. Also notice the T2 hyperintense lesion in the lower thoracic spinal cord (*straight arrow*). This lesion turned out to represent multiple sclerosis.

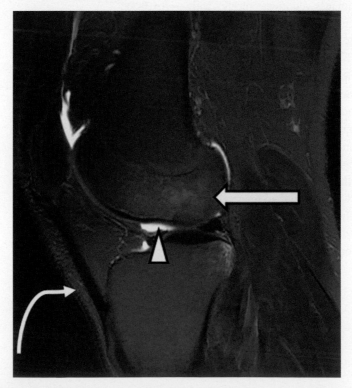

FIGURE 5–3. Sagittal T2-weighted fat saturated image of the knee. Notice that the normal patellar ligament is very hypointense (*curved arrow*). Compare this to the partially torn and edematous anterior cruciate ligament (*arrow head*). Also, note the hyperintense signal in the femoral condyle, which appears to be a bone contusion (*straight arrow*).

Proton Density–Weighted Images

6

In proton density (PD)–weighted images, the signal intensity is derived from the density of protons within the imaged tissue. PD images use a long TR and a short TE. Because of these parameters, a dual-echo or multiecho sequence can acquire both PD and T2-weighted images simultaneously. PD is sometimes referred to as an intermediate-weighted image, with characteristics of both T1- and T2-weighted images.

One of the benefits of using this sequence is the high signal-to-noise ratio. This allows a detailed view of minute anatomy. This characteristic lends itself to musculoskeletal imaging when evaluating small ligaments and menisci is crucial. Similar to T1- and T2-weighted imaging, PD imaging is often used with fat suppression to better show fluid and edema. Let's take a look at some images to see how normal tissue and diseased tissue appear on PD–weighted images (Figures 6–1 to 6–3).

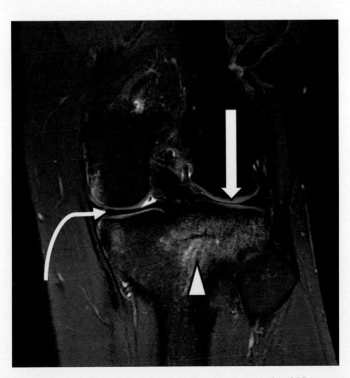

FIGURE 6–1. Coronal PD fat saturation image of the knee. First, notice the exquisite detail PD images allow you to see. The high intrinsic signal-to-noise ratio allows better detail than conventional T1- and T2-weighted spin echo sequences. This patient was diagnosed with an anterior cruciate ligament tear and bone contusions. The fat suppression allows us to see the edema from the injury, illustrated by the arrowhead. The curved arrow points to the medial meniscus. Notice the different PD appearance of the meniscus and the articular cartilage shown with the straight arrow.

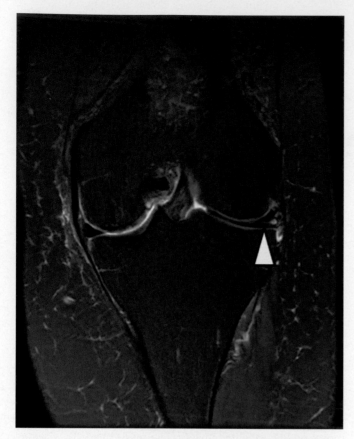

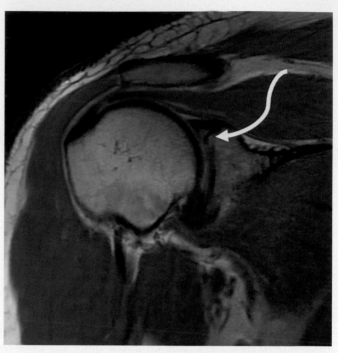

FIGURE 6–3. Coronal PD sequence of the shoulder without fat suppression. This patient was diagnosed with a superior labrum anterior to posterior (SLAP) tear. The glenoid labrum exhibits a region of hyperintensity shown by the curved arrow, representing the tear.

FIGURE 6–2. Coronal PD fat saturation image of the knee of a different patient. This patient was diagnosed with a meniscal tear, shown by the arrowhead. The horizontal white line represents fluid in the middle of the meniscus, which should be hypointense. The excellent spatial resolution and detail allowed by PD make this a relatively easy diagnosis.

Diffusion-Weighted Imaging

7

Understanding diffusion-weighted imaging (DWI) necessitates an understanding of the way water molecules move in space. Water molecules move in a random fashion called Brownian motion. In a free and open space (imagine a glass of water), molecules will move randomly in all dimensions; this is referred to as diffusion. At every point within the glass, the molecules will have similar diffusion characteristics because there are no barriers to restrict the movement of the molecules.

In the body, there are several barriers to random diffusion of water. In the brain, cell membranes act as a barrier to diffusion. Water will therefore be restricted to diffuse either within or outside the cell. In general, water will be able to move more freely outside the cell than inside it. In certain conditions in the brain, such as ischemia or infarction, the cells will swell. Therefore, within a voxel containing ischemic tissue, there will be a higher proportion of intracellular water than the surrounding healthy tissue. Going back to our discussion on diffusion characteristics, this will mean the water in this area will diffuse less than the water in normal tissue, where a higher proportion of water molecules are extracellular and freer to move.

These sequences are extremely important for neuroimaging. They allow the detection of ischemic stroke within minutes of onset, with images exhibiting restricted or decreased diffusion in the affected area. This is in contrast to CT, which takes hours to show changes after an ischemic stroke. Several tumors and cystic lesions have specific diffusion characteristics as well.

The apparent diffusion coefficient (ADC) map is generated to show a map of the rate of diffusion in the imaged tissue. The intensity is directly proportional to the amount of diffusion within each voxel. Therefore, on ADC, an area of restricted diffusion will be hypointense. On the DWI sequence, the foci of restricted diffusion will exhibit hyperintensity. However, the DWI is susceptible to T2 shine-through effect. Areas with very high T2 signal, such as cerebrospinal fluid (CSF), can exhibit high intensity on DWI, mimicking pathology. Referring to the ADC map will clarify the finding. If the region is hyperintense on both DWI and ADC, it is likely to be a result of T2 shine-through effect and not reflect pathology. If the region is hyperintense on DWI and hypointense on ADC, the region truly is exhibiting restricted diffusion. Now let's apply this knowledge to some images (Figures 7–1 to 7–3).

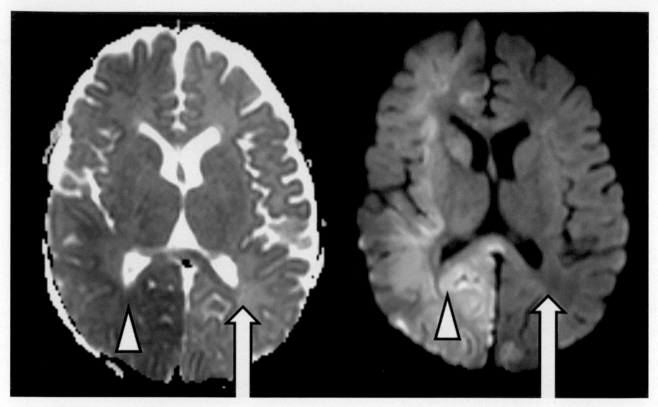

FIGURE 7–1. Two axial DWI images of the brain. The image on the left is an axial ADC map of the brain. The image on the right is an axial DWI of the brain at the same level. Notice the increased signal intensity from the right cerebral hemisphere on the DWI image on the right. This corresponds to a decreased (*darker*) value on the ADC map on the left (*arrowheads*). This means there is decreased diffusion of water in those areas. This patient suffered a large ischemic stroke on the right, evidenced by these findings. The left hemisphere is normal (*straight arrows*).

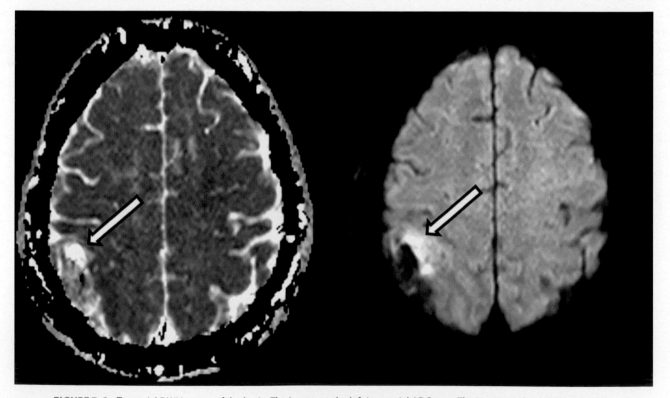

FIGURE 7–2. Two axial DWI images of the brain. The image on the left is an axial ADC map. The image on the right is the axial DWI. This patient had an intraparenchymal hemorrhage in the right parietal lobe. At first glance of the DWI, one might think there is associated restricted diffusion and infarct because of the hyperintense signal anterior to the bleed (*straight arrows*). However, upon review of the ADC map, we see that this area is hyperintense. If it were true restricted diffusion, the area of interest would be dark on the ADC map. Therefore, this area represents a T2 shine-through artifact.

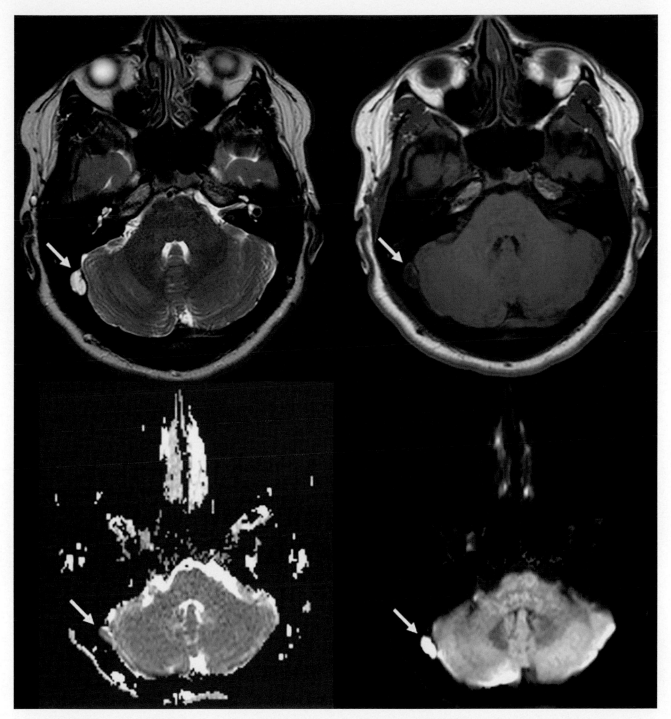

FIGURE 7–3. Four axial DWI images of the cerebellum. This case illustrates the beauty of MRI in characterizing lesions (*arrows*) based on their various physical properties. The image on the top left is a T2-weighted image. The image on the top right is a T1-weighted image. The image on the bottom left is the ADC map. The image on the bottom right is the DWI. The important finding is the smoothly marginated, extra-axial, lobular lesion lateral to the right cerebellar hemisphere. It is isointense to cerebrospinal fluid on the T1- and T2-weighted images. The diagnostic considerations for this finding based solely on the T1 and T2 characteristics are an epidermoid cyst or an arachnoid cyst. If we only had these 2 sequences, we would not be able to differentiate. However, this lesion exhibits restricted diffusion because it is hyperintense on the DWI sequence and dark on the ADC map. This lets us confidently make the diagnosis of an epidermoid cyst.

Gradient Echo

8

Gradient echo (GRE or GE) sequences have several interesting properties that make them very valuable in diagnostic imaging. GRE sequences fundamentally differ from spin echo sequences. Instead of paired radiofrequency pulses, a GRE sequence applies a single radiofrequency pulse and a subsequent gradient reversal. TR and TE are very short. Also, GRE sequences utilize a flip angle (FA), which indicates how far the net magnetization (M) is moved away from the Mz toward the Mxy. These characteristics let GRE sequences be obtained in a very short time. This is beneficial for many reasons, including patient comfort and minimization of motion artifact. There are numerous different possible parameters for GRE sequences with a diverse range of image characteristics.

One of the basic differences between spin echo and GRE sequences is the lack of phase refocusing to account for magnetic field inhomogeneities. This makes these sequences highly susceptible to artifacts. While this may seem like a disadvantage, we actually use these properties to detect tiny hemorrhages that would otherwise be undetectable on conventional spin echo sequences. These sequences are sometimes referred to as T2*. Another benefit of GRE sequences is a principle referred to as inflow enhancement. This allows inflowing blood to appear hyperintense, allowing an accurate view of blood vessels without the need for intravenous contrast.

Yet another potential characteristic of GRE sequences is the ability to image in and out of phase. Briefly, fat and water have different resonant frequencies. Imaging at the moment when water and fat are directly out of phase is called "out of phase." Imaging when both are in phase simultaneously is termed "in phase." Let's think about a single voxel for a moment to understand this principle. If there is a relatively equal amount of water and fat within a single voxel, the signals will be canceled out if imaged out of phase. When imaged in phase, both water and fat will be in the same phase and give off a high signal. This is useful when trying to determine if certain organs or tumors contain fat. For instance, the liver can sometimes become pathologically infiltrated with fat, a condition called steatosis. When imaged in phase, the liver will appear normal. However, when imaged out of phase, the water from the normal liver and the microscopic fat (both within the same voxel) will cancel each other out and render a hypointense signal. The out-of-phase images are characterized by an artifact called the India ink artifact. This manifests as dark lines outlining organs within the abdomen, separating them from adjacent fat. This is due to water from organs and the fat from the mesentery both occupying one voxel and the signal therefore being canceled.

The various MRI manufacturers have different terminology for GRE sequences, and unfortunately, there are a plethora of various sequences and abbreviations when it comes to GRE sequences. Table 8–1 will hopefully clarify some of the confusion that may result.

Let's review GRE images (Figures 8–1 to 8–3).

TABLE 8–1 • Manufacturer Abbreviations

Sequence	Philips	GE	Siemens	Hitachi	Toshiba
Gradient echo	FFE	GRE	GRE	GE	FE
Spoiled gradient echo	T1 FFE	SPGR/MPSPGR	FLASH	RSSG	RF spoiled/FE
Ultrafast gradient echo	T1 FFE T2 FFE	FGRE, fast SPGR	TurboFLASH	SARGE	Fast FE
Volume interpolated gradient echo	THRIVE	FAME/LAVA/LAVA XV	VIBE		
Balanced gradient echo	BFFE	FIESTA	TRUE FISP		TRUE SSFP
Steady-state gradient echo	FFE	MPGR, GRE	FISP	TRSG	FE
Contrast-enhanced steady-state gradient echo	T2 FFE	SSFP	PSIF		FE

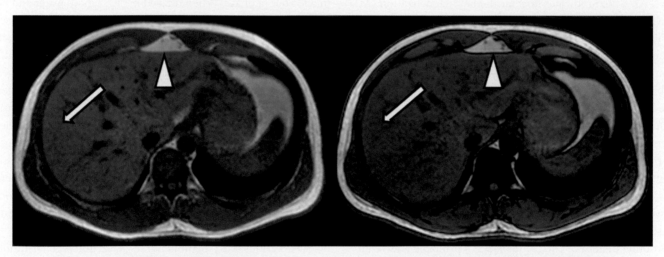

FIGURE 8–1. Axial GRE images of the abdomen. The left image is the in-phase image. The right image is the out-of-phase image. You can tell because of the India ink artifact (*arrowhead*). The liver is darker on the out-of-phase image. This is due to increased fat within the liver, decreasing the signal of the water in the liver due to fat and water molecules being out of phase at the time of imaging. In the in-phase images, both fat and water give off signal in phase and are additive, rendering a more intense signal (*straight arrows*). This patient was diagnosed with steatosis, or fatty liver.

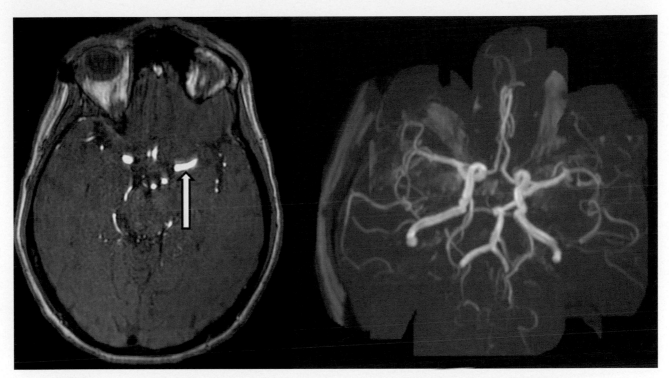

FIGURE 8-2. Magnetic resonance angiography (MRA) of the brain. These images exhibit the usefulness of inflow enhancement used with GRE sequences. Please note these images are obtained without contrast. On the left image, the left middle cerebral artery is indicated by the straight arrow on the axial GRE slice through the brain. A 3-dimensional reconstruction (*right image*) was formed of the high-intensity vessels to allow easier inspection.

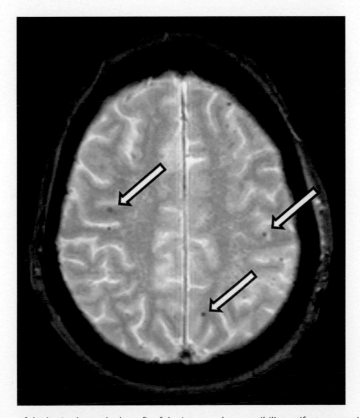

FIGURE 8-3. Axial image of the brain shows the benefit of the increased susceptibility artifacts seen with some GRE sequences. This sequence is also referred to as T2*. The punctate foci of hypointensity (*straight arrows*) represent microhemorrhages in this patient with hypertension. These are created due to magnetic field inhomogeneity from iron containing hemoglobin.

9

Inversion Recovery Sequences

Inversion recovery (IR) sequences are commonly used in several MRI applications. The main advantage of IR sequences is the ability to null signal from certain tissues. Briefly, a 180-degree radiofrequency (RF) pulse is delivered, inverting the magnetization, followed by a 90-degree RF pulse, which directs the magnetization into the transverse plane. The time between the 180-degree pulse and the 90-degree pulse is the inversion time (TI). In addition to nulling signal from certain tissues, IR sequences have a higher dynamic range, allowing easier detection of subtle differences in signal characteristics. A disadvantage of IR sequences is a decreased signal-to-noise ratio, leading to a noisier image. IR sequences are also more susceptible to flow effects and require longer scan times.

The fluid-attenuated inversion recovery (FLAIR) sequence is one of the most commonly used and most useful sequences in neuroradiology. Neuroradiology applications typically use T2-FLAIR, rendering the cerebrospinal fluid (CSF) dark with the brain parenchyma retaining T2 signal characteristics. This sequence is also referred to as turbo dark field on Siemens, but most will probably refer to it as FLAIR. This sequence nulls the cerebrospinal fluid signal, with a typical TI of 2000 milliseconds.

This allows for easier visualization of brain edema and other parenchymal pathologic processes, especially those found near the periphery of the cerebrum or lateral ventricles. (Most brain metastases are found peripherally at the gray-white junction; most multiple sclerosis plaques are found in the periventricular white matter, making FLAIR a helpful sequence for detection of these common pathologies.)

Another important application of IR sequences is the short tau inversion recovery (STIR) sequence. This sequence is a very effective fat-suppression technique using a short T1 IR. In fact, STIR is one of the only ways to obtain adequate fat suppression in older low field strength magnets. The TI for fat suppression is typically around 140 milliseconds. STIR fat suppression is less dependent of the homogeneity of the magnetic field than the traditional T1 fat-suppression techniques and offers a more global suppression of fat. It is important to note that STIR cannot be used with gadolinium contrast, as the enhanced tissues will have a shortened T1 and will be nulled by the short TI. Thus, T1 fat-suppressed sequences are still the mainstay for fat-suppressed postcontrast imaging.

Let's review IR images (Figures 9–1 to 9–3).

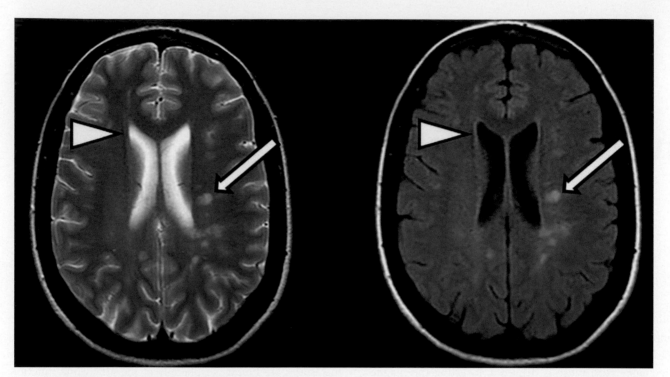

FIGURE 9–1. Two axial images of the brain. The image on the left is an axial T2-weighted sequence of the brain. The image on the right is an axial FLAIR sequence of the brain. First, notice the difference in the signal of the cerebrospinal fluid (CSF) marked with the arrowhead. In the FLAIR sequence, the fluid has been nulled and is dark. In the T2-weighted sequence, the fluid signal is intense. Both sequences reveal several periventricular multiple sclerosis plaques (*straight arrows*).

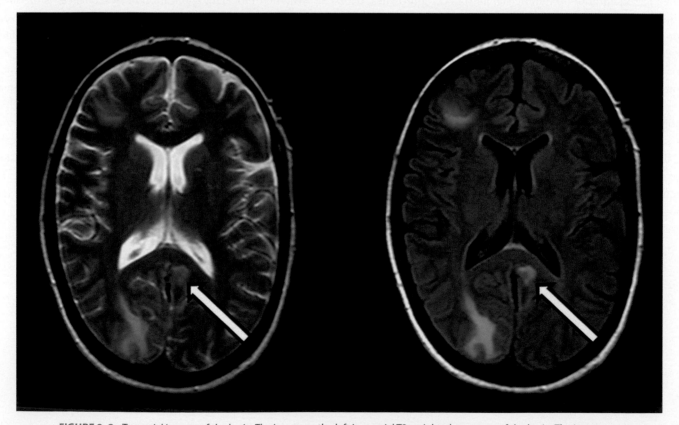

FIGURE 9–2. Two axial images of the brain. The image on the left is an axial T2-weighted sequence of the brain. The image on the right is an axial FLAIR sequence of the brain. This patient had multiple brain metastases, most of them quite easily seen. However, take notice of the small metastasis in the left occipital lobe shown by the straight arrows. If this were the only lesion, it would be difficult to recognize on the T2-weighted image alone due to the adjacent intense signal from the CSF. Look how much more easily seen the lesion is on the FLAIR sequence with the adjacent CSF signal nulled. This case highlights the usefulness of FLAIR in neuroimaging.

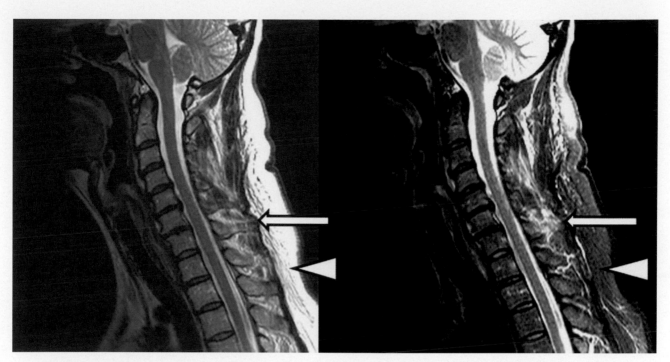

FIGURE 9–3. Two midline sagittal images of the cervical and superior thoracic spine. The image on the left is a sagittal T2-weighted sequence. The image on the right is a sagittal STIR sequence. This patient sustained a hyperflexion cervical spine injury, with injury to the interspinous ligaments at the C6-C7 level, shown by the straight arrows. The injury results in regional edema. Although the edema does result in hyperintense signal on both the T2-weighted image and the STIR image, the edema is much more easily seen on the STIR sequence due to fat signal suppression (*arrowheads*). A more subtle injury may have been missed completely on the T2 sequence if the STIR sequence had not been obtained.

10

Multi-Echo Spin Echo and Fast Spin Echo Sequences

Multi-echo and fast spin echo sequences (also known as rapid acquisition with relaxation enhancement [RARE]) are similar in concept to the traditional spin echo sequences discussed in previous chapters. They differ in the fact that they use multiple sequential 180-degree pulses, generally to obtain more information in a shorter amount of time. Advantages of these sequences are their short acquisition time and their low sensitivity to susceptibility artifact and heterogeneities in the magnetic field.

Another advantage of the multi-echo sequence is its ability to obtain protein density (PD) and T2-weighted images simultaneously (both have long TR, but PD has a short TE and T2 has a long TE).

The terminology of these sequences differs among the various manufacturers. Table 10–1 summarizes the various terminology.

TABLE 10–1 • Manufacturer Abbreviations

Sequence Type	Philips	GE	Siemens	Hitachi	Toshiba
Multi-echo spin echo	Multi SE	SE	Multi-echo/MS	SE	Multi-echo
Fast spin echo	TSE	FSE	Turbo SE	Fast SE	Fast SE

11

Ultrafast Spin Echo Sequences

Ultrafast spin echo sequences are sequences usually used to image noncirculating liquid structures in the body. The most common application is probably Magnetic Resonance Cholangiopancreatography (MRCP). Briefly, the sequences are obtained quickly by applying a single 90-degree pulse and subsequent application of several 180-degree pulses. A single slice may be generated within one second. These lead to very heavily T2-weighted images. This is advantageous in viewing structures such as the gallbladder or pancreatic duct (as in MRCP). However, generally, the signal-to-noise ratio is lower than in more commonly used sequences. Maximum intensity projection (MIP) images are then constructed from these slices.

TABLE 11–1 • Manufacturer Abbreviations

Sequence Type	Philips	GE	Siemens	Hitachi	Toshiba
Ultrafast spin echo	SSH TSE	SS-FSE	SSTSE/ HASTE	FSE-ADA	(SUPER) FASE-DIET

The various manufacturers have several names for these sequences, listed in Table 11–1.

Let's take a look at a look at an example (Figure 11–1).

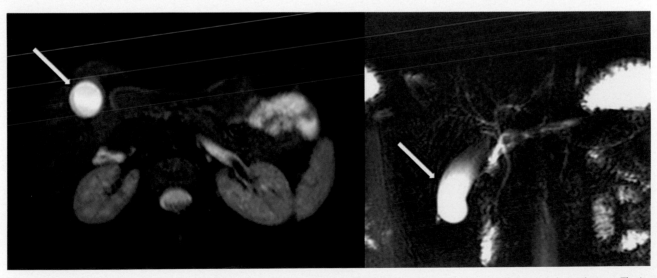

FIGURE 11–1. Two images of the abdomen. The image on the left is an axial slice through the abdomen using an ultrafast spin echo technique. The image on the right is the maximum intensity projection (MIP) reconstruction in the coronal plane. Notice how heavily T2-weighted these images are, with fluid in the gallbladder and stomach yielding the only intense signal. The gallbladder is indicated with arrows. Also notice the aliasing artifact seen on the coronal MIP image, with a portion of the stomach appearing on the left side of the image.

PART II

Imaging Applications

12

Introduction to Imaging Applications

The following imaging applications are intended to provide a general concept of an MRI protocol (image application) for a given MRI examination. Specific imaging applications may vary depending on a variety of factors, such as type of MRI scanner, specific hardware and software, radiologist, referrer preference, and patient factors. Note that the field of view at your facility may be slightly larger or smaller than what is shown in this section.

LEXICON

Terminology of the various pulse sequences used in MRI differs among the various manufacturers. Figure 12–1 summarizes the various terminologies.

Sequence Type	Philips	Siemens	GE	Toshiba	Hitachi
Spin Echo (SE)	SE	SE	SE	SE	SE
Multi Spin Echo	Multi SE	Multi Echo/MS	SE	Multi Echo	SE
Fast Spin Echo	TSE (Turbo SE)	Turbo SE	FSE (Fast SE)	Fast SE	Fast SE
Ultra Fast Spin Echo	SSH TSE	SSTSE/HASTE	SS-FSE	(SUPER) FASE-DIET	FSE-ADA
Inversion Recovery	IR	IR/IRM	IR	IR	IR
Fast Inversion Recovery	IR TSE	Turbo IR/TIRM	FSE-IR	FAST IR	FIR
Short Tau Inversion Recovery (STIR)	STIR	STIR	STIR	STIR	STIR
Fluid Attenuated Inversion Recovery (FLAIR)	FLAIR	Turbo Dark Fluid	FLAIR	FLAIR	FLAIR
Gradient Echo	FFE	GRE	GRE	FE	GE
Spoiled Gradient Echo	T1 FFE	FLASH	SPGR/MPSPGR	RF Spoiled/FE	RSSG
Ultra Fast Gradient Echo	T1-TFE , T2-TFE	TurboFLASH	FGRE, Fast SPGR	Fast FE	SARGE
Ultra Fast 3D Gradient Echo	3D TFE	MPRAGE	3D FGRE, 3D Fast SPGR		MPRAGE
Ultrafast Gradient Echo with Magnetization Preparation	IR TFE	T1/T2 Turbo FLASH	IR-Prepped/DE-SPGR/ FSPGR	Fast FE	
Volume Interplated Gradient Echo	THRIVE	VIBE	FAME/LAVA/LAVA XV		
Steady State Gradient Echo	FFE	FISP	MPGR.GRE	FE	TRSG
Contrast Enhanced Steady State Gradient Echo	T2 FFE	PSIF	SSFP	FE	
Balanced Gradient Echo	BFFE	TRUE FISP	FIESTA	TRUE SSFP	BASG
Fast Balanced Gradient Echo	BTFE				
Spin Echo -Echo Planar	SE-EPI	EPI SE	SE EPI	SE EPI	SE EPI
Gradient Echo - Echo Planar	FFE-EPI	EPI Perf, EPIFI	GRE EPI	FE-EPI	SG-EPI
Hybrid Echo	GRASE	Turbo GSE		Hybrid EPI	
Multi Echo	Mffe	Medic	Merge/Cosmic		
Spin Echo Black Blood	Black Blood Pre-Pulse	Dark-Blood Prepared TSE, TASTE, FLASH	Double IR FSE		
Spin Echo Black Blood Fat Nulled	Black Blood Pre-Pulse with SPIR or SPAIR	TRIM	Triple IR FSE, FSE-XL IR with Blood Suppression		
Single Shot Black Blood	BB-SSh	Single Shot 2D True FISP			
Coronary Imaging with Navigation	B-TFE or TFE with PB Navigators	PACE	T2 Prep SSFP with Navigators		
Motion Correction Techniques	MultiVane	BLADE	Propeller		RADAR
Time-of-Flight (TOF) MRA	Inflow MRA	TOF	TOF		TOF
T1 3D with Fat Suppression Bilateral Sagittals	BLISS	VIEWS	VIBRANT		
4D Time Resolved T1 3D with Fat Suppression	4D BLISS				
T1 3D with Fat Suppression	THRIVE, eTHRIVE	VIBE	LAVA, LAVA XV		Tigre
T2 3D	VISTA	Space	CUBE		
Time Resolved TOF with Contrast	TRACS/4D TRACK	TWIST	TRICKS		TRAQ
Contrast Enhanced MRA	Bolus Track	Care Bolus	Fluoro Trigger	Visual Prep	Flute
Non-Contrast Angiography	TRANCE	NATIVE		FBI/CIA	VASC
CE MRA with Moving Table	MobiTrack, Mobi Flex	Tim CT Angio	SmartStep		
Real Time Interactive Scan	Interactive	CARE	iDRIVE		
Susceptibility Weighted Imaging	Venous BOLD	Susceptibility Weighted	SWAN		

FIGURE 12–1. MRI lexicon. (From Philips Healthcare.)

Brain and Head Positioning

13

The patient's body should be positioned in a manner in which the requested anatomical structure may be imaged. Most MRI procedures will be performed with the patient in the supine position. Once the patient is safely on the MRI scanning table, it is suggested that the patient be positioned as straight as possible. To assist with performing this task, a review of key anatomic structures is useful. These structures may include the glabella, nasion, and mental point of the patient's face (Figure 13–1). Other anatomic structures along the midline of the patient and associated with the chest, abdomen, and pelvis, such as the jugular notch and xiphoid process of the sternum, and the umbilicus and the midpoint of the pelvis (pubic symphysis) are helpful landmarks to use in assuring that the patient is straight on the patient couch.

When imaging the brain or other head-related structures, accurate positioning of the patient's head is important so that the internal anatomic structures are symmetrically presented. As shown on Figure 13–1, the frontal view demonstrates key landmarks such as the glabella, nasion, and mental point. Further, the interpupillary line should be perpendicular to the midsagittal plane of the patient's face. This will help to assure there is less rotation and tilting of the internal anatomic structures and improve the comparison of left-sided versus right-sided structures. As shown on Figure 13–2, the lateral view demonstrates key lines for alignment such as the orbitomeatal line (OML) and the supraorbital meatal line (SOML).

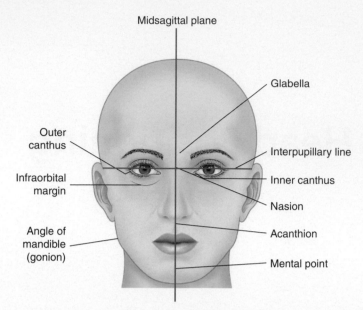

Midsagittal plane

Glabella

Outer
canthus

Interpupillary line

Infraorbital
margin

Inner canthus

Nasion

Angle of
mandible
(gonion)

Acanthion

Mental point

FIGURE 13-1. Frontal view showing key anatomic structures used for positioning of the head. Midline structures such as the glabella, nasion, acanthion, and mental point are used to define the midsagittal plane. Using the midline structures, align so they are straight and without rotation. The interpupillary line identifies a line between the pupils of the patient's eyes. To avoid tilt of the patient's head when positioning, align the interpupillary line to be perpendicular to the midsagittal plane. Make sure this line is not angled. In doing so, the resultant anatomy when comparing the left side and right side should appear similar. When positioned properly, the axial images should not demonstrate any signs of rotation or tilt. (Reproduced with permission from Jennifer Jones, Long BW, Rollins JH, Smith BJ. *Merrill's Atlas of Radiographic Positioning and Procedures.* 13th ed, Vol 2. Elsevier; 2016.)

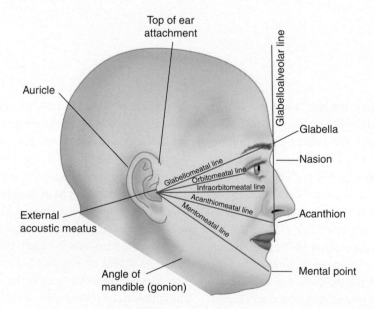

Top of ear
attachment

Glabelloalveolar line

Auricle

Glabella

Nasion

Glabellomeatal line
Orbitomeatal line
Infraorbitomeatal line
Acanthiomeatal line
Mentomeatal line

External
acoustic meatus

Acanthion

Angle of
mandible (gonion)

Mental point

FIGURE 13-2. Lateral view showing key anatomic structures used to assist in positioning the head for an MRI exam. If possible, position the patient's head with the orbitomeatal line (OML) perpendicular to the table. The OML is defined as a line between the outer canthus of the eye to the external auditory meatus. This line may also be referred to as the outer canthomeatal line or just the canthomeatal line. (Reproduced with permission from Jennifer Jones, Long BW, Rollins JH, Smith BJ. *Merrill's Atlas of Radiographic Positioning and Procedures.* 13th ed, Vol 2. Elsevier; 2016.)

14

Routine Brain

COIL SELECTION

- Primary coil: Head coil
- Secondary coil: Head and neck coil

PATIENT/PART POSITIONING AND CENTERING

- The patient is positioned supine, headfirst in the MRI table.
- Make sure the patient is comfortable.
- Position the patient so that the orbitomeatal line is perpendicular to the z-axis of the MRI unit. The interpupillary line should be parallel to the orbitomeatal line (see Figures 13–1 and 13–2).

- The head should be at isocenter.
- Position the patient's head so the midsagittal plane is parallel to the z-axis of the MRI unit and there is no rotation (see Figure 13–2).
- Center on the glabella (see Figure 13–2).
- Instruct the patient to lie still and not move any part of their body, especially the head.
- Instruct the patient to not cross their arms and legs.

SLICE ALIGNMENT AND SCAN RANGE

Axial Sequence Acquisition

Slice Alignment

- There are 2 methods that may be used when aligning the slice overlay for an axial image.
    1. Align the slice overlay parallel to a line extending from the anterior commissure to the posterior commissure line (AC/PC) on the sagittal scout (Figure 14–1).
    2. Align the slice overlay to be parallel with the hard palate (orbitomeatal line) (see Figure 14–1).
- On the coronal scout, align the slice overlay to be perpendicular to the longitudinal fissure (Figure 14–2).
- Extend the slice overlay from the foramen magnum to the vertex.
- The field of view must include the brain, including cerebellar tonsils (Figure 14–3).

Phase and Frequency Orientation

- Phase: Anteroposterior
- Frequency: Right to left
- Phase and frequency orientations may be swapped.

Saturation Band Placement

- A saturation band may be used to eliminate or reduce motion and/or magnetic susceptibility artifact from the face.
- If used, the saturation band should be placed in a line extending from the glabella to the second cervical vertebra (C2).

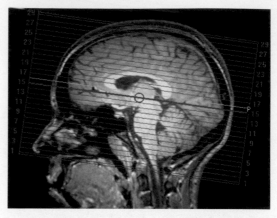

FIGURE 14–1. Midline sagittal scout image showing image slice overlay for an axial sequence. Note that the slice overlay is positioned parallel with the anterior commissure–posterior commissure (AC/PC) line.

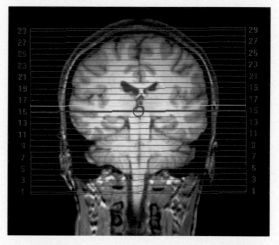

FIGURE 14–2. Coronal scout image showing image slice overlay position perpendicular to the midline for an axial sequence. Note the symmetrical positioning of the head.

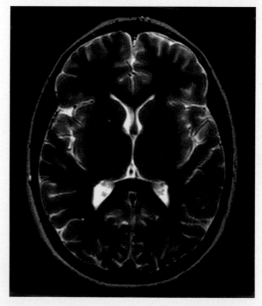

FIGURE 14–3. Axial T2-weighted image. Note the good symmetrical positioning of the head. Also, note the anatomic structures such as the basal ganglia and lateral ventricles.

Sagittal Sequence Acquisition

Slice Alignment

- Using the axial and coronal scout images, align the slice overlay to be parallel to the longitudinal fissure (Figures 14–4 and 14–5).
- An odd number of slices should be used to allow for a midsagittal slice (Figure 14–6).
- Place the midsagittal slice over the longitudinal fissure.
- Slices cover the entire brain, from temporal lobe to temporal lobe.
- The field of view should extend to the level of C2 (see Figure 14–6).

Phase and Frequency Orientation

- Phase: Anteroposterior
- Frequency: Superior to inferior
- Phase and frequency orientations may be swapped.

Saturation Band Placement

- A saturation band may be used to eliminate or reduce motion and/or magnetic susceptibility artifact from the face.
- If used, the saturation band should be placed in a line extending from the glabella to C2.

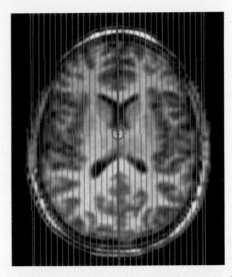

FIGURE 14–4. Axial scout image showing image slice overlay for a sagittal sequence. Note that there is an odd number of slices in this example, so the middle slice would be a midline sagittal image. All other images would be parasagittal either on the left side or the right side.

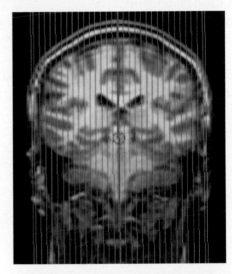

FIGURE 14–5. Coronal scout image showing image slice overlay for a sagittal sequence. Note that there is an odd number of slices in this example, so the middle slice would be a midsagittal image.

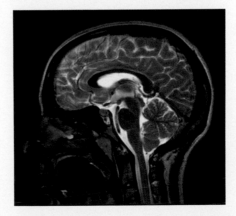

FIGURE 14–6. Midline sagittal T2-weighted image. Note that the midline anatomic structures, such as the corpus callosum, lateral ventricle, fourth ventricle, midbrain, pons, medulla oblongata, cerebellum, basilar artery, straight sinus, and superior sagittal sinus, are very well seen due to patient positioning and slice overlay.

Coronal Sequence Acquisition

Slice Alignment

- Using the axial scout image position, the slice overlay should be perpendicular to the anatomy in the midline such as the longitude fissure or the third ventricle (Figure 14–7).
- On the sagittal scout image, align the slice overlay to be parallel to the brainstem (Figure 14–8).
- Slices cover the entire brain, from the frontal lobes to the occipital lobes.
- The field of view should extend from the vertex to the level of C2 (Figure 14–9).

Phase and Frequency Orientation

- Phase: Right to left
- Frequency: Superior to inferior
- Phase and frequency orientations may be swapped.

Saturation Band Placement

- A saturation band may be used to eliminate or reduce motion and/or magnetic susceptibility artifact from the face.
- If used, the saturation band should be placed in a line extending from the glabella to C2.

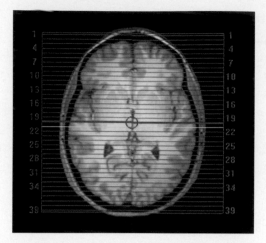

FIGURE 14–7. Axial scout image showing image slice overlay for a coronal sequence. Note that the slice overlay is perpendicular to the midline.

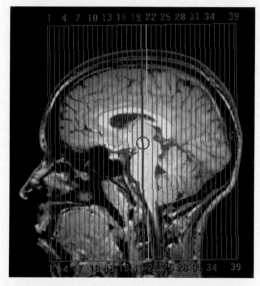

FIGURE 14–8. Midline sagittal scout image showing image slice overlay for a coronal sequence.

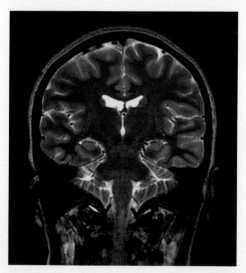

FIGURE 14–9. Coronal T2-weighted image. Note the good symmetrical positioning of the head. Also, note the anatomic structures such as the basal ganglia, lateral ventricles, body of the corpus callosum, and brainstem.

IMAGING APPLICATION

TABLE 14–1 • General Sequences

General Sequences	TR		TE		TI		FA (degrees)		NEX		SLT/GAP (in millimeters)	
	1.5 T	3.0 T	1.5 T	3.0 T	1.5 T	3.0 T	1.5 T	3.0 T	1.5 T	3.0 T	1.5 T	3.0 T
T1 SE	500	800	15	13	N/A	N/A	90	90	1	1	5/1	5/1
T2 SE	4500	3000	90	80	N/A	N/A	90	90	2	2	5/1	5/1
T2 GRE	700	600	12	14	N/A	N/A	18	15	1	3	5/1	5/1
DWI	4500	4500	50	60	N/A	N/A	90	90	3	2	5/1	5/1
FLAIR	6000	11,000	120	125	2000	2800	90	90	2	1	5/1	5/1
T1 SE post C+	500	750	15	13	N/A	N/A	90	90	1	1	5/1	5/1

Abbreviations: DWI, diffusion weighted imaging; FLAIR, fluid-attenuated inversion recovery; GRE, gradient echo; N/A, not applicable; SE, spin echo.

SUGGESTED PROTOCOL VARIATIONS

Seizure

A coronal short tau inversion recovery (STIR) sequence aligned with the temporal lobes of the brain may be helpful in the evaluation of a patient with a history of seizures and/or epilepsy (see Chapter 23).

Trauma

The attending radiologist and/or the requesting physician may ask for additional sequences or orthogonal planes depending on the traumatic injury.

Stroke

The diffusion-weighted image (DWI) sequence is important in determining whether an ischemic stroke or hemorrhage as occurred (see Chapter 18). The T2 gradient echo sequence is of particular significance due to its inherent susceptibility and ability to detect hemorrhagic lesions. A time-of-flight (TOF) or phase-contrast (PC) magnetic resonance angiography (MRA) sequence would depict ischemia, infarction, or a ruptured cerebral artery (see Chapter 15). A susceptibility-weighted image (SWI) may further aid in the diagnosis and analysis of a stroke (see Chapter 21).

Tumor

A tumor protocol may require sequences in addition to the routine brain protocol. Additional pre- and postcontrast sequences may be included. Three-orthogonal-plane postcontrast sequences may be of benefit to the radiologist. A spectroscopy sequence may be added to evaluate the chemical makeup of a tumor or lesion (see Chapter 22). The technologist should follow the protocol provided at their facility.

Surgery Planning

An exam may be performed for computer-assisted surgical planning (also known as image-guided surgery, computer-aided surgery, or computer-assisted intervention). Many different health care corporations (eg, Medtronic, Stryker) have developed these systems. Acquired MRI images may be changed or manipulated at a separate workstation to meet the needs of the surgeon. This system allows for precise surgery. In planning these sequences, technologists should follow the protocol provided at their facility.

After Operation

A postoperation protocol may require sequences in addition to the routine brain protocol. Additional pre- and postcontrast sequences may be included. Three-orthogonal-planes postcontrast sequences may be of benefit to the radiologist. The technologist should follow the protocol provided at their facility.

15

Cerebral Angiography (Circle of Willis [COW]) (Magnetic Resonance Angiography Brain [MRA Brain])

COIL SELECTION

- Primary coil: Head coil
- Secondary coil: Head and neck coil

PATIENT/PART POSITIONING AND CENTERING

- The patient is positioned supine, headfirst in the MRI table.
- Make sure the patient is comfortable.
- Position the patient so that the orbitomeatal line is perpendicular to the z-axis of the MRI unit. The interpupillary line should be parallel to the orbitomeatal line (see Figures 13–1 and 13–2).

- The head should be at isocenter.
- Position the patient's head so the midsagittal plane is parallel to the z-axis of the MRI unit and there is no rotation (see Figure 13–2).
- Center on the glabella (see Figure 13–2).
- Instruct the patient to lie still and not move any part of their body, especially the head.
- Instruct the patient to not cross their arms and legs.

SLICE ALIGNMENT AND SCAN RANGE

Slice Alignment

- Align the slice overlay parallel to a line extending from the anterior commissure to the posterior commissure (AC/PC) on the sagittal scout (Figure 15–1).
- On the coronal scout, align the slice overlay to be perpendicular to the longitudinal fissure (Figure 15–2).
- Extend the slice overlay from a point just superior of the body of the corpus callosum to the foramen magnum (see Figures 15–1 and 15–2).

Phase and Frequency Orientation

- Phase: Right to left
- Frequency: Anteroposterior
- Phase and frequency orientations may be swapped.

Saturation Band Placement

- A saturation band is placed superior and outside the field of view (see Figures 15–1 and 15–2).
- The saturation band will saturate venous flow.

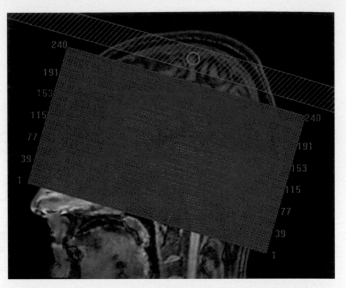

FIGURE 15–1. Midline sagittal scout image showing slice overlay for an axial magnetic resonance angiography (MRA) sequence. Note the 240 planned slices and that the saturation band (the *blue band*) is placed superior of the field of view. The band is placed superior to the planned slices to saturate hydrogen protons in the venous blood, specifically the superior sagittal sinus, thereby eliminating venous signal. Also note the thin slice thickness and gap.

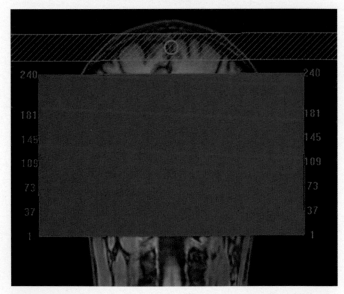

FIGURE 15–2. Coronal scout image showing slice overlay for an axial MRA sequence. Note the 240 planned slices and that the saturation band (the *blue band*) is placed superior of the field of view. Also note the thin slice thickness and gap.

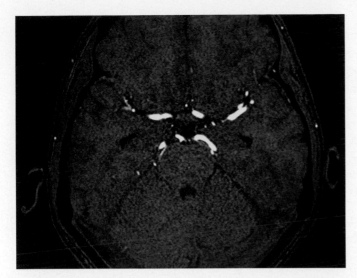

FIGURE 15–3. Axial image. Note that this is one of the 240 planned slices and will be reconstructed to form a maximum intensity projection (MIP)of the cerebral arteries.

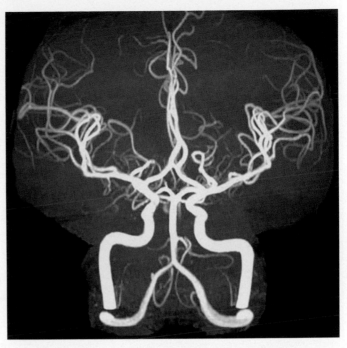

FIGURE 15–4. Coronal maximum intensity projection (MIP). Note the anatomic structures such as the vertebral arteries, basilar artery, internal carotids, posterior cerebral arteries, middle cerebral arteries, anterior cerebral arteries, anterior communicating arteries, and posterior communicating arteries. Compare how these anatomic structures are demonstrated on the coronal (this figure), axial (Figure 15–5), and sagittal (Figure 15–6) MIPs.

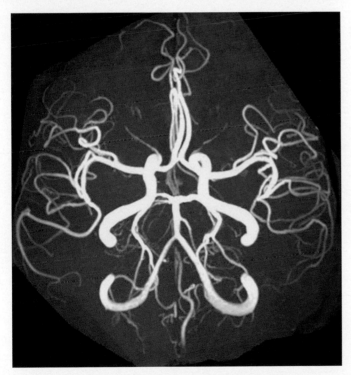

FIGURE 15–5. Axial maximum intensity projection(MIP). Note the symmetry of the Circle of Willis and middle cerebral arteries.

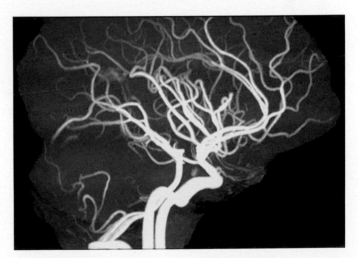

FIGURE 15–6. Sagittal maximum intensity projection (MIP).

IMAGING APPLICATION

General Sequences	TR		TE		TI		FA (degrees)		NEX		SLT/GAP (in millimeters)	
	1.5 T	3.0 T	1.5 T	3.0 T	1.5 T	3.0 T	1.5 T	3.0 T	1.5 T	3.0 T	1.5 T	3.0 T
Time of flight (TOF)	25	20	7	5	N/A	N/A	20	20	1	1	1/0	1/0
Phase contrast (PC)	15	20	5	5	N/A	N/A	15	15	2	2	40/0	40/0
Contrast enhanced (CE)	5	10	2	5	N/A	N/A	40	40	1	1	4/1	4/1

TABLE 15–1 • General Sequences

Abbreviation: N/A, not applicable.

16

Brain Venography (Magnetic Resonance Venography Brain [MRV Brain])

COIL SELECTION

- Primary coil: Head coil
- Secondary coil: Head and neck coil

PATIENT/PART POSITIONING AND CENTERING

- The patient is positioned supine, headfirst in the MRI table.
- Make sure the patient is comfortable.
- Position the patient so that the orbitomeatal line is perpendicular to the z-axis of the MRI unit. The interpupillary line should be parallel to the orbitomeatal line (see Figures 13–1 and 13–2).
- The head should be at isocenter.
- Position the patient's head so the midsagittal plane is parallel to the z-axis of the MRI unit and there is no rotation (see Figure 13–2).
- Center on the glabella (see Figure 13–2).
- Instruct the patient to lie still and not move any part of their body, especially the head.
- Instruct the patient to not cross their arms and legs.

SLICE ALIGNMENT AND SCAN RANGE

Slice Alignment

- Align the slice overlay parallel to a line extending from the anterior commissure to the posterior commissure (AC/PC) on the sagittal scout (Figure 16–1).
- On the coronal scout, align the slice overlay to be perpendicular to the longitudinal fissure (see Figure 16–2).
- Extend the slice overlay from the foramen magnum to the vertex, so that the head is covered (see Figure 16–1).

Phase and Frequency Orientation

- Phase: Anteroposterior
- Frequency: Right to left
- Phase and frequency orientations may be swapped.

Saturation Band Placement

- A saturation band is placed inferior of the field of view (see Figures 16–1 and 16–2).
- The saturation band will saturate arterial flow.

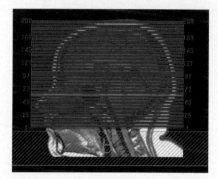

FIGURE 16–1. Midline sagittal scout image showing slice overlay for an axial magnetic resonance venography sequence. Note the 200 planned slices (*red lines*) and the saturation band (*blue band*) is placed inferior of the field of view. The band is placed inferior of the planned slices to saturate hydrogen protons in the blood, prior to entering into the brain, thereby eliminating arterial signal. Also note the thin slice thickness and gap.

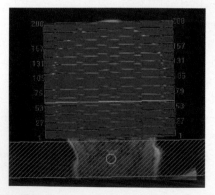

FIGURE 16–2. Coronal scout image showing slice overlay for an axial magnetic resonance venography sequence. Note the 200 planned slices and that the saturation band (the *blue band*) is placed inferior of the field of view. Also note the thin slice thickness and gap.

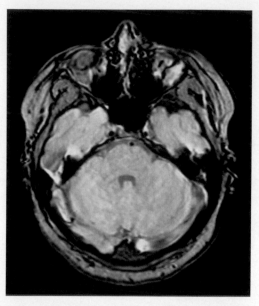

FIGURE 16–3. Axial image. Note that this is one of the 200 planned slices and will be reconstructed to form a maximum intensity projection of the venous flow.

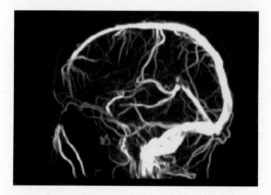

FIGURE 16–4. Sagittal maximum intensity projection (MIP). Note the anatomic structures such as the superior sagittal sinus, confluence of sinuses, straight sinus, transverse sinuses, and sigmoid sinuses. Compare how these anatomic structures are demonstrated on the sagittal (this figure) and coronal (Figure 16–5) MIPs.

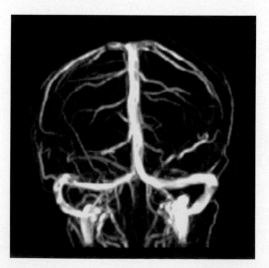

FIGURE 16–5. Coronal maximum intensity projection (MIP). Note the good positioning of the head and symmetry of the left and right transverse sinuses.

IMAGING APPLICATION

TABLE 16–1 • General Sequences

General Sequences	TR		TE		TI		FA (degrees)		NEX		SLT/GAP (in millimeters)	
	1.5 T	3.0 T	1.5 T	3.0 T	1.5 T	3.0 T	1.5 T	3.0 T	1.5 T	3.0 T	1.5 T	3.0 T
3-Dimensional time of flight	25	20	7	5	N/A	N/A	20	20	1	1	2/1	2/1

Abbreviation: N/A, not applicable.

17

Pituitary

COIL SELECTION

- Primary coil: Head coil
- Secondary coil: Head and neck coil

PATIENT/PART POSITIONING AND CENTERING

- The patient is positioned supine, headfirst in the MRI table.
- Make sure the patient is comfortable.
- Position the patient so that the orbitomeatal line is perpendicular to the z-axis of the MRI unit. The interpupillary line should be parallel to the orbitomeatal line (see Figures 13–1 and 13–2).
- The head should be at isocenter.
- Position the patient's head so the midsagittal plane is parallel to the z-axis of the MRI unit and there is no rotation (see Figure 13–2).
- Center on the glabella (see Figure 13–2).
- Instruct the patient to lie still and not move any part of their body, especially the head.
- Instruct the patient to not cross their arms and legs.

SLICE ALIGNMENT AND SCAN RANGE

Coronal Sequence Acquisition

Slice Alignment

- On the sagittal scout image, align the slice overlay to be parallel to the brainstem and cover the pituitary region (Figure 17–1).
- On the axial scout image, align the slice overlay to be perpendicular to the longitudinal fissure (Figure 17–2).
- The left-to-right field of view should extend from one side of the calvarium to the other side (see Figure 17–2).
- The anteroposterior field of view should extend anterior of the genu of the corpus callosum to the pons (see Figure 17–1).
- The superior-to-inferior field of view should be superior of the corpus callosum to the level of the first cervical vertebra (see Figure 17–1).
- The pituitary stalk (infundibulum) is seen on Figures 17–3 and 17–4.

Phase and Frequency Orientation

- Phase: Right to left
- Frequency: Superior to inferior
- Phase and frequency orientations may be swapped.

Saturation Band Placement

- A saturation band may be used to eliminate or reduce motion and/or magnetic susceptibility artifact from the face.
- If used, the saturation band should be placed inferior of the field of view.

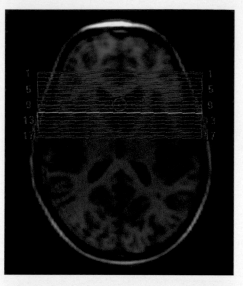

FIGURE 17–2. Axial scout image showing image slice overlay for a coronal sequence. Note that the slice overlay is perpendicular to the longitudinal fissure.

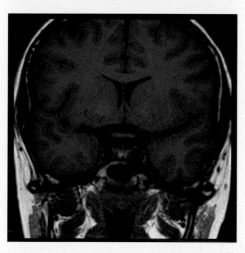

FIGURE 17–3. Coronal T1-weighted image. Note that the anatomic structures such as the pituitary and pituitary stalk (infundibulum) are very well seen due to patient positioning and slice overlay.

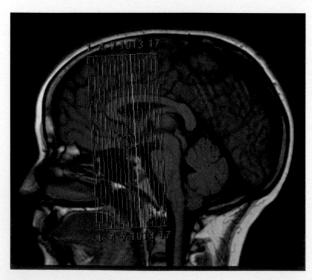

FIGURE 17–1. Midline sagittal scout image showing image slice overlay for a coronal sequence. Note that the slice overlay is parallel to the brainstem. Also, the red box indicates the field-of-view.

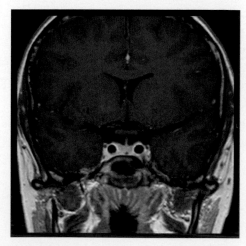

FIGURE 17–4. Coronal postcontrast T1-weighted image. Note the hyperintense contrast and the difference between the pre-contrast coronal T1-weighted image (Figure 17–3) and the postcontrast T1-weighted image (this figure).

Sagittal Sequence Acquisition

Slice Alignment

- On the coronal and axial scout images, align the slice overlay parallel to the longitudinal fissure and brainstem (Figures 17–5 and 17–6).
- An odd number of slices should be used to allow for a midsagittal slice.
- Place the midsagittal slice over the longitudinal fissure (see Figures 17–5 and 17–6).
- The left-to-right field of view should extend to include the frontal horns of the lateral ventricles.
- The anteroposterior field of view should extend from the orbit to the cerebellum (Figure 17–7).
- The superior-to-inferior field of view should extend from above the corpus callosum to the level of the first cervical vertebra (C1) (see Figure 17–7).
- Sagittal images of the pituitary stalk are seen on Figures 17–8 and 17–9.

Phase and Frequency Orientation

- Phase: Anteroposterior
- Frequency: Superior to inferior
- Phase and frequency orientations may be swapped.

Saturation Band Placement

- A saturation band may be used to eliminate or reduce motion and/or magnetic susceptibility artifact from the face.
- If used, the saturation band should be placed inferior of the field of view.

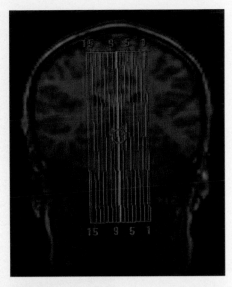

FIGURE 17–5. Coronal scout image showing image slice overlay for a sagittal sequence. Note that there is an odd number of slices in this example, so the middle slice would be a midsagittal image.

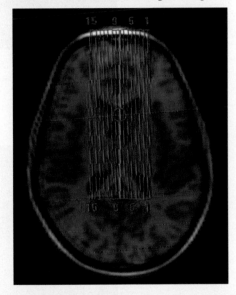

FIGURE 17–6. Axial scout image showing image slice overlay for a sagittal sequence. Note that there is an odd number of slices in this example, so the middle slice would be a midsagittal image.

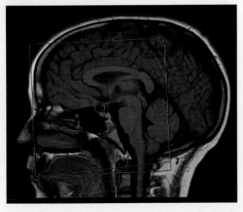

FIGURE 17–7. Sagittal scout image showing image slice overlay for a sagittal sequence. Note that this image is included to demonstrate the field of view. The field of view may be decreased, but it is important to maintain a proper amount of signal so the resultant image will be of sufficient quality.

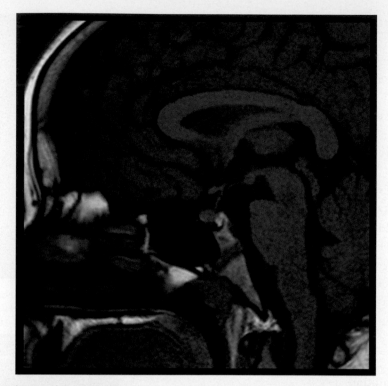

FIGURE 17–8. Sagittal T1-weighted image. Note that the anatomic structures, such as the pituitary, pituitary stalk (infundibulum), sella turcica, clivus, and basilar artery (which is not seen, but located anterior to the pons), are very well seen due to patient positioning and slice overlay.

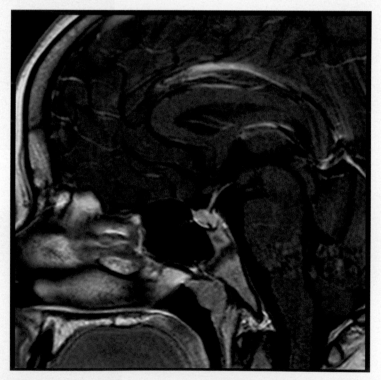

FIGURE 17–9. Sagittal postcontrast T1-weighted image. Note the hyperintense contrast and the difference between the precontrast sagittal T1-weighted image (Figure 17–8) and the postcontrast T1-weighted image (this figure). Positioning the patient and slice overlay allow us to see the very thin pituitary stalk (infundibulum).

IMAGING APPLICATION

TABLE 17–1 • General Sequences											
General Sequences	**TR**		**TE**		**TI**		**FA (degrees)**		**NEX**		**SLT/GAP (in millimeters)**
	1.5 T	**3.0 T**	**1.5 T**	**3.0 T**	**1.5 T**	**3.0 T**	**1.5 T**	**3.0 T**	**1.5 T**	**3.0 T**	**1.5 T**	**3.0 T**
T1 SE	450	450	15	15	N/A	N/A	90	90	4	2	3/0.3	3/0.3
T1 SE post C+	450	450	15	15	N/A	N/A	90	90	4	2	3/0.3	3/0.3

Abbreviations: N/A, not applicable; SE, spin echo.

SUGGESTED PROTOCOL VARIATIONS

Dynamic

A dynamic sequence may be helpful in detecting pituitary lesions (Table 17–2).

Tumor

A tumor protocol may require additional sequences and a larger field of view to include the lesion. Additional pre- and postcontrast sequences may be included. Three-orthogonal-plane postcontrast sequences may be beneficial.

TABLE 17–2 • Dynamic Sequences											
Dynamic Sequence	**TR**		**TE**		**TI**		**FA (degrees)**		**NEX**		**SLT/GAP**
	1.5 T	**3.0 T**	**1.5 T**	**3.0 T**	**1.5 T**	**3.0 T**	**1.5 T**	**3.0 T**	**1.5 T**	**3.0 T**	**1.5 T**	**3.0 T**
T1 RARE	400	500	10	12	N/A	N/A	90	90	1	1	3/0.3	3/0.3

Abbreviations: N/A, not applicable; RARE, rapid acquisition with relaxation enhancement.

18

Brain Diffusion–Weighted Imaging (DWI)

COIL SELECTION

- Primary coil: Head coil
- Secondary coil: Head and neck coil

PATIENT/PART POSITIONING AND CENTERING

- The patient is positioned supine, headfirst in the MRI table.
- Make sure the patient is comfortable.

- Position the patient so that the orbitomeatal line is perpendicular to the z-axis of the MRI unit. The interpupillary line should be parallel to the orbitomeatal line (see Figures 13–1 and 13–2).
- The head should be at isocenter.
- Position the patient's head so the midsagittal plane is parallel to the z-axis of the MRI unit and there is no rotation (see Figure 13–2).
- Center on the glabella (see Figure 13–2).
- Instruct the patient to lie still and not move any part of their body, especially the head.
- Instruct the patient to not cross their arms and legs.

SLICE ALIGNMENT AND SCAN RANGE

Axial Sequence Acquisition

Slice Alignment

- There are 2 methods that may be used when aligning the slice overlay for an axial image.
    1. Align the slice overlay parallel to a line extending from the anterior commissure to the posterior commissure (AC/PC) on the sagittal scout (Figure 18–1).
    2. Align the slice overlay to be parallel hard palate (orbito-meatal line) (see Figure 18–1).
- On the coronal scout, align the slice overlay to be perpendicular to the longitudinal fissure (Figure 18–2).
- Extend the slice overlay from the foramen magnum to the vertex.
- The field of view must include the brain, including cerebellar tonsils (Figure 18–3).

Phase and Frequency Orientation

- Phase: Anteroposterior
- Frequency: Right to left
- Phase and frequency orientations may be swapped.

Saturation Band Placement

- A saturation band may be used to eliminate or reduce motion and/or magnetic susceptibility artifact from the face.
- If used, the saturation band should be placed in a line extending from the glabella to the second cervical vertebra (C2).

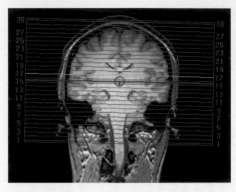

FIGURE 18–2. Coronal scout image showing image slice overlay position perpendicular to the midline for an axial sequence. Note the symmetrical positioning of the head.

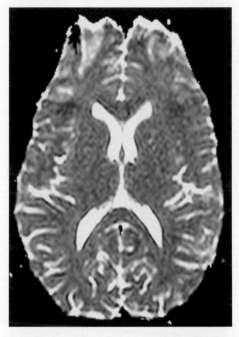

FIGURE 18–3. Axial apparent diffusion coefficient map.

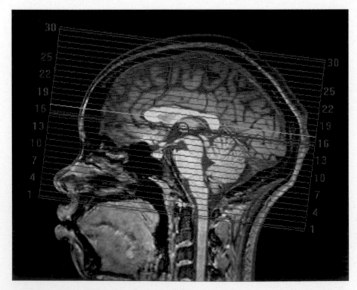

FIGURE 18–1. Midline sagittal scout image showing image slice overlay for an axial sequence. Note that the slice overlay is positioned along the anterior commissure–posterior commissure line.

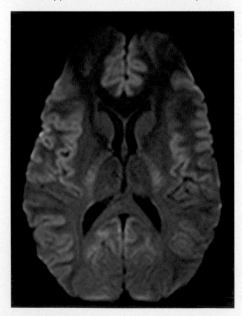

FIGURE 18–4. Axial b1000. Note that the b value may be changed, but typically, the b value is set at 1000.

Sagittal Sequence Acquisition (if Requested)

Slice Alignment

- See Figures 14–4 to 14–6 for more information.
- Using the axial and coronal scout images, align the slice overlay to be parallel to the longitudinal fissure.
- An odd number of slices should be used to allow for a midsagittal slice.
- Place the midsagittal slice over the longitudinal fissure.
- Slices cover the entire brain, from temporal lobe to temporal lobe.
- The field of view should extend to the level of C2.

Phase and Frequency Orientation

- Phase: Anteroposterior
- Frequency: Superior to inferior
- Phase and frequency orientations may be swapped.

Saturation Band Placement

- A saturation band may be used to eliminate or reduce motion and/or magnetic susceptibility artifact from the face.
- If used, the saturation band should be placed in a line extending from the glabella to C2.

Coronal Sequence Acquisition (if Requested)

Slice Alignment

- See Figures 14–7 to 14–9 for more information.
- Using the axial scout image, position the slice overlay to be perpendicular to the anatomy in the midline such as the longitude fissure or the third ventricle.
- On the sagittal scout image, align the slice overlay to be parallel to the brainstem.
- Slices cover the entire brain, from the frontal lobes to the occipital lobes.
- The field of view should extend from the vertex to the level of C2.

Phase and Frequency Orientation

- Phase: Right to left
- Frequency: Superior to inferior
- Phase and frequency orientations may be swapped.

Saturation Band Placement

- A saturation band may be used to eliminate or reduce motion and/or magnetic susceptibility artifact from the face.
- If used, the saturation band should be placed in a line extending from the glabella to C2.

IMAGING APPLICATION

The b value may be changed, but typically the b value is 1000.

TABLE 18-1 • General Sequences

General Sequences	TR		TE		TI		FA (degrees)		NEX		SLT/GAP (in millimeters)	
	1.5 T	3.0 T	1.5 T	3.0 T	1.5 T	3.0 T	1.5 T	3.0 T	1.5 T	3.0 T	1.5 T	3.0 T
DWI	4500	4500	50	60	N/A	N/A	90	90	3	2	5/1	5/1

Abbreviations: DWI, diffusion-weighted imaging; N/A, not applicable.

19

Brain Diffusion Tensor Imaging (DTI)

COIL SELECTION

- Primary coil: Head coil
- Secondary coil: Head and neck coil

PATIENT/PART POSITIONING AND CENTERING

- The patient is positioned supine, headfirst in the MRI table.
- Make sure the patient is comfortable.
- Position the patient so that the orbitomeatal line is perpendicular to the z-axis of the MRI unit. The interpupillary line should be parallel to the orbitomeatal line (see Figures 13–1 and 13–2).

- The head should be at isocenter.
- Position the patient's head so the midsagittal plane is parallel to the z-axis of the MRI unit and there is no rotation (see Figure 13–2).
- Center on the glabella (see Figure 13–2).
- Instruct the patient to lie still and not move any part of their body, especially the head.
- Instruct the patient to not cross their arms and legs.

SLICE ALIGNMENT AND SCAN RANGE

Axial Sequence Acquisition

Slice Alignment

- There are 2 methods that may be used when aligning the slice overlay for an axial image.
    1. Align the slice overlay parallel to a line extending from the anterior commissure to the posterior commissure (AC/PC) on the sagittal scout.
    2. Align the slice overlay to be parallel hard palate (orbitomeatal line).
- On the coronal scout, align the slice overlay to be perpendicular to the longitudinal fissure.
- Extend the slice overlay from the foramen magnum to the vertex.
- The field of view must include the brain, including cerebellar tonsils.
- See Figures 14–1 to 14–3 for more information.
- Protocols and diffusion tensor imaging (DTI) sequences may be different at each facility. Note that Figures 19–1 to 19–6 were acquired using a different DTI sequence than Figure 19–7.

Phase and Frequency Orientation

- Phase: Anteroposterior
- Frequency: Right to left
- Phase and frequency orientations may be swapped.

Saturation Band Placement

- A saturation band may be used to eliminate or reduce motion and/or magnetic susceptibility artifact from the face.
- If used, the saturation band should be placed in a line extending from the glabella to the second cervical vertebra (C2).

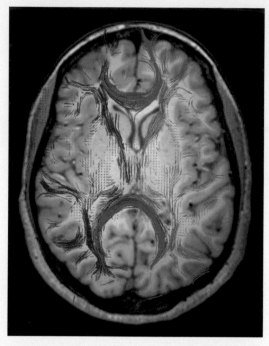

FIGURE 19–1. Axial T1 image with DTI fiber tracking. Note that the left-side fibers are blue and the right-side fibers are red. Notice the communication between the hemispheres of the brain.

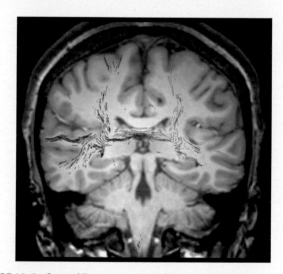

FIGURE 19–2. Coronal T1 image with DTI fiber tracking. Note that the left-side fibers are blue and the right-side fibers are red. Notice the communication between the hemispheres of the brain.

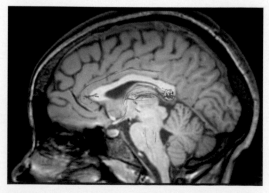

FIGURE 19–3. Sagittal T1 image with DTI fiber tracking.

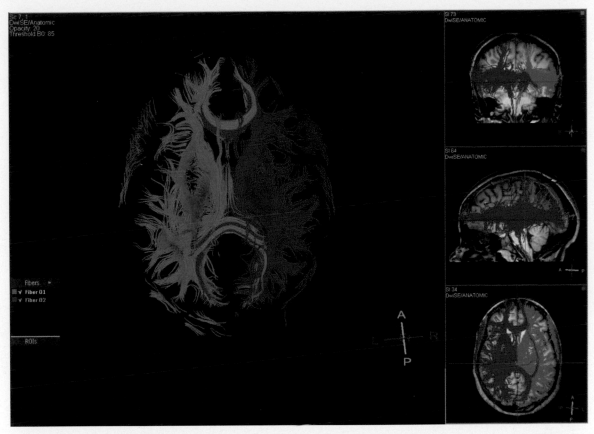

FIGURE 19–4. Axial DTI fiber tracking image without an image overlay. Note that the left-side fibers are blue and the right-side fibers are red. Notice the communication between the hemispheres of the brain.

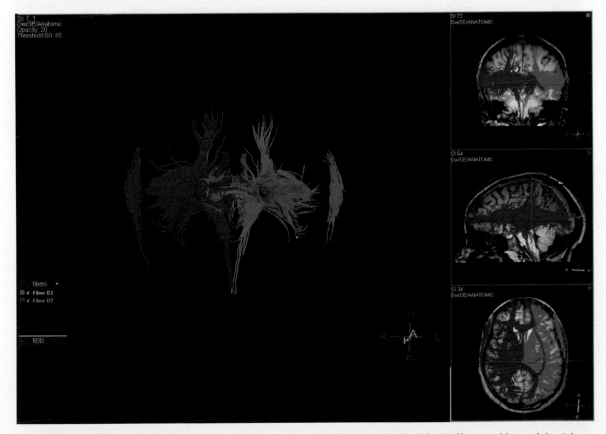

FIGURE 19–5. Coronal DTI fiber tracking image without an image overlay. Note that the left-side fibers are blue and the right-side fibers are red. Notice the communication between the hemispheres of the brain.

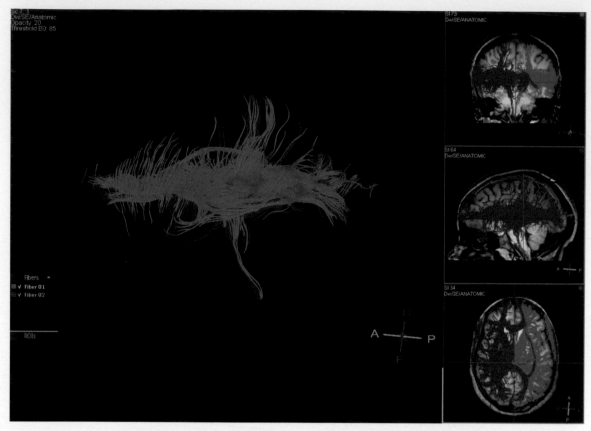

FIGURE 19–6. Sagittal DTI fiber tracking image without an image overlay. Note that the left-side fibers are blue and the right-side fibers are red.

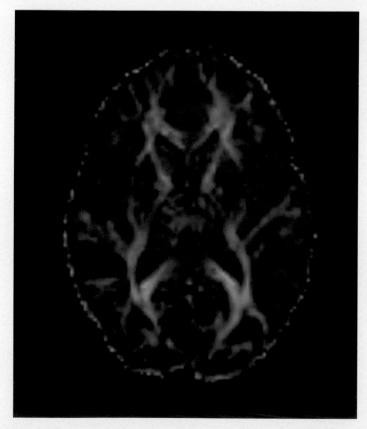

FIGURE 19–7. Axial DTI image demonstrating fiber tracking. Notice the communication between the hemispheres of the brain. Note: Figures 19–1 to 19–6 were acquired using a different DTI sequence than Figure 19–7. Figure 19–7 is included to demonstrate the difference in DTI sequences.

Sagittal Sequence Acquisition (if Requested)

Slice Alignment

- See Figures 14–4 to 14–6 for more information.
- Using the axial and coronal scout images, align the slice overlay to be parallel to the longitudinal fissure.
- An odd number of slices should be used to allow for a midsagittal slice.
- Place the midsagittal slice over the longitudinal fissure.
- Slices cover the entire brain, from temporal lobe to temporal lobe.
- The field of view should extend to the level of C2.

Phase and Frequency Orientation

- Phase: Anteroposterior
- Frequency: Superior to inferior
- Phase and frequency orientations may be swapped.

Saturation Band Placement

- A saturation band may be used to eliminate or reduce motion and/or magnetic susceptibility artifact from the face.
- If used, the saturation band should be placed in a line extending from the glabella to C2.

Coronal Sequence Acquisition (if Requested)

Slice Alignment

- See Figures 14–7 to 14–9 for more information.
- Using the axial scout image, position the slice overlay to be perpendicular to the anatomy in the midline such as the longitude fissure or the third ventricle.
- On the sagittal scout image, align the slice overlay to be parallel to the brainstem.
- Slices cover the entire brain, from the frontal lobes to the occipital lobes.
- The field of view should extend from the vertex to the level of C2.

Phase and Frequency Orientation

- Phase: Right to left
- Frequency: Superior to inferior
- Phase and frequency orientations may be swapped.

Saturation Band Placement

- A saturation band may be used to eliminate or reduce motion and/or magnetic susceptibility artifact from the face.
- If used, the saturation band should be placed in a line extending from the glabella to C2.

Brain Perfusion Imaging

COIL SELECTION

- Primary coil: Head coil
- Secondary coil: Head and neck coil

PATIENT/PART POSITIONING AND CENTERING

- The patient is positioned supine, headfirst in the MRI table.
- Make sure the patient is comfortable.

- Position the patient so that the orbitomeatal line is perpendicular to the z-axis of the MRI unit. The interpupillary line should be parallel to the orbitomeatal line (see Figures 13–1 and 13–2).
- The head should be at isocenter.
- Position the patient's head so the midsagittal plane is parallel to the z-axis of the MRI unit and there is no rotation (see Figure 13–2).
- Center on the glabella (see Figure 13–2).
- Instruct the patient to lie still and not move any part of their body, especially the head.
- Instruct the patient to not cross their arms and legs.

SLICE ALIGNMENT AND SCAN RANGE

Axial Sequence Acquisition

Slice Alignment

- There are 2 methods that may be used when aligning the slice overlay for an axial image.
  1. Align the slice overlay parallel to a line extending from the anterior commissure to the posterior commissure (AC/PC) on the sagittal scout (Figure 20–1).
  2. Align the slice overlay to be parallel hard palate (orbito-meatal line) (see Figure 20–1).
- On the coronal scout, align the slice overlay to be perpendicular to the longitudinal fissure (Figure 20–2).
- Extend the slice overlay from the foramen magnum to the vertex.
- The field of view must include the brain, including the cerebellar tonsils (Figure 20–3).

- Protocols and perfusion sequences may be different at each facility. Note that Figures 20–1 and 20–2 were acquired using a different perfusion sequence than Figures 20–3 and 20–4. Figures 20–1 and 20–2 required selecting 2 regions of interest (ROI) and comparing them. Figures 20–3 and 20–4 were acquired using a perfusion sequence that scanned the entire brain, much like a standard axial sequence.

Phase and Frequency Orientation

- Phase: Anteroposterior
- Frequency: Right to left
- Phase and frequency orientations may be swapped.

Saturation Band Placement

- A saturation band may be used to eliminate or reduce motion and/or magnetic susceptibility artifact from the face.
- If used, the saturation band should be placed in a line extending from the glabella to the second cervical vertebra (C2).

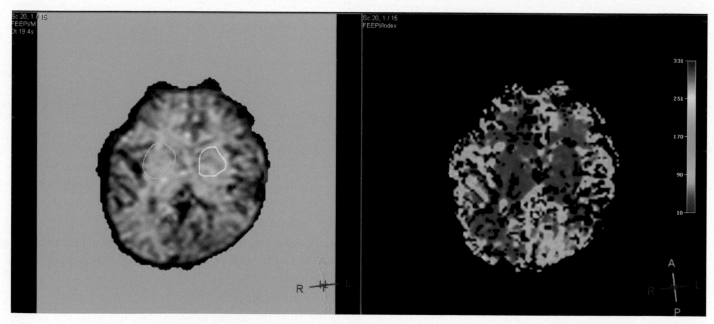

FIGURE 20–1. Two axial T1 perfusion sequences. Note in the left image that 2 regions of interest (ROIs) have been selected.

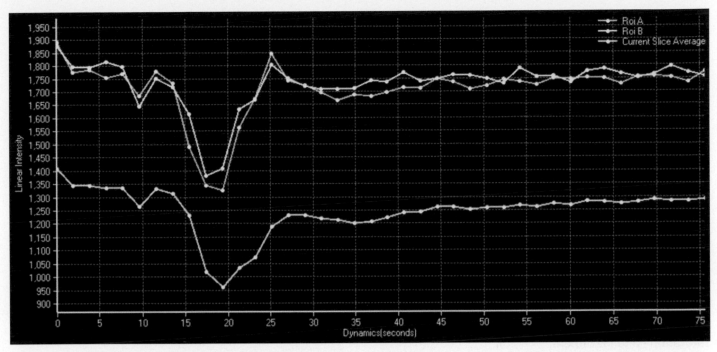

FIGURE 20–2. Chart comparing the regions of interest (ROIs) from Figure 20–1.

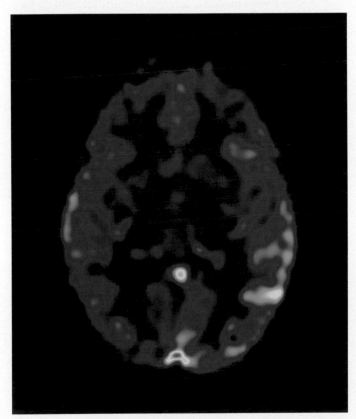

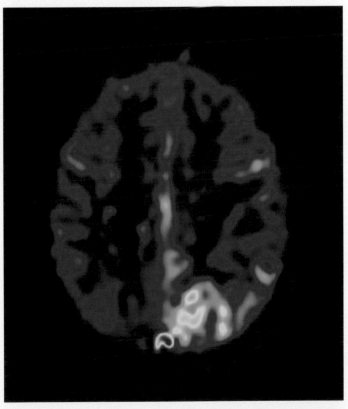

FIGURE 20–3. Axial pseudo-continuous arterial spin–labeled (pCASL) perfusion sequence. Note the color map and relative cerebral blood flow. Areas colored blue demonstrate somewhat normal perfusion, whereas areas that are green, yellow, orange, and red demonstrate areas of increased perfusion. Figures 20–3 and 20–4 were acquired on the same patient.

FIGURE 20–4. Axial pseudo-continuous arterial spin–labeled (pCASL) perfusion sequence. Note, this is the same patient as demonstrated in Figure 20–3, but the slice is at a different level. Notice the areas of increased perfusion in the left cerebral hemisphere. The areas of increased perfusion are shown as green, yellow, orange, and red. This patient was diagnosed with an arteriovenous malformation (AVM).

Sagittal Sequence Acquisition (if Requested)

Slice Alignment
- See Figures 14–4 to 14–6 for more information.
- Using the axial and coronal scout images, align the slice overlay to be parallel to the longitudinal fissure.
- An odd number of slices should be used to allow for a mid-sagittal slice.
- Place the midsagittal slice over the longitudinal fissure.
- Slices cover the entire brain, from temporal lobe to temporal lobe.
- The field of view should extend to the level of C2.

Phase and Frequency Orientation
- Phase: Anteroposterior
- Frequency: Superior to inferior
- Phase and frequency orientations may be swapped.

Saturation Band Placement
- A saturation band may be used to eliminate or reduce motion and/or magnetic susceptibility artifact from the face.
- If used, the saturation band should be placed in a line extending from the glabella to C2.

Coronal Sequence Acquisition (if Requested)

Slice Alignment
- See Figures 14–7 to 14–9 for more information.
- Using the axial scout image, position the slice overlay to be perpendicular to the anatomy in the midline such as the longitude fissure or the third ventricle.
- On the sagittal scout image, align the slice overlay to be parallel to the brainstem.
- Slices cover the entire brain, from the frontal lobes to the occipital lobes.
- The field of view should extend from the vertex to the level of C2.

Phase and Frequency Orientation
- Phase: Right to left
- Frequency: Superior to inferior
- Phase and frequency orientations may be swapped.

Saturation Band Placement
- A saturation band may be used to eliminate or reduce motion and/or magnetic susceptibility artifact from the face.
- If used, the saturation band should be placed in a line extending from the glabella to C2.

21

Brain Susceptibility–Weighted Imaging (SWI)

COIL SELECTION

- Primary coil: Head coil
- Secondary coil: Head and neck coil

PATIENT/PART POSITIONING AND CENTERING

- The patient is positioned supine, headfirst in the MRI table.
- Make sure the patient is comfortable.
- Position the patient so that the orbitomeatal line is perpendicular to the z-axis of the MRI unit. The interpupillary line should be parallel to the orbitomeatal line (see Figures 13–1 and 13–2).
- The head should be at isocenter.
- Position the patient's head so the midsagittal plane is parallel to the z-axis of the MRI unit and there is no rotation (see Figure 13–2).
- Center on the glabella (see Figure 13–2).
- Instruct the patient to lie still and not move any part of their body, especially the head.
- Instruct the patient to not cross their arms and legs.

SLICE ALIGNMENT AND SCAN RANGE

Axial Sequence Acquisition

Slice Alignment

- There are 2 methods that may be used when aligning the slice overlay for an axial image.
  1. Align the slice overlay parallel to a line extending from the anterior commissure to the posterior commissure (AC/PC) on the sagittal scout.
  2. Align the slice overlay to be parallel hard palate (orbitomeatal line).
- On the coronal scout, align the slice overlay to be perpendicular to the longitudinal fissure (Figure 14–2).
- Extend the slice overlay from the foramen magnum to the vertex.
- The field of view must include the brain, including cerebellar tonsils.
- See Figures 14–1 to 14–3 for more information.

Phase and Frequency Orientation

- Phase: Anteroposterior
- Frequency: Right to left
- Phase and frequency orientations may be swapped.

Saturation Band Placement

- A saturation band may be used to eliminate or reduce motion and/or magnetic susceptibility artifact from the face.
- If used, the saturation band should be placed in a line extending from the glabella to the second cervical vertebra (C2).

Sagittal Sequence Acquisition (if Requested)

Slice Alignment

- See Figures 14–4 to 14–6 for more information.
- Using the axial and coronal scout images, align the slice overlay to be parallel to the longitudinal fissure.
- An odd number of slices should be used to allow for a midsagittal slice.
- Place the midsagittal slice over the longitudinal fissure.
- Slices cover the entire brain, from temporal lobe to temporal lobe.
- The field of view should extend to the level of C2.

Phase and Frequency Orientation

- Phase: Anteroposterior
- Frequency: Superior to inferior
- Phase and frequency orientations may be swapped.

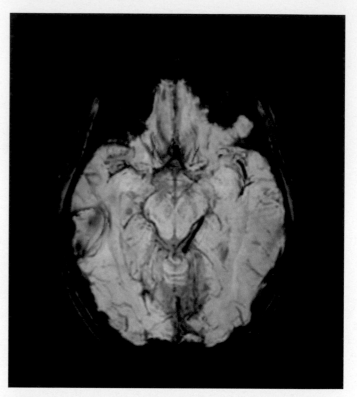

FIGURE 21–1. Axial susceptibility-weighted (SWI) image. Note the hypointense blood vessels.

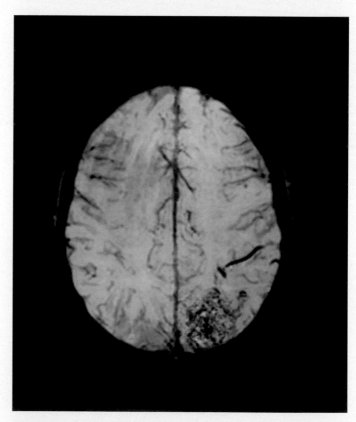

FIGURE 21–2. Axial susceptibility-weighted (SWI) image. Note that this is the same patient as demonstrated in Figure 21–1, but this slice is at a different level. Further, note the collection of blood vessels in the left posterior cerebral hemisphere. This demonstrates an arteriovenous malformation (AVM).

Saturation Band Placement

- A saturation band may be used to eliminate or reduce motion and/or magnetic susceptibility artifact from the face.
- If used, the saturation band should be placed in a line extending from the glabella to C2.

Coronal Sequence Acquisition (If Requested)

Slice Alignment

- See Figures 14–7 to 14–9 for more information.
- Using the axial scout image, position the slice overlay to be perpendicular to the anatomy in the midline such as the longitude fissure or the third ventricle.
- On the sagittal scout image, align the slice overlay to be parallel to the brainstem.

- Slices cover the entire brain, from the frontal lobes to the occipital lobes.
- The field of view should extend from the vertex to the level of C2.

Phase and Frequency Orientation

- Phase: Right to left
- Frequency: Superior to inferior
- Phase and frequency orientations may be swapped.

Saturation Band Placement

- A saturation band may be used to eliminate or reduce motion and/or magnetic susceptibility artifact from the face.
- If used, the saturation band should be placed in a line extending from the glabella to C2.

IMAGING APPLICATION

TABLE 21–1 • General Sequences

General Sequences	TR		TE		TI		FA (degrees)		NEX		SLT/GAP (in millimeters)	
	1.5 T	3.0 T	1.5 T	3.0 T	1.5 T	3.0 T	1.5 T	3.0 T	1.5 T	3.0 T	1.5 T	3.0 T
T2* 3D GRE	20	17	15	29	N/A	N/A	7	7	1	1	5/0	5/0

Abbreviations: 3D, 3-dimensional; GRE, gradient echo; N/A, not applicable.

22

Brain Spectroscopy

COIL SELECTION

- Primary coil: Head coil
- Secondary coil: Head and neck coil

PATIENT/PART POSITIONING AND CENTERING

- The patient is positioned supine, headfirst in the MRI table.
- Make sure the patient is comfortable.
- Position the patient so that the orbitomeatal line is perpendicular to the z-axis of the MRI unit. The interpupillary line should be parallel to the orbitomeatal line (see Figures 13–1 and 13–2).
- The head should be at isocenter.
- Position the patient's head so the midsagittal plane is parallel to the z-axis of the MRI unit and there is no rotation (see Figure 13–2).
- Center on the glabella (see Figure 13–2).
- Instruct the patient to lie still and not move any part of their body, especially the head.
- Instruct the patient to not cross their arms and legs.

SLICE ALIGNMENT AND SCAN RANGE

A region of interest (ROI) is placed in an area of abnormal signal and normal signal. Ask the attending radiologist where they want the ROIs placed. Typically, if the abnormal signal is localized to one area of the brain, an ROI is placed only in the abnormal area. No portion of the ROI should touch normal brain tissue. The other ROI is placed in normal signal so the abnormal and normal ROIs are mirror images. For example, if a patient has a mass in the left temporal lobe, an ROI should be placed in the mass and another in the right temporal lobe. Separate spectroscopy graphs should be created for the abnormal area and normal area. This will create a useful chemical comparison between the normal and abnormal areas of the brain. Figures 22–1 to 22–10 below demonstrate placement of ROI and subsequent chemical composition graphs.

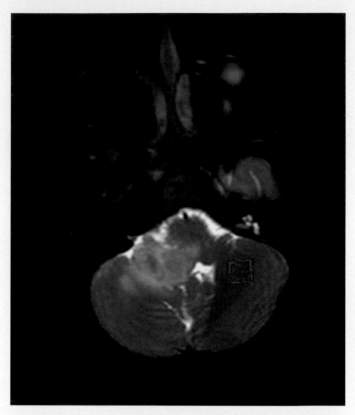

FIGURE 22–1. Axial scout image showing a single-voxel ROI in normal brain tissue.

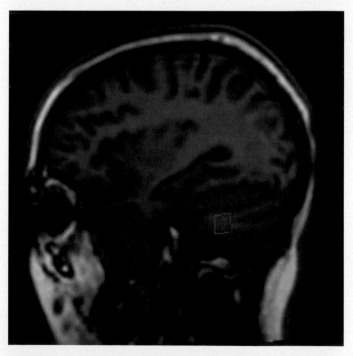

FIGURE 22–2. Sagittal scout image showing a single-voxel ROI in normal brain tissue.

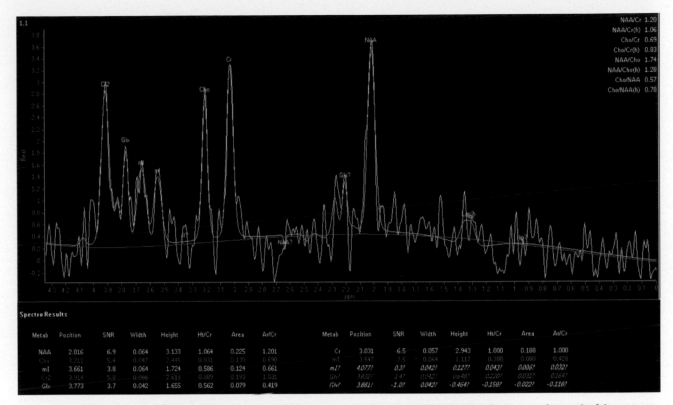

NAA/Cr	1.20
NAA/Cr(h)	1.06
Cho/Cr	0.69
Cho/Cr(h)	0.83
NAA/Cho	1.74
NAA/Cho(h)	1.28
Cho/NAA	0.57
Cho/NAA(h)	0.78

Spectro Results

Metab	Position	SNR	Width	Height	Ht/Cr	Area	Ar/Cr	Metab	Position	SNR	Width	Height	Ht/Cr	Area	Ar/Cr
NAA	2.016	6.9	0.064	3.133	1.064	0.225	1.201	Cr	3.031	6.5	0.057	2.943	1.000	0.188	1.000
Cho	3.212	5.4	0.047	2.445	0.831	0.130	0.690	mI	3.547	2.5	0.064	1.117	0.380	0.080	0.428
mI	3.661	3.8	0.064	1.724	0.586	0.124	0.661	mI?	4.077?	0.3?	0.042?	0.127?	0.043?	0.006?	0.032?
Cr2	3.914	5.8	0.066	2.618	0.889	0.193	1.031	Glx?	3.832?	1.4?	0.042?	0.648?	0.220?	0.031?	0.164?
Glx	3.773	3.7	0.042	1.655	0.562	0.079	0.419	Glx?	3.881?	-1.0?	0.042?	-0.464?	-0.158?	-0.022?	-0.118?

FIGURE 22–3. Graph of the chemical composition of the single-voxel ROI in normal brain tissue. Compare to the graph of the ROI in brain tumor tissue (Figure 22–6).

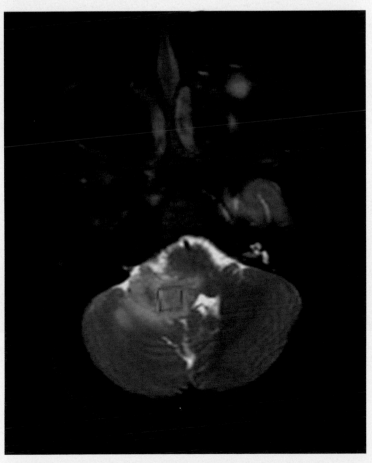

FIGURE 22–4. Axial scout image showing a single-voxel ROI in brain tumor tissue.

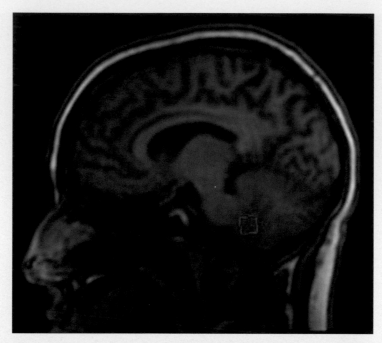

FIGURE 22–5. Sagittal scout image showing a single-voxel ROI in brain tumor tissue.

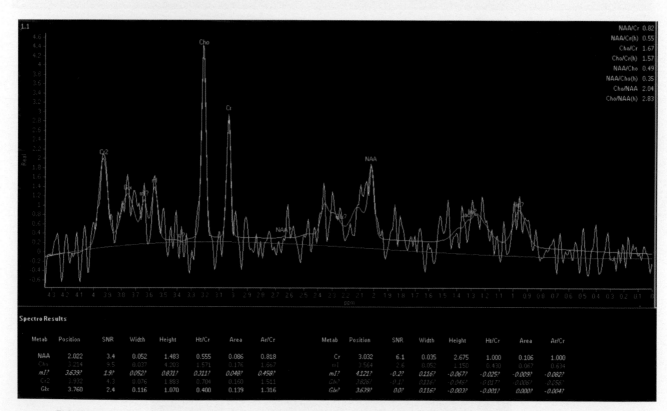

FIGURE 22–6. Graph of the chemical composition of the single-voxel ROI in brain tumor tissue. Compare to the graph of the ROI in normal brain tissue (Figure 22–3).

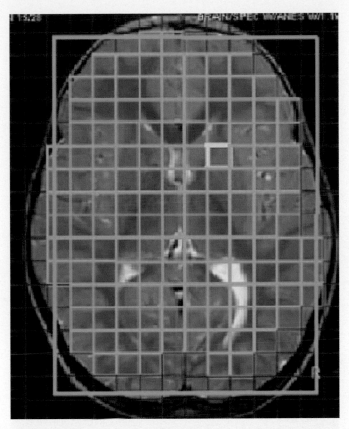

FIGURE 22–7. Multivoxel axial scout image showing a single-voxel ROI in the left basal ganglia. Compare to Figure 22–9.

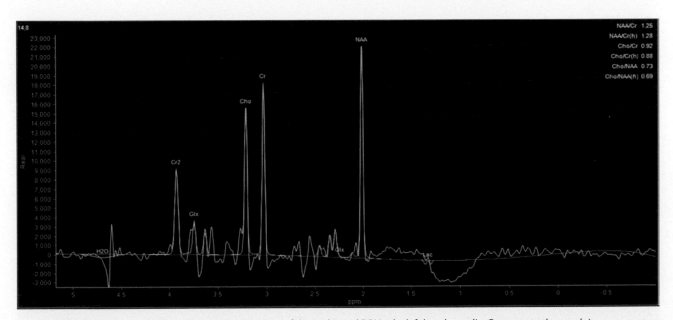

FIGURE 22–8. Graph of the chemical composition of the multivoxel ROI in the left basal ganglia. Compare to the graph in Figure 22–10.

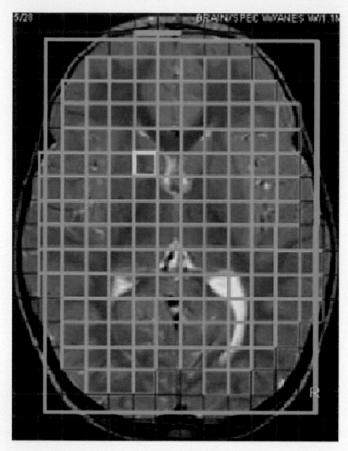

FIGURE 22–9. Multivoxel axial scout image showing a single-voxel ROI in the right basal ganglia. Compare to Figure 22–7.

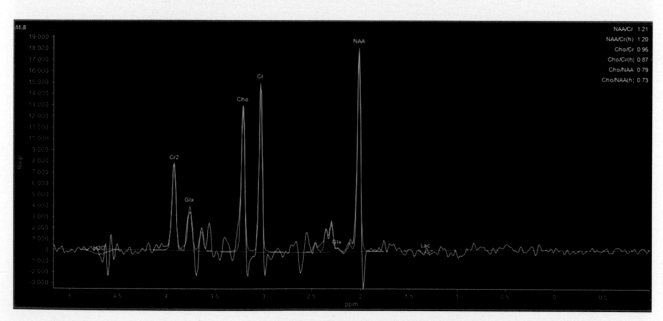

FIGURE 22–10. Graph of the chemical composition of the multivoxel ROI in the right basal ganglia. Compare to the graph in Figure 22–8.

23

Temporal Lobes

COIL SELECTION

- Primary coil: Head coil
- Secondary coil: Head and neck coil

PATIENT/PART POSITIONING AND CENTERING

- The patient is positioned supine, headfirst in the MRI table.
- Make sure the patient is comfortable.
- Position the patient so that the orbitomeatal line is perpendicular to the z-axis of the MRI unit. The interpupillary line should be parallel to the orbitomeatal line (see Figures 13–1 and 13–2).
- The head should be at isocenter.
- Position the patient's head so the midsagittal plane is parallel to the z-axis of the MRI unit and there is no rotation (see Figure 13–2).
- Center on the glabella (see Figure 13–2).
- Instruct the patient to lie still and not move any part of their body, especially the head.
- Instruct the patient to not cross their arms and legs.

SLICE ALIGNMENT AND SCAN RANGE

A coronal short tau inversion recovery (STIR) aligned with the temporal lobes of the brain may be helpful in the evaluation of a patient with a history of seizures and/or epilepsy. Temporal lobe sequences, such as the coronal STIR, may be added to the routine brain protocol. The technologist should follow the protocol provided at their facility. The slice alignment and scan range below are for any coronal sequences, aligned with the temporal lobes.

Slice Alignment

- Slices are perpendicular to the temporal horns of the lateral ventricles (Figure 23–1).
- Slices cover the entire temporal lobes (see Figures 23–1 and 23–2).
- The field of view should cover all of the temporal lobes but may also be extended to include the entire brain. Please consult the protocol used at your facility.

Phase and Frequency Orientation

- Phase: Right to left
- Frequency: Superior to inferior
- Phase and frequency orientations may be swapped to reduce motion artifact.

Saturation Band Placement

- A saturation band may be used to eliminate or reduce motion and/or magnetic susceptibility artifact from the face.
- If used, the saturation band should be placed in a line extending from the glabella to cervical vertebra 2 (C2).

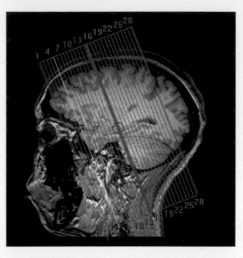

FIGURE 23–1. Parasagittal scout image showing image slice overlay for a coronal sequence of the temporal lobes. Note that the slices are perpendicular to the long axis of the temporal lobes. Also, the field of view may be extended to cover the entire brain.

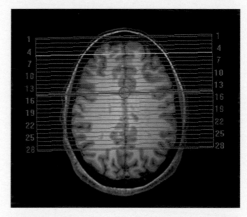

FIGURE 23–2. Axial scout image showing image slice overlay for a coronal sequence of the temporal lobes. Note that the slices are perpendicular to the temporal lobes. As a side note, you would want to use a slightly inferior axial image that demonstrates the temporal lobes.

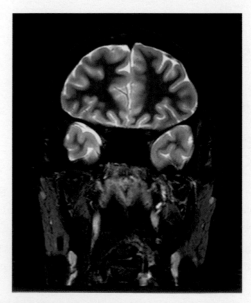

FIGURE 23–3. Coronal STIR of the temporal lobes. Note that the slices are perpendicular (short-axis) to the temporal lobes.

IMAGING APPLICATION

TABLE 23–1 • Seizure Sequence

Seizure Sequence	TR		TE		TI		FA (degrees)		NEX		SLT/GAP (in millimenters)	
	1.5 T	3.0 T	1.5 T	3.0 T	1.5 T	3.0 T	1.5 T	3.0 T	1.5 T	3.0 T	1.5 T	3.0 T
STIR	3000	6000	60	75	150	220	90	90	3	3	3/1	3/1

Abbreviation: STIR, short tau inversion recovery.

Orbits

COIL SELECTION

- Primary coil: Head coil
- Secondary coil: Head and neck coil

PATIENT/PART POSITIONING AND CENTERING

- The patient is positioned supine, headfirst in the MRI table.
- Make sure the patient is comfortable.
- Position the patient so that the orbitomeatal line is perpendicular to the z-axis of the MRI unit. The interpupillary line

is to be parallel to the orbitomeatal line (see Figures 13–1 and 13–2).

- The head should be at isocenter.
- Position the patient's head so the midsagittal plane is parallel to the z-axis of the MRI unit and there is no rotation (see Figure 13–2).
- Center on the glabella (see Figure 13–2).
- Instruct the patient to lie still and not move any part of their body, especially the head.
- Instruct the patient to not cross their arms and legs.

SLICE ALIGNMENT AND SCAN RANGE

Axial Sequence Acquisition

Slice Alignment

- On the sagittal and coronal scout images, align the slice overlay to be parallel to the optic nerve (Figures 24–1 and 24–2). Use an odd number of slices so the center slice shows the optic nerve on its long axis.
- The superior-to-inferior field of view must include the rectus muscles (see Figure 24–1).
- The left-to-right field of view must include the rectus muscles of the orbits.
- The anteroposterior field of view should extend from the lens of the orbit to the brainstem so that the optic chiasm is included (Figures 24–3 and 24–4).

Phase and Frequency Orientation

- Phase: Anteroposterior
- Frequency: Right to left
- Phase and frequency orientations may be swapped.

Saturation Band Placement

- A saturation band may be used to eliminate or reduce motion and/or magnetic susceptibility artifact from the face.
- If used, the saturation band should be placed inferior to the field of view.

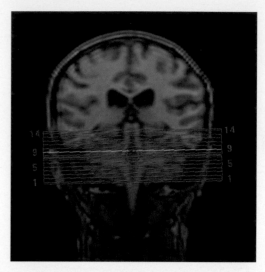

FIGURE 24–2. Coronal scout image showing image slice overlay for an axial sequence.

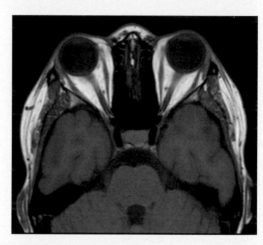

FIGURE 24–3. Axial T1-weighted image. Note that the anatomic structures, such as the globe, lens, optic nerves, medial rectus muscles, and lateral rectus muscles, are very well seen due to patient positioning and slice overlay.

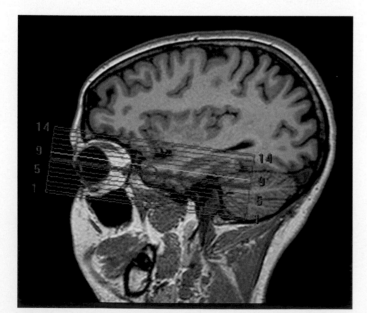

FIGURE 24–1. Sagittal scout image showing image slice overlay for an axial sequence. Note the parallel alignment with the optic nerve.

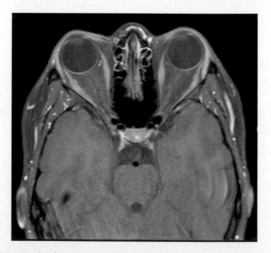

FIGURE 24–4. Axial postcontrast T1-weighted fat-saturated image. This image is included to demonstrate the difference between a T1-weighted image (Figure 24–3) and a postcontrast T1-weighted fat-saturated image (Figure 24–4). Note that the image is at a slightly different level than Figure 24–3 due to patient movement following the administration of contrast. This sequence was set up to be a postcontrast mirror of Figure 24–3.

Coronal Sequence Acquisition

Slice Alignment

- On the sagittal scout, align the slice overlay to be perpendicular to the optic nerve (Figure 24–5).
- On the axial scout, extend the slice overlay from the lens of the orbit to the brainstem so that the optic chiasm is included (Figure 24–6).
- The anatomy of the optic nerves should be symmetrical (unless pathology is present) (Figures 24–7 to 24–9).
- The left-to-right field of view must include the rectus muscles.
- The superior-to-inferior field of view must include the rectus muscles.
- If imaging each orbit individually, use the axial and sagittal scout images to align the slices perpendicular to the optic nerve.

Phase and Frequency Orientation

- Phase: Right to left
- Frequency: Superior to inferior
- Phase and frequency orientations may be swapped.

Saturation Band Placement

- A saturation band may be used to eliminate or reduce motion and/or magnetic susceptibility artifact from the face.
- If used, the saturation band should be placed inferior to the field of view.

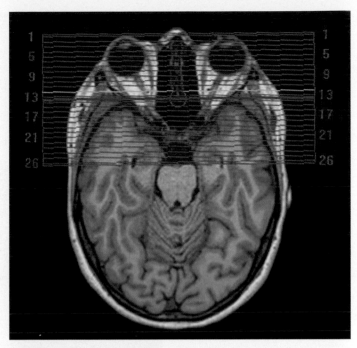

FIGURE 24–6. Axial scout image showing image slice overlay for a coronal sequence. Note that the slice overlay is perpendicular to the midline of the patient's head.

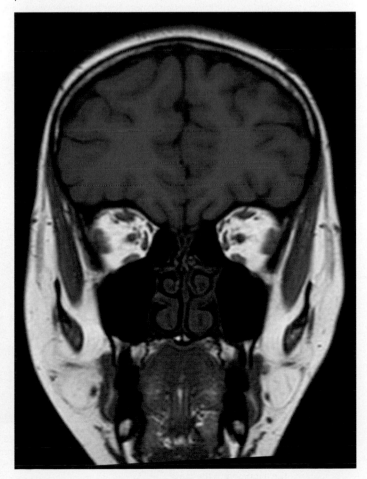

FIGURE 24–7. Coronal T1-weighted image. Note the anatomic structures such as the optic nerves, medial rectus muscles, lateral rectus muscles, superior rectus muscles, superior oblique rectus muscles, and inferior rectus muscles. This is an example of a retro-orbital image of the orbital area. Muscles are hypointense while the fat is hyperintense.

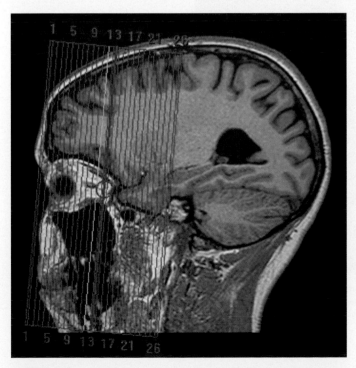

FIGURE 24–5. Parasagittal scout image showing image slice overlay for a coronal sequence. Note the perpendicular alignment with the optic nerve.

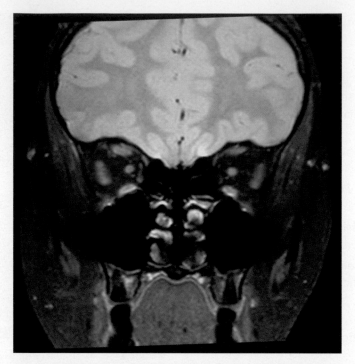

FIGURE 24–8. Coronal proton density (PD) fat-saturated image. This image is included to demonstrate the difference between a T1-weighted image (Figure 24–7), PD fat-saturated image (Figure 24–8), and postcontrast T1-weighted fat-saturated image (Figure 24–9). It is important to note that this sequence was planned to have a smaller field of view than Figure 24–7, but the alignment is the same.

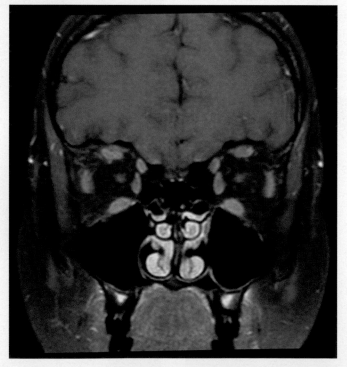

FIGURE 24–9. Coronal postcontrast T1-weighted fat-saturated image. Image is included to demonstrate the difference between a T1-weighted image (Figure 24–7), PD fat-saturated image (Figure 24–8), and postcontrast T1-weighted fat-saturated image (Figure 24–9). It is important to note that this sequence was planned to have a smaller field of view than Figure 24–7, but the alignment is the same.

Sagittal Sequence Acquisition (if Requested)

Slice Alignment

- Sagittal sequences may not be required; consult the attending radiologist and/or requesting physician.
- Use the axial and coronal scout images to align the slices parallel to the optic nerve (see Figure 24–10 for resultant image).
- The left-to-right field of view must include the rectus muscles.
- The anteroposterior field of view should extend from the lens of the orbit to the brainstem.
- The superior-to-inferior field of view must include the rectus muscles.

Phase and Frequency Orientation

- Phase: Anteroposterior
- Frequency: Superior to inferior
- Phase and frequency orientations may be swapped.

Saturation Band Placement

- A saturation band may be used to eliminate or reduce motion and/or magnetic susceptibility artifact from the face.
- If used, the saturation band should be placed inferior to the field of view.

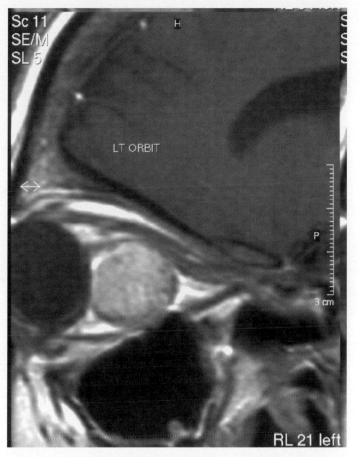

FIGURE 24–10. Sagittal oblique T1-weighted image angled along the long axis of the optic nerve. Note that the retrobulbar cavernous hemangioma (round and slightly hyperintense) is seen displacing the optic nerve superiorly. (Reprinted from Grey ML, Ailinani JM. *CT & MRI Pathology: A Pocket Atlas*. 3rd ed. McGraw-Hill; 2018, with permission from The McGraw-Hill Professional.)

IMAGING APPLICATION

TABLE 24–1 • General Sequences												

General Sequences	TR		TE		TI		FA (degrees)		NEX		SLT/GAP (in millimeters)	
	1.5 T	3.0 T	1.5 T	3.0 T	1.5 T	3.0 T	1.5 T	3.0 T	1.5 T	3.0 T	1.5 T	3.0 T
T1 SE	550	450	10	12	N/A	N/A	90	90	4	3	3/0.3	3/0.3
PD	2500	2000	30	15	N/A	N/A	90	90	3	2	3/0.3	3/0.3
T1 SE post C+	550	450	10	12	N/A	N/A	90	90	4	3	3/0.3	3/0.3

Abbreviations: N/A, not available; PD, proton density; SE, spin echo.

SUGGESTED PROTOCOL VARIATIONS

Trauma

The attending radiologist and/or the requesting physician may ask for additional sequences or orthogonal planes depending on the traumatic injury.

Tumor

A tumor protocol may require sequences in addition to the routine orbit protocol and a larger field of view to include the lesion. Additional pre- and postcontrast sequences may be included. Three-orthogonal-plane postcontrast sequences may be of benefit to the radiologist. The technologist should follow the protocol provided at their facility.

Face

COIL SELECTION

- Primary coil: Head coil
- Secondary coil: Head and neck coil

PATIENT/PART POSITIONING AND CENTERING

- The patient is positioned supine, headfirst in the MRI table.
- Make sure the patient is comfortable.
- Position the patient so that the orbitomeatal line is perpendicular to the z-axis of the MRI unit. The interpupillary line is to be parallel to the orbitomeatal line (see Figures 13–1 and 13–2).
- The head should be at isocenter.
- Position the patient's head so the midsagittal plane is parallel to the z-axis of the MRI unit and there is no rotation (see Figure 13–2).
- Center on the nasion (see Figure 13–2).
- Instruct the patient to lie still and not move any part of their body, especially the head.
- Instruct the patient to not cross their arms and legs.

SLICE ALIGNMENT AND SCAN RANGE

Axial Sequence Acquisition

Slice Alignment

- On the sagittal scout, align the slice overlay parallel to the hard palate (Figure 25–1).
- Slices are perpendicular to a line extending from the frontal sinus to mandibular symphysis (Figures 25–1 and 25–2).
- The superior-to-inferior field of view should extend from the frontal sinus to the thyroid cartilage (see Figure 25–1).
- The left-to-right field of view should extend from one zygomatic arch to the other zygomatic arch.
- The anteroposterior field of view should extend from the nose to spinal cord (see Figure 25–1).
- Slices should include the soft tissue immediately inferior to the mandible, nose, and cheeks (Figure 25–3).

Phase and Frequency Orientation

- Phase: Anteroposterior
- Frequency: Right to left
- Phase and frequency orientations may be swapped to reduce motion artifact.

Saturation Band Placement

- A saturation band may be used to eliminate or reduce motion artifact from the thorax.
- If used, the saturation band should be placed inferior to the field of view.

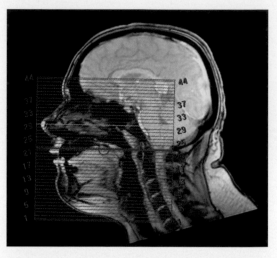

FIGURE 25–1. Midline sagittal scout image showing image slice overlay for an axial sequence.

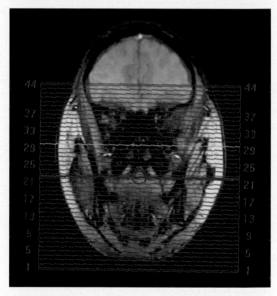

FIGURE 25–2. Coronal scout image showing image slice overlay for an axial sequence.

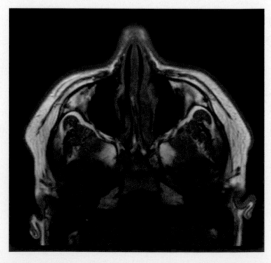

FIGURE 25–3. Axial T1-weighted image of the face. Note the symmetry of the left and right side of the face.

Coronal Sequence Acquisition

Slice Alignment

- On the sagittal scout, align the slice overlay parallel to a line extending from the frontal sinus to mandibular symphysis (Figure 25–4).
- Slices are perpendicular to the hard palate (see Figure 25–4).
- The superior-to-inferior field of view should extend from the frontal sinus to the thyroid cartilage (see Figure 25–4)
- The left-to-right field of view should extend from one zygomatic arch to the other zygomatic arch (Figure 25–5).
- The anteroposterior field of view should extend from the nose to spinal cord (see Figure 25–4).
- Slices should include the soft tissue immediately inferior to the mandible, nose, and cheeks (Figure 25–6).

Phase and Frequency Orientation

- Phase: Right to left
- Frequency: Superior to inferior
- Phase and frequency orientations may be swapped to reduce motion artifact.

Saturation Band Placement

- A saturation band may be used to eliminate or reduce motion artifact from the thorax.
- If used, the saturation band should be placed inferior to the field of view.

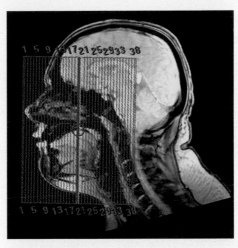

FIGURE 25–4. Midline sagittal scout image showing image slice overlay for a coronal sequence of the face.

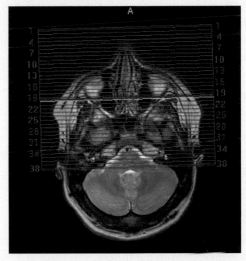

FIGURE 25–5. Axial scout image showing image slice overlay for a coronal sequence. Note that the slice overlay is perpendicular to the midline.

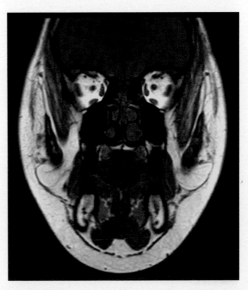

FIGURE 25–6. Coronal T1-weighted image. Note the anatomic structures such as the orbits, rectus muscles, optic nerves, nasal septum, turbinates, maxillary sinuses, mandible, and tongue.

Sagittal Sequence Acquisition

Slice Alignment

- Slices are parallel to the longitudinal fissure, bony nasal septum, and mandibular symphysis on the axial (Figure 25–7) and coronal (Figure 25–8) planning images.

- An odd number of slices should be used to allow for a midsagittal slice.

- Place the midsagittal slice over the longitudinal fissure, bony nasal septum, and mandibular symphysis.

- The superior-to-inferior field of view should extend from the frontal sinus to the thyroid cartilage.

- The left-to-right field of view should extend from one zygomatic arch to the other zygomatic arch.

- The anteroposterior field of view should extend from the nose to spinal cord.

- Slices should include the soft tissue immediately inferior to the mandible, nose, and cheeks. It is helpful to use a sagittal survey image to check the field of view and be sure all soft tissue is covered (Figure 25–9).

Phase and Frequency Orientation

- Phase: Anteroposterior
- Frequency: Superior to inferior
- Phase and frequency orientations may be swapped to reduce motion artifact.

Saturation Band Placement

- A saturation band may be used to eliminate or reduce motion artifact from the thorax.
- If used, the saturation band should be placed inferior to the field of view.

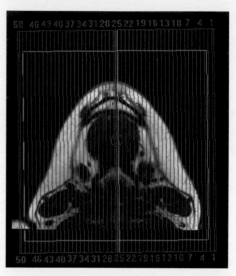

FIGURE 25–7. Axial scout image showing image slice overlay for a sagittal sequence. Note that there is an odd number of slices in this example, so the middle slice would be a midsagittal image.

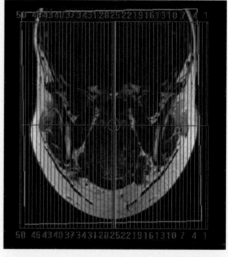

FIGURE 25–8. Coronal scout image showing image slice overlay for a sagittal sequence. Note that there is an odd number of slices in this example, so the middle slice would be a midsagittal image.

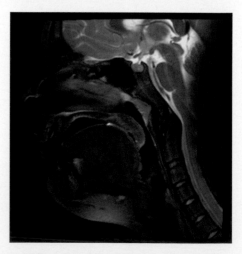

FIGURE 25–9. Midline sagittal T2-weighted fat-saturated image. Note the anatomic structures shown such as the basilar artery, pituitary gland, pituitary stalk (infundibulum) hard palate, soft palate, nasal septum, tongue, sphenoid sinus, and frontal sinus.

IMAGING APPLICATION

TABLE 25–1 • General Sequences

General Sequences	TR		TE		TI		FA (degrees)		NEX		SLT/GAP (in millimeters)	
	1.5 T	3.0 T	1.5 T	3.0 T	1.5 T	3.0 T	1.5 T	3.0 T	1.5 T	3.0 T	1.5 T	3.0 T
T1 SE	600	500	10	10	N/A	N/A	90	90	3	2	3/0.3	3/0.3
T2 SE	6000	3500	100	80	N/A	N/A	90	90	3	2	3/0.3	3/0.3
STIR	6000	5000	30	80	135	200	90	90	3	2	3/0.3	3/0.3
T1 SE post C+	600	500	10	10	N/A	N/A	90	90	3	2	3/0.3	3/0.3

Abbreviations: N/A, not applicable; SE, spin echo; STIR, short tau inversion recovery.

SUGGESTED PROTOCOL VARIATIONS

Trauma

The attending radiologist and/or the requesting physician may ask for additional sequences or orthogonal planes depending on the traumatic injury.

Tumor

A tumor protocol may require sequences in addition to the routine face protocol and a larger field of view to include the lesion. Additional pre- and postcontrast sequences may be included. Three-orthogonal-plane postcontrast sequences may be of benefit to the radiologist. The technologist should follow the protocol provided at their facility.

26

Internal Auditory Canals (IACs)

COIL SELECTION

- Primary coil: Head coil
- Secondary coil: Head and neck coil

PATIENT/PART POSITIONING AND CENTERING

- The patient is positioned supine, headfirst in the MRI table.
- Make sure the patient is comfortable.
- Position the patient so that the orbitomeatal line is perpendicular to the z-axis of the MRI unit. The interpupillary line should be parallel to the orbitomeatal line (see Figures 13–1 and 13–2).
- The head should be at isocenter.
- Position the patient's head so the midsagittal plane is parallel to the z-axis of the MRI unit and there is no rotation (see Figure 13–2).
- Center on the glabella (see Figure 13–2).
- Instruct the patient to lie still and not move any part of their body, especially the head.
- Instruct the patient to not cross their arms and legs.

SLICE ALIGNMENT AND SCAN RANGE

Axial Sequence Acquisition

Slice Alignment
- Slices should be aligned according to a line drawn from cochlea to cochlea. Angle the slices so that they enter each cochlea at the same point (Figure 26–1).
- Slices are perpendicular to the brainstem (Figures 26–1 and 26–2).
- The field of view (FOV) must include the left and right mastoid regions (Figures 26–3 and 26–4).
- The anatomy on each side of the image should correspond to the other side so that it is a mirror image (unless pathology is present) (see Figure 26–4).

Phase and Frequency Orientation
- Phase: Anteroposterior
- Frequency: Right to left
- Phase and frequency orientations may be swapped.

Saturation Band Placement
- A saturation band may be used to eliminate or reduce motion and/or magnetic susceptibility artifact from the face.
- If used, the saturation band should be placed in a line extending from the glabella to the second cervical vertebra (C2) and anterior to the FOV.

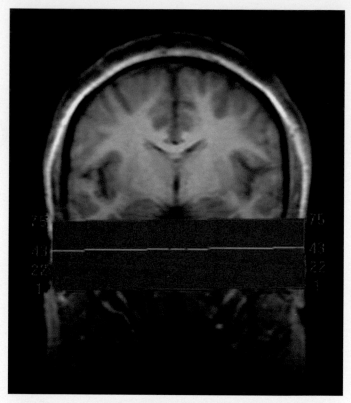

FIGURE 26–1. Coronal scout image showing image slice overlay for an axial sequence. Note the 75 planned slices with thin slice thickness and gap.

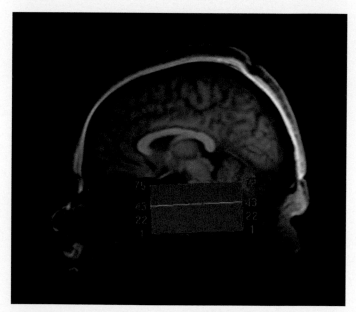

FIGURE 26–2. Sagittal scout image showing image slice overlay for an axial sequence. The slices are perpendicular to the brainstem. Note the 75 planned slices with thin slice thickness and gap. As a side note, a parasagittal scout of the IAC should be used.

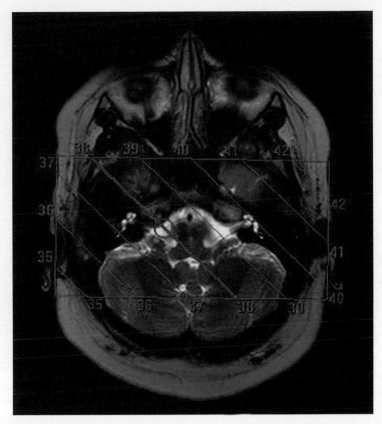

FIGURE 26–3. Axial scout image showing image slice overlay for an axial sequence. This image is included to demonstrate the field of view, which is shown as the perimeter box. Note that the field of view may be decreased, but it is important to maintain a proper amount of signal so the resultant image will be of sufficient quality and all pertinent anatomy must be included.

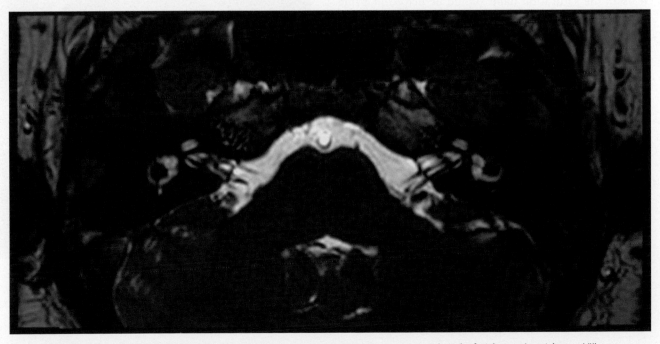

FIGURE 26–4. Axial balanced fast field echo (BFFE) image. Note the anatomic structures such as the facial nerve (cranial nerve VII), vestibulocochlear nerve (cranial nerve VIII), semicircular canals, and cochlea.

Coronal Sequence Acquisition

Slice Alignment

- On the axial scout, align the slice overlay to parallel a line drawn between the left cochlea and right cochlea. Angle the slices so that they enter each cochlea at the same point (Figure 26–5).

- The sagittal scout demonstrates the FOV for the coronal images (Figure 26–6).

- The anatomy on each side of the image should correspond to the other side so that it is a mirror image (unless pathology is present).

- The FOV must include the left and right mastoid region (Figures 26–7 and 26–8).

- If imaging each internal auditory canal (IAC) individually, use the axial coronal scouts to align parallel to cranial nerves VII and VIII (see Figure 26–8).

Phase and Frequency Orientation

- Phase: Right to left
- Frequency: Superior to inferior
- Phase and frequency orientations may be swapped.

Saturation Band Placement

- A saturation band may be used to eliminate or reduce motion and/or magnetic susceptibility artifact from the face.

- If used, the saturation band should be placed in a line extending from the glabella to C2 and anterior to the FOV.

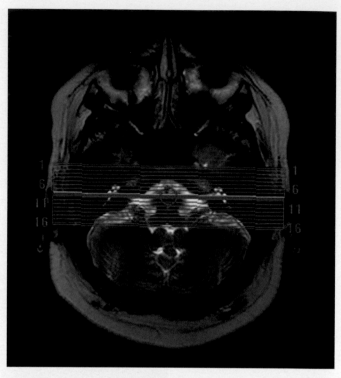

FIGURE 26–5. Axial scout image showing image slice overlay for a coronal sequence. Note the alignment with the IACs.

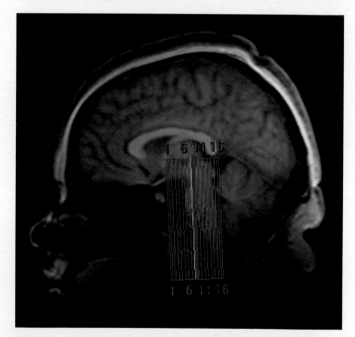

FIGURE 26–6. Sagittal scout image showing image slice overlay for a coronal sequence.

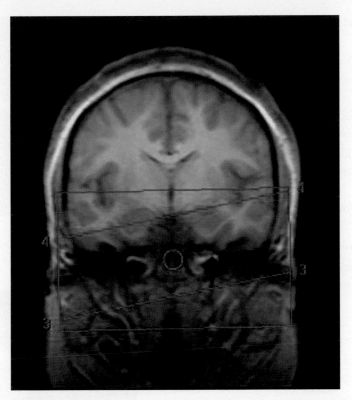

FIGURE 26–7. Coronal scout image showing image slice overlay for a coronal sequence. This image is included to demonstrate the field of view, which is shown as the perimeter box.

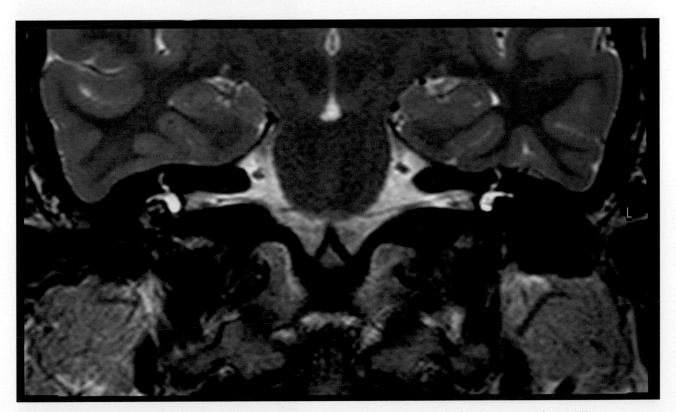

FIGURE 26–8. Coronal T2-weighted image. Note that the anatomic structures, such as the facial nerve (cranial nerve VII), vestibulocochlear nerve (cranial nerve VIII), semicircular canals, and cochlea, are very well seen due to patient positioning and slice overlay.

Sagittal Sequence Acquisition

Slice Alignment

- On the axial (Figure 26–9) and coronal (Figure 26–10) scout images, align the slice overlay perpendicular to cranial nerves VII and VIII.

- The left-to-right FOV should extend from the tympanic membrane to the medulla oblongata (see Figure 26–10).

- If imaging each IAC individually, use the axial coronal scouts to align parallel to cranial nerves VII and VIII.

Phase and Frequency Orientation

- Phase: Anteroposterior
- Frequency: Superior to inferior
- Phase and frequency orientations may be swapped.

Saturation Band Placement

- A saturation band may be used to eliminate or reduce motion and/or magnetic susceptibility artifact from the face.

- If used, the saturation band should be placed in a line extending from the glabella to C2 and anterior to the FOV.

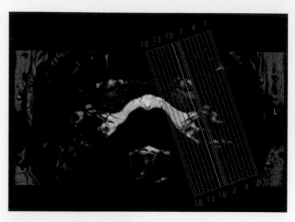

FIGURE 26–9. Axial scout image showing image slice overlay for a sagittal oblique sequence of the left IAC. Note the alignment perpendicular to cranial nerve VII and cranial nerve VIII.

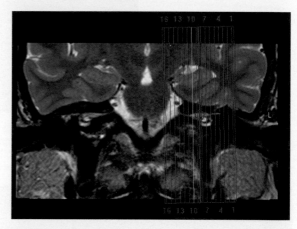

FIGURE 26–10. Coronal scout image showing image slice overlay for a sagittal sequence of the left IAC. Note the alignment perpendicular to cranial nerve VII and cranial nerve VIII.

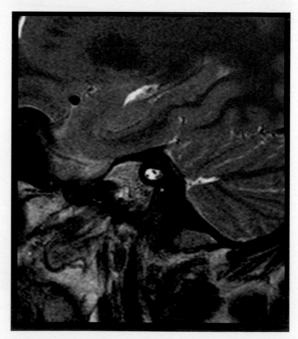

FIGURE 26–11. Parasagittal T2-weighted image (short axis) of the left IAC. Note the anatomic structures such as the facial nerve (cranial nerve VII) and vestibulocochlear nerve (cranial nerve VIII).

IMAGING APPLICATION

TABLE 26–1 • General Sequences

General Sequences	TR		TE		TI		FA (degrees)		NEX		SLT/GAP (in millimeters)	
	1.5 T	3.0 T	1.5 T	3.0 T	1.5 T	3.0 T	1.5 T	3.0 T	1.5 T	3.0 T	1.5 T	3.0 T
T1 SE	500	650	15	10	N/A	N/A	90	90	3	3	2/0.2	2/0.2
T2 SE	3500	3000	100	80	N/A	N/A	90	90	4	3	2/0.2	2/0.2
3D balanced GRE	8	7	4	3	N/A	N/A	50	45	2	3	2/0.2	2/0.2
T1 SE post C+	500	650	15	10	N/A	N/A	90	90	3	3	2/0.2	2/0.2

Abbreviations: 3D, 3-dimensional; GRE, gradient echo; N/A, not applicable; SE, spin echo.

SUGGESTED PROTOCOL VARIATIONS

Trauma

The attending radiologist and/or the requesting physician may ask for additional sequences or orthogonal planes depending on the traumatic injury.

Tumor

A tumor protocol may require sequences in addition to the routine IAC protocol and a larger FOV to include the lesion. Additional pre- and postcontrast sequences may be included. Three-orthogonal-plane postcontrast sequences may be of benefit to the radiologist. The technologist should follow the protocol provided at their facility.

Temporomandibular Joints (TMJs)

27

COIL SELECTION

- Primary coil: Temporomandibular joint (TMJ) surface coil
- Secondary coil: Head coil or head and neck coil

PATIENT/PART POSITIONING AND CENTERING

- The patient is positioned supine, headfirst in the MRI table.
- Make sure the patient is comfortable.
- Position the patient so that the orbitomeatal line is perpendicular to the z-axis of the MRI unit. The interpupillary line should be parallel to the orbitomeatal line (see Figures 13–1 and 13–2).
- The head should be at isocenter.
- Position the patient's head so the midsagittal plane is parallel to the z-axis of the MRI unit and there is no rotation (see Figure 13–2).
- Center on the nasion (see Figure 13–2).

- Instruct the patient to lie still and not move any part of their body, especially the head.
- Instruct the patient to not cross their arms and legs.

SLICE ALIGNMENT AND SCAN RANGE

The attending radiologist and/or the requesting physician will most likely ask for closed and open mouth TMJ sequences. Closed and open mouth examples are shown in the figures in this chapter. Gauze or a spacer may be placed in the anterior portion of the patient's mouth. The radiologist may require the patient to open their mouth a specified amount. If not, have the patient open their mouth as much as comfortably possible. It is important to note that the patient must remain motionless for several sequences with gauze in their mouth and that this is a very uncomfortable position. Also, be sure to wear gloves when placing and removing gauze in the patient's mouth. When the open mouth sequences are complete, remove the gauze, compress the gauze, measure the thickness of the gauze in millimeters, and document the thickness. This measurement will tell the radiologist how far the patient opened their mouth.

Sagittal (Oblique) Sequence Acquisition

Slice Alignment

- Using the axial scout images, align the slice overlay perpendicular to the mandibular condyles (Figure 27–1).

- On the coronal scout images, align the slice overlay parallel to the mandibular rami (Figure 27–2).

- Adjust the field of view (FOV) to cover the TMJ capsule.

- A closed mouth sagittal image of the TMJ is seen on Figure 27–3.

- An open mouth sagittal image of the TMJ is seen on Figure 27–4. The open mouth sequence is acquired using the same slice alignment and scan range as the closed mouth sequence.

Phase and Frequency Orientation

- Phase: Anteroposterior
- Frequency: Superior to inferior
- Phase and frequency orientations may be swapped.

Saturation Band Placement

- A saturation band may be used to eliminate or reduce motion and/or magnetic susceptibility artifact from the face.

- If used, the saturation band should be placed in a line extending from the glabella to the second cervical vertebra (C2) and anterior to the FOV.

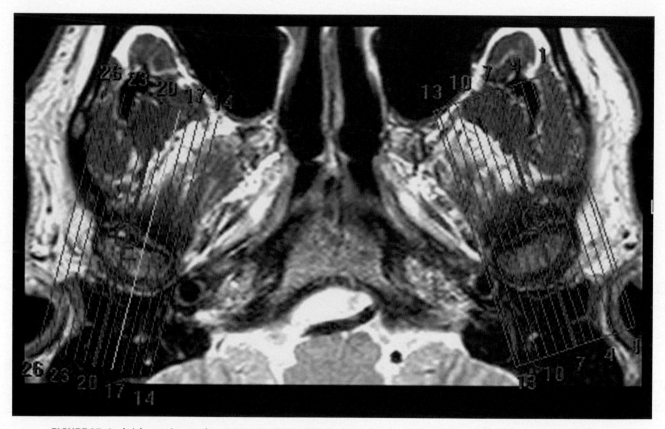

FIGURE 27–1. Axial scout image showing image slice overlay for left and right sagittal oblique closed mouth sequence. Note that the slice overlay is aligned to each TMJ separately.

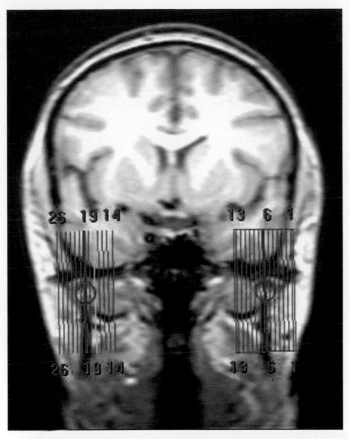

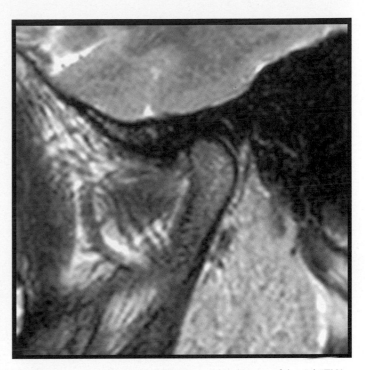

FIGURE 27–3. Closed mouth sagittal T2-weighted image of the right TMJ. Note the anatomic structures such as the joint capsule, condylar head, and condylar neck.

FIGURE 27–2. Coronal scout image showing image slice overlay for a sagittal closed mouth sequence. Note that the slice overlay is aligned to each TMJ separately.

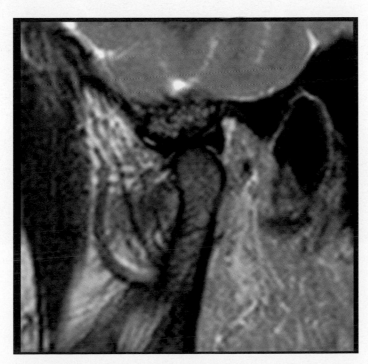

FIGURE 27–4. Open mouth sagittal T2-weighted image of the right TMJ. Note that the patient's mouth was open 20 mm. Compare the closed mouth (Figure 27–3) and open mouth images (Figure 27–4), and notice the different position of the articular disk, mandibular fossa, condylar head, and condylar neck.

Coronal Sequence Acquisition

Coronal images may be acquired using two different methods. The first method is an oblique coronal, which is parallel to the mandibular rami. The second method is a straight coronal, which is aligned to the left and right mandibular rami and includes both TMJ joints. Usually only one of these methods should be performed in an exam, so check with your facility to determine which method to perform.

Option One: Slice Alignment for Oblique Coronal

- Using the axial scout images, align the slice overlay to be parallel to the mandibular condyles (Figure 27–5).
- On the coronal scout images, align the slice overlay parallel to the mandibular rami (Figure 27–6).
- Adjust the FOV to cover the TMJ capsule.
- A closed mouth coronal image of the TMJ is seen on Figure 27–8.
- An open mouth coronal image of the TMJ is seen on Figure 27–9. The open mouth sequence is acquired using the same slice alignment and scan range as the closed mouth sequence.

Option Two: Slice Alignment for Straight Coronal

- Slices should be aligned according to a line drawn from mandibular condyle to condyle. Angle the slices so that they enter each condyle at the same point.
- The anatomy on each side of the image should correspond to the other side, so that it is a mirror image (unless pathology is present).
- Adjust the FOV to cover the TMJ capsules.

Phase and Frequency Orientation

- Phase: Right to left
- Frequency: Superior to inferior
- Phase and frequency orientations may be swapped.

Saturation Band Placement

- A saturation band may be used to eliminate or reduce motion and/or magnetic susceptibility artifact from the face.
- If used, the saturation band should be placed in a line extending from the glabella to C2 and anterior to the FOV.

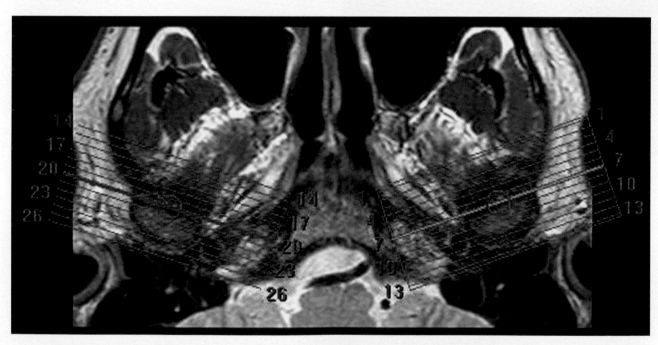

FIGURE 27–5. Axial scout image showing image slice overlay for left and right coronal oblique closed mouth image. Note that the slice overlay is aligned to each TMJ separately.

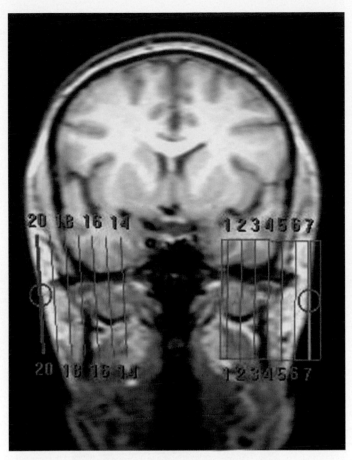

FIGURE 27-6. Coronal scout image showing image slice overlay for a coronal oblique closed mouth image. Note that the slice overlay is aligned to each TMJ separately.

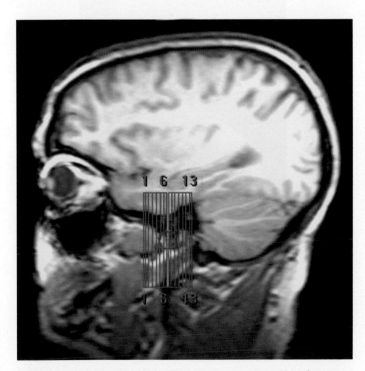

FIGURE 27-7. Sagittal scout image showing image slice overlay for a coronal oblique closed mouth image. As a side note, you should use a parasagittal scout showing the rami.

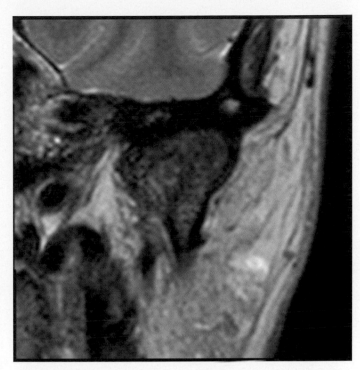

FIGURE 27-8. Closed mouth coronal T2-weighted image of the left TMJ. Note the anatomic structures such as the joint capsule, condylar head, and condylar neck.

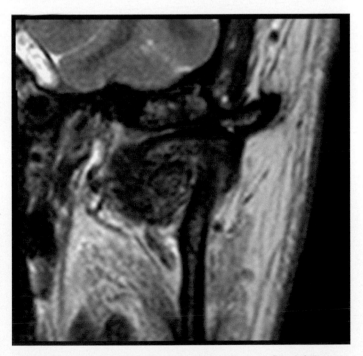

FIGURE 27-9. Open mouth coronal T2-weighted image of the left TMJ. Note that the patient's mouth was open 20 mm. Compare the closed mouth (Figure 27-8) and open mouth images (Figure 27-9) and notice the different position of the articular disk, condylar head, and condylar neck.

Axial Sequence Acquisition

Slice Alignment

- Using the coronal and sagittal scout images, align the slice overlay to cover the left and right mandibular condyles. Angle the slices so that they enter each condyle at the same point (Figures 27–10 and 27-11).

- The left-to-right FOV should extend from one TMJ capsule to the other TMJ capsule (Figures 27-10 and 27–12).

- The superior-to-inferior FOV should be superior to the zygomatic arch to the superior portion of the mandibular rami (see Figure 27–10).

- The anteroposterior FOV must include the TMJ capsules (Figure 27–11).

- A closed mouth axial image of the TMJ is seen on Figure 27–13.

- An open mouth axial image of the TMJ is seen on Figure 27–14. The open mouth sequence is acquired using the same slice alignment and scan range as the closed mouth sequence.

- Note: The axial sequence acquisition above describes the slice alignment and scan range for a large axial acquisition of both TMJs. Separate axial sequences may be acquired of each individual TMJ capsule.

Phase and Frequency Orientation

- Phase: Anteroposterior
- Frequency: Right to left
- Phase and frequency orientations may be swapped.

Saturation Band Placement

- A saturation band may be used to eliminate or reduce motion and/or magnetic susceptibility artifact from the face.

- If used, the saturation band should be placed in a line extending from the glabella to C2 and anterior to the FOV.

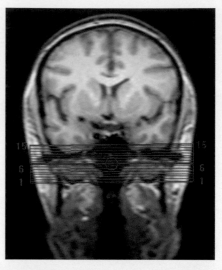

FIGURE 27–10. Coronal scout image showing image slice overlay for an axial closed mouth sequence.

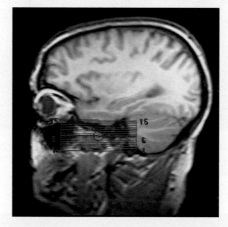

FIGURE 27–11. Sagittal scout image showing image slice overlay for an axial closed mouth sequence.

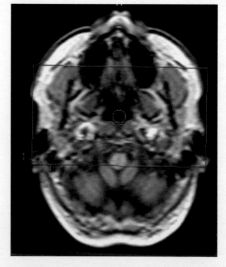

FIGURE 27–12. Axial scout image showing image slice overlay for an axial closed mouth sequence. This image is included to demonstrate the FOV, which is shown as the perimeter box. Note the FOV may be decreased, but it is important to maintain a proper amount of signal so the resultant image will be of sufficient quality.

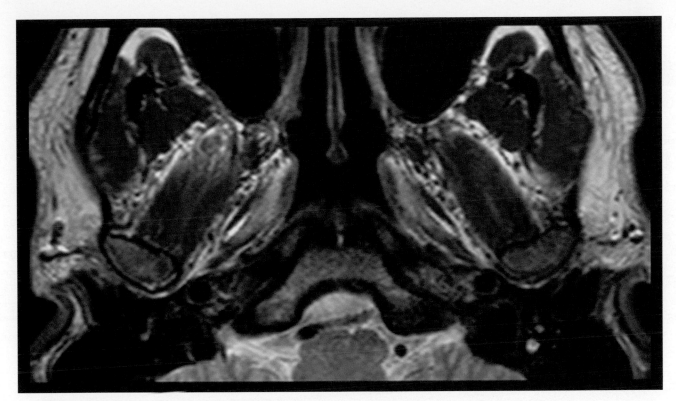

FIGURE 27–13. Closed mouth axial T2-weighted image. Note the condylar head.

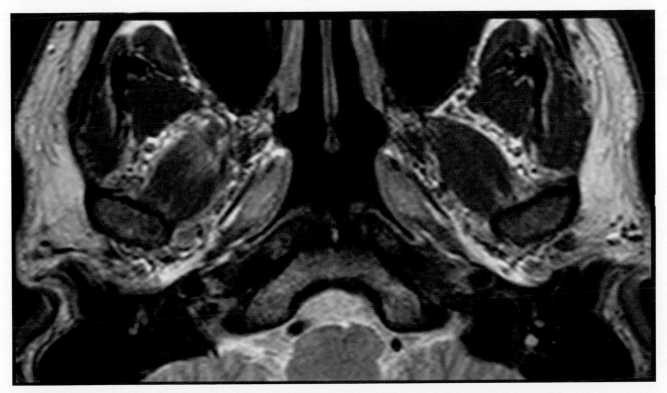

FIGURE 27–14. Open mouth axial T2-weighted image. Note that the patient's mouth was open 20 mm. Compare the closed mouth (Figure 27–13) and open mouth images (Figure 27–14).

IMAGING APPLICATION

TABLE 27–1 • General Sequences

General Sequences	TR		TE		TI		FA (degrees)		NEX		SLT/GAP (in millimeters)	
	1.5 T	3.0 T	1.5 T	3.0 T	1.5 T	3.0 T	1.5 T	3.0 T	1.5 T	3.0 T	1.5 T	3.0 T
T1 SE	550	650	15	15	N/A	N/A	90	90	4	3	3/0.3	3/0.3
T2 SE	3000	4000	90	80	N/A	N/A	90	90	4	3	3/0.3	3/0.3
PD	1700	1300	30	30	N/A	N/A	90	90	3	3	3/0.3	3/0.3
T1 SE post C+	550	650	15	15	N/A	N/A	90	90	4	3	3/0.3	3/0.3

Abbreviations: N/A, not applicable; PD, proton density; SE, spin echo.

SUGGESTED PROTOCOL VARIATIONS

Arthrogram

The injection of contrast media and/or gas in the capsular space may be requested. The requested media will be injected, usually under the guidance of fluoroscopy. The patient will then be imaged in MRI. Additional sequences to the routine protocol may be requested by the radiologist.

Trauma

The attending radiologist and/or the requesting physician may ask for additional sequences or orthogonal planes depending on the traumatic injury.

Tumor

A tumor protocol may require sequences in addition to the routine TMJ protocol and a larger FOV to include the lesion. Additional pre- and postcontrast sequences may be included. Three-orthogonal-plane postcontrast sequences may be of benefit to the radiologist. The technologist should follow the protocol provided at their facility.

Spines

28

Cervical Spine

COIL SELECTION

- Primary coil: Spine coil
- Secondary coil: Head and neck coil

PATIENT/PART POSITIONING AND CENTERING

- The patient is positioned supine and headfirst on the MRI table or patient couch.
- Make the patient comfortable.
- Position the patient so that the spine is parallel to the z-axis of the MRI unit. The spine should be as flat and straight on the coil as possible.
- Center on the thyroid cartilage or the fourth to fifth cervical vertebrae (C4-C5) so that the cervical spine is at isocenter.
- Instruct the patient to lie still and not move any part of their body.
- Instruct the patient to not cross their arms and legs.

SLICE ALIGNMENT AND SCAN RANGE

Sagittal Sequence Acquisition

Slice Alignment

- On the coronal scout image, align the slice overlay to be parallel to the spinal cord and spinous process (Figure 28–1).

- On the axial scout image, align the slice overlay vertical, or parallel with the spinous processes (Figure 28–2).

- Use an odd number of slices to allow for a midline sagittal slice. Extend the slice overlay to include the entire transverse processes.

- The superior-to-inferior field of view (FOV) should extend from the cerebellum to the level of the first thoracic vertebra (T1), making sure the C7/T1 is included. A saturation band may be placed anterior to the FOV to help reduce motion (Figure 28–3).

- The left-to-right FOV must include the transverse processes (see Figures 28–1 and 28–2).

- The anteroposterior FOV should extend from the vertebral bodies to the muscle posterior to the spinous processes.

- A midline sagittal image showing good position of the patient and slice overlay is shown in Figure 28–4.

Phase and Frequency Orientation

- Phase: Anteroposterior
- Frequency: Superior to inferior
- Phase and frequency orientations may be swapped to reduce motion artifact.

Saturation Band Placement

- A saturation band may be used to eliminate or reduce motion artifact from the face, throat, and thorax.

- If used, the saturation band should be placed anterior to the FOV.

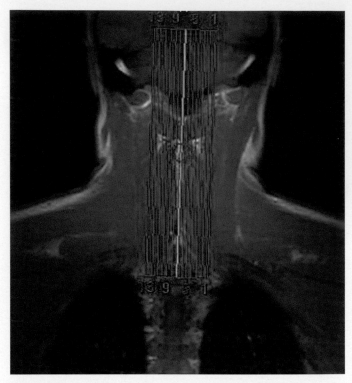

FIGURE 28–1. Coronal scout image showing image slice overlay for a sagittal sequence. Note that there is an odd number of slices in this example, so the middle slice would be a midsagittal image.

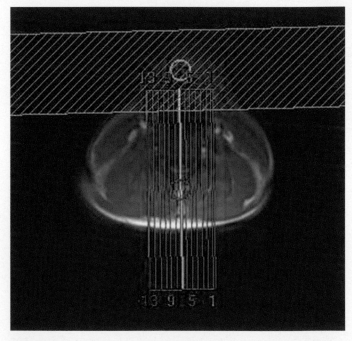

FIGURE 28–2. Axial scout image showing image slice overlay for a sagittal sequence. Note that the saturation band overlay (the blue band) is anterior to the cervical spine so that motion artifact will be reduced.

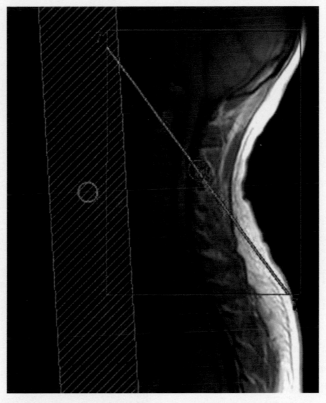

FIGURE 28–3. Sagittal scout image showing image slice overlay for a sagittal sequence. Note that the saturation band overlay (the blue band) is anterior to the cervical spine so that motion and flow artifacts will be reduced. This scout image is included to demonstrate the FOV and is shown as a red perimeter box.

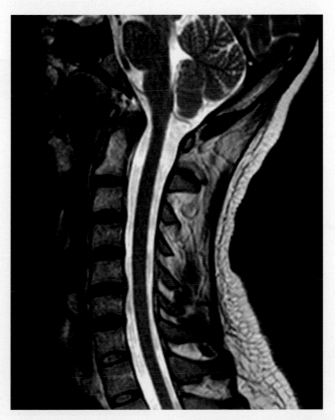

FIGURE 28–4. Midsagittal T2-weighted image. Note that the anatomic structures, such as the spinal cord, cerebrospinal fluid, vertebral bodies, intervertebral disks, and spinous processes, are very well seen due to patient positioning and slice overlay. Also, notice that the area where the saturation band was placed is dark and motion artifact is greatly reduced.

Axial Sequence Acquisition

Option One: Slice Alignment for One Field of View

- On a sagittal scout image, align the slice overlay perpendicular to the spinal cord.
- The superior-to-inferior FOV should extend from the level of C1 to the level of T1, making sure C7/T1 is included (Figure 28–5).
- On the coronal scout image, align the slice overlay perpendicular to the spinal cord (Figure 28–6).
- The left-to-right FOV must include the transverse processes.
- The anteroposterior FOV should extend from the vertebral bodies to the muscle posterior to the spinous processes (Figure 28–7).
- An axial image of the cervical spine is shown in Figure 28–8.

Option Two: Slice Alignment for Intervertebral Disc Acquisition Only

- Slices are perpendicular to the spinal cord.
- Slices are parallel to the intervertebral discs.
- Extend the slice overlay from the lower third of the vertebra above the disc to the upper third of the vertebra below each disc space.
- An odd number of slices should be used to allow for a mid-intervertebral disk slice.
- Place the mid-intervertebral disc slice in the center of the intervertebral disk.
- Several stacks of slices may be used, but avoid cross-talk artifact in useful anatomy.
- The superior-to-inferior FOV should extend from the level of C1 to the level of T1, making sure the C7/T1 is included.
- The left-to-right FOV must include the transverse processes.
- The anteroposterior FOV should extend from the vertebral bodies to the muscle posterior to the spinous processes.

Phase and Frequency Orientation

- Phase: Anteroposterior
- Frequency: Right to left
- Phase and frequency orientations may be swapped to reduce motion artifact.

Saturation Band Placement

- A saturation band may be used to eliminate or reduce motion artifact from the face, throat, and thorax.
- If used, the saturation band should be placed anterior to the FOV.

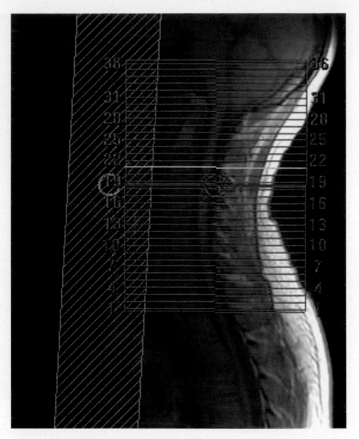

FIGURE 28–5. Midline sagittal scout image showing image slice overlay for an axial sequence. Note that the saturation band overlay (the blue band) is anterior to the cervical spine so that motion and flow artifacts will be reduced.

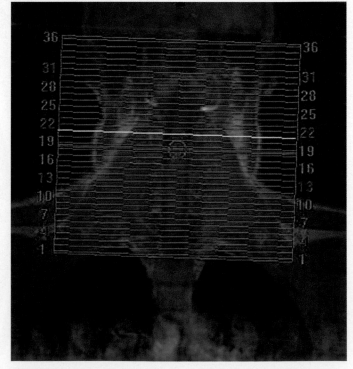

FIGURE 28–6. Coronal scout image showing image slice overlay for an axial sequence.

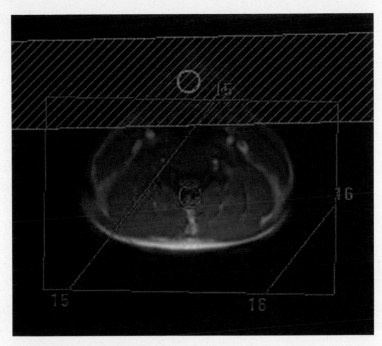

FIGURE 28–7. Axial scout image showing image slice overlay for an axial sequence. Note that the axial scout is included to demonstrate the FOV and is useful in placing the saturation band overlay (the blue band) so that it is not impeding upon pertinent anatomy. The red box demonstrates the field-of-view.

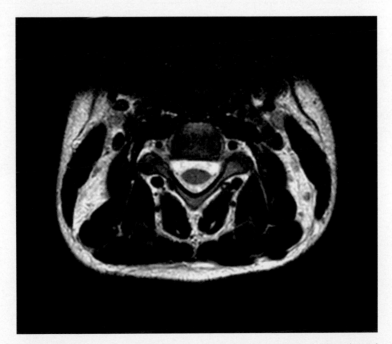

FIGURE 28–8. Axial T2-weighted image. Note that the anatomic structures such as the spinal cord, cerebrospinal fluid, vertebral body, transverse process, facet joints, and laminae. Also, notice that the area where the saturation band was placed is dark and motion artifact is greatly reduced. The FOV may be decreased, but it is important to maintain a proper amount of signal so the resultant image will be of sufficient quality and all pertinent anatomy must be included.

Coronal Sequence Acquisition (if Requested)

Slice Alignment

- Slices are parallel to the transverse processes.
- The superior-to-inferior FOV should extend from the level of C1 to the level of T1, making sure the C7/T1 is included.
- The left-to-right FOV must include the vertebral bodies.
- The anteroposterior FOV should extend from the vertebral bodies to the muscle posterior to the spinous processes.

Phase and Frequency Orientation

- Phase: Right to left
- Frequency: Superior to inferior
- Phase and frequency orientations may be swapped to reduce motion artifact.

Saturation Band Placement

- A saturation band may be used to eliminate or reduce motion artifact from the face, throat, and thorax.
- If used, the saturation band should be placed anterior to the FOV.

IMAGING APPLICATION

TABLE 28–1 • General Sequences

General Sequences	TR		TE		TI		FA (degrees)		NEX		SLT/GAP (in millimeters)	
	1.5 T	3.0 T	1.5 T	3.0 T	1.5 T	3.0 T	1.5 T	3.0 T	1.5 T	3.0 T	1.5 T	3.0 T
T1 SE	500	500	8	8	N/A	N/A	90	90	6	2	3/0.3	3/0.3
T2 SE	4000	2000	120	80	N/A	N/A	90	90	6	2	3/0.3	3/0.3
STIR	2500	3000	70	70	170	200	90	90	4	3	3/0.3	3/0.3
T1 SE post C+	500	500	8	8	N/A	N/A	90	90	6	2	3/0.3	3/0.3

Abbreviations: SE, spin echo; STIR, short tau inversion recovery.

SUGGESTED IMAGING APPLICATION VARIATIONS

Trauma

The attending radiologist and/or the requesting physician may ask for additional sequences or orthogonal planes depending on the traumatic injury (Table 28–2).

Scoliosis

A scoliosis protocol may require additional sequences in the coronal plane. Coronal sequences will allow for the evaluation of abnormal left curvature (levoscoliosis) and/or right curvature (dextroscoliosis) of the spine.

Tumor

A tumor protocol may require sequences in addition to the routine spine protocol and a larger FOV to include the lesion. Additional pre- and postcontrast sequences may be included. Three-orthogonal-plane postcontrast sequences may be of benefit to the radiologist. The technologist should follow the protocol provided at their facility.

TABLE 28–2 • Trauma Sequences

Trauma Sequences	TR		TE		TI		FA (degrees)		NEX		SLT/GAP (in millimeters)	
	1.5 T	3.0 T	1.5 T	3.0 T	1.5 T	3.0 T	1.5 T	3.0 T	1.5 T	3.0 T	1.5 T	3.0 T
T2 GRE out-of-phase (fat suppression)	350	150	16	6	N/A	N/A	25	25	4	4	3/0.3	3/0.3

Abbreviations: GRE, gradient echo; N/A, not applicable.

Thoracic Spine

29

COIL SELECTION

- Primary coil: Spine coil

PATIENT/PART POSITIONING AND CENTERING

- The patient is positioned supine and headfirst on the MRI table or patient couch.
- Make the patient comfortable.

- Position the patient so that the spine is parallel to the z-axis of the MRI unit. The spine should be as flat and straight on the coil as possible.
- Center at mid-sternum or approximately the seventh thoracic vertebra (T7) so that the thoracic spine is at isocenter.
- Instruct the patient to lie still and not move any part of their body.
- Instruct the patient to not cross their arms and legs.

SLICE ALIGNMENT AND SCAN RANGE

Sagittal Sequence Acquisition

Slice Alignment

- On the coronal scout image, align the slice overlay to be parallel to the spinal cord and spinous process (Figure 29–1).

- On the axial scout image, align the slice overlay vertical (Figure 29–2).

- Use an odd number of slices to allow for a midline sagittal slice. Extend the slice overlay to include the transverse processes.

- The superior-to-inferior field of view (FOV) should extend from the level of the seventh cervical vertebra (C7) to the level of the first lumbar vertebra (L1), making sure to include C7/L1 (Figure 29–3).

- The left-to-right FOV must include the transverse processes.

- The anteroposterior FOV should extend from the vertebral bodies to the muscle posterior to the spinous processes.

- A midline sagittal image showing good position of the patient and slice overlay is shown in Figure 29–4.

Phase and Frequency Orientation

- Phase: Anteroposterior

- Frequency: Superior to inferior

- Phase and frequency orientations may be swapped to reduce motion artifact.

Saturation Band Placement

- A saturation band may be used to eliminate or reduce motion artifact from the thorax.

- If used, the saturation band should be placed anterior to the FOV.

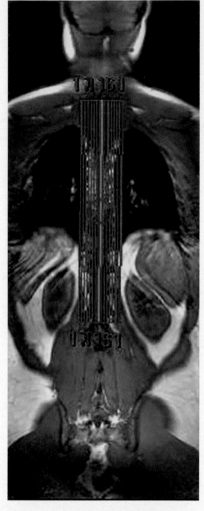

FIGURE 29–1. Coronal scout image showing image slice overlay for a sagittal sequence. Note that there are an odd number of slices in this example, so the middle slice would be a midsagittal image.

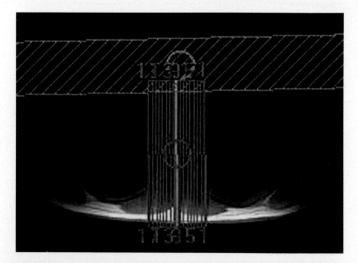

FIGURE 29–2. Axial scout image showing image slice overlay for a sagittal sequence. Note that the saturation band overlay (the *blue band*) is anterior to the thoracic spine so that motion and flow artifacts will be reduced.

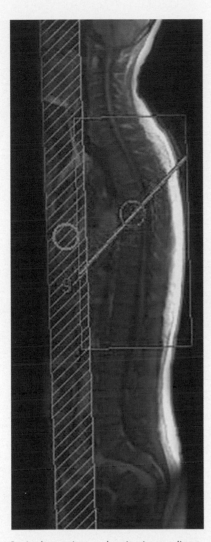

FIGURE 29-3. Sagittal scout image showing image slice overlay for a sagittal sequence. Note that the saturation band overlay (the *blue band*) is anterior of the thoracic spine so that motion and flow artifacts will be reduced. This scout image is included to demonstrate the FOV and is shown as a red perimeter box.

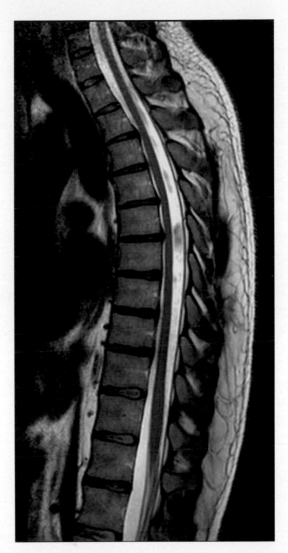

FIGURE 29-4. Midsagittal T2-weighted image. Note that the anatomic structures, such as the spinal cord, cerebrospinal fluid, conus medullaris, cauda equina, vertebral bodies, intervertebral discs, and spinous processes, are very well seen due to patient positioning and slice overlay. Also, notice that the area where the saturation band was placed is dark and motion artifact is greatly reduced.

Axial Sequence Acquisition

Option One: Slice Alignment for One Field of View

- On a sagittal scout image, align the slice overlay to be perpendicular to the spinal cord.
- Slices are parallel to the intervertebral disks (Figure 29–5)
- Several stacks of slices may be used, but avoid cross-talk artifact in useful anatomy (see Figure 29–5).
- On a coronal scout image, align the slice overlay to be perpendicular to the vertebra (Figure 29–6).
- The superior-to-inferior FOV should extend from C7 to L1, making sure to include C7/L1 (see Figure 29–5).
- The left-to-right FOV must include the transverse processes.
- The anteroposterior FOV should extend from the vertebral bodies to the muscle posterior to the spinous processes (see Figure 29–5).
- An axial image of the thoracic spine is shown in Figure 29–7.

Option Two: Slice Alignment for Intervertebral Disc Acquisition Only

- Slices are perpendicular to the spinal cord.
- Slices are parallel to the intervertebral discs.
- An odd number of slices should be used to allow for a mid-intervertebral disc slice.
- Place the mid-intervertebral disk slice in the center of the intervertebral disc.
- The left-to-right FOV must include the transverse processes.
- The superior-to-inferior FOV only covers the intervertebral disc spaces from the level of C7 to L1.
- The anteroposterior FOV should extend from the vertebral bodies to the muscle posterior to the spinous processes.

Phase and Frequency Orientation

- Phase: Anteroposterior
- Frequency: Right to left
- Phase and frequency orientations may be swapped to reduce motion artifact.

Saturation Band Placement

- A saturation band may be used to eliminate or reduce motion artifact from the thorax.
- If used, the saturation band should be placed anterior to the FOV.

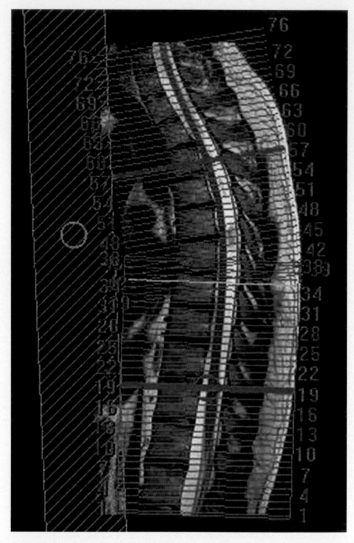

FIGURE 29–5. Midline sagittal scout image showing image slice overlay for an axial sequence. Note the 2 sets of slice overlays, which are perpendicular to the spine. If you use more than one set of slice overlays that overlap, then you must take steps to avoid cross-talk artifact. You may have to split the sets into separate series or, in other words, perform each set of slice overlays separately. Another remedy is to interleave the slices. Also, notice the saturation band overlay (the *blue band*) is anterior to the thoracic spine so that motion and flow artifacts will be reduced.

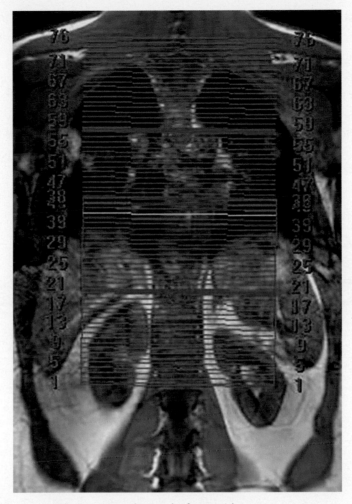

FIGURE 29–6. Coronal scout image showing image slice overlay for an axial sequence.

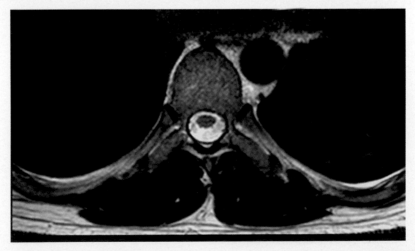

FIGURE 29–7. Axial T2-weighted image. Note the anatomic structures such as the spinal cord, cerebrospinal fluid, vertebral body, transverse process, laminae, costophrenic joints, costotransverse joints, ribs, and lungs. Also, notice that the area where the saturation band was placed is dark and motion artifact is greatly reduced. The FOV may be decreased, but it is important to maintain a proper amount of signal so the resultant image will be of sufficient quality and all pertinent anatomy must be included.

Coronal Sequence Acquisition (if Requested)

Slice Alignment

- Slices are parallel to the transverse processes.
- The superior-to-inferior FOV should extend from C7 to L1.
- The left-to-right FOV must include the vertebral bodies.
- The anteroposterior FOV should extend from the vertebral bodies to the muscle posterior of the spinous processes.

Phase and Frequency Orientation

- Phase: Right to left
- Frequency: Superior to inferior
- Phase and frequency orientations may be swapped to reduce motion artifact.

Saturation Band Placement

- A saturation band may be used to eliminate or reduce motion artifact from the thorax.
- If used, the saturation band should be placed anterior of the FOV.

IMAGING APPLICATION

TABLE 29–1 • General Sequences

General Sequences	TR		TE		TI		FA (degrees)		NEX		SLT/GAP (in millimeters)	
	1.5 T	3.0 T	1.5 T	3.0 T	1.5 T	3.0 T	1.5 T	3.0 T	1.5 T	3.0 T	1.5 T	3.0 T
T1 SE	500	500	8	8	N/A	N/A	90	90	6	2	3/0.3	3/0.3
T2 SE	4000	2000	120	80	N/A	N/A	90	90	6	2	3/0.3	3/0.3
STIR	2500	3000	70	70	170	200	90	90	4	3	3/0.3	3/0.3
T1 SE post C+	500	500	8	8	N/A	N/A	90	90	6	2	3/0.3	3/0.3

Abbreviations: N/A, not applicable; SE, spin echo; STIR, short tau inversion recovery.

SUGGESTED IMAGING APPLICATION VARIATIONS

Trauma

The attending radiologist and/or the requesting physician may ask for additional sequences or orthogonal planes depending on the traumatic injury (Table 29–2).

Scoliosis

A scoliosis protocol may require additional sequences in the coronal plane. Coronal sequences will allow for the evaluation of abnormal left curvature (levoscoliosis) and/or right curvature (dextroscoliosis) of the spine.

Tumor

A tumor protocol may require sequences in addition to the routine spine protocol and a larger FOV to include the lesion. Additional pre- and postcontrast sequences may be included. Three-orthogonal-plane postcontrast sequences may be of benefit to the radiologist. The technologist should follow the protocol provided at their facility.

TABLE 29–2 • Trauma Sequences

Trauma Sequences	TR		TE		TI		FA (degrees)		NEX		SLT/GAP (in millimeters)	
	1.5 T	3.0 T	1.5 T	3.0 T	1.5 T	3.0 T	1.5 T	3.0 T	1.5 T	3.0 T	1.5 T	3.0 T
T2 GRE out-of-phase (fat suppression)	350	150	16	6	N/A	N/A	25	25	4	4	3/0.3	3/0.3

Abbreviations: GRE, gradient echo; N/A, not applicable.

30

Lumbar Spine

COIL SELECTION

- Primary coil: Spine coil

PATIENT/PART POSITIONING AND CENTERING

- The patient is positioned supine and headfirst on the MRI table or patient couch.
- Make the patient comfortable.

- Position the patient so that the spine is parallel to the z-axis of the MRI unit. The spine should be as flat and straight on the coil as possible.
- Center 2 inches superior to the iliac crest or approximately the third lumbar vertebra (L3) so that the lumbar spine is at isocenter.
- Instruct the patient to lie still and not move any part of their body.
- Instruct the patient to not cross their arms and legs.

SLICE ALIGNMENT AND SCAN RANGE

Sagittal Sequence Acquisition

Slice Alignment

- On the coronal scout image, align the slice overlay to be parallel to the spinal cord and spinous process (Figure 30–1).
- On the axial scout image, align the slice overlay vertical (Figure 30–2).
- Use an odd number of slices to allow for a midline sagittal slice. Extend the slice overlay to include the entire transverse processes.
- Place the midsagittal slice on a line extending from the middle of the vertebral body through the middle of the spinous process.
- The superior-to-inferior field of view (FOV) should extend from the level of the 12th thoracic vertebra (T12) to the level of the fused second sacral vertebra (S2). If imaging the lumbosacral spine, then extend the inferior FOV to include the sacrum (Figure 30–3).
- The left-to-right FOV must include the transverse processes.
- The anteroposterior FOV should extend from the vertebral bodies to the muscle posterior to the spinous processes.
- A midline sagittal image showing good position of the patient and slice overlay is shown in Figure 30–4.

Phase and Frequency Orientation

- Phase: Anteroposterior
- Frequency: Superior to inferior
- Phase and frequency orientations may be swapped to reduce motion artifact.

Saturation Band Placement

- A saturation band may be used to eliminate or reduce motion artifact from the abdomen.
- If used, the saturation band should be placed anterior to the FOV.

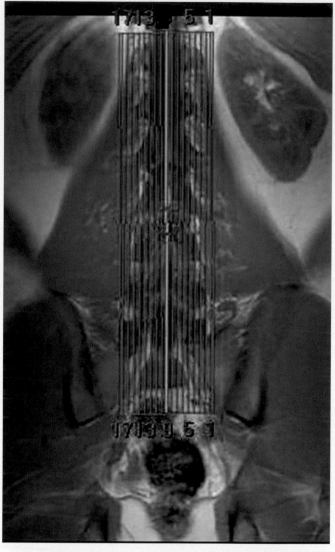

FIGURE 30–1. Coronal scout image showing image slice overlay for a sagittal sequence. Note that there is an odd number of slices in this example, so the middle slice would be a midsagittal image.

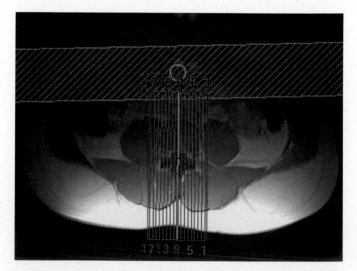

FIGURE 30–2. Axial scout image showing image slice overlay for a sagittal sequence. Note that the saturation band overlay (the *blue band*) is anterior to the lumbar spine so that motion artifact will be reduced.

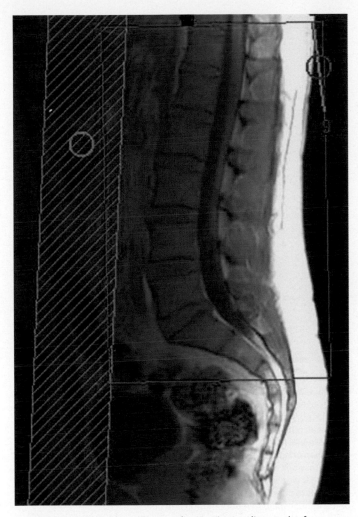

FIGURE 30–3. Sagittal scout image showing image slice overlay for a sagittal sequence. Note that the saturation band overlay (the *blue band*) is anterior to the lumbar spine so that motion and flow artifacts will be reduced. This scout image is included to demonstrate the FOV and is shown as a red perimeter box.

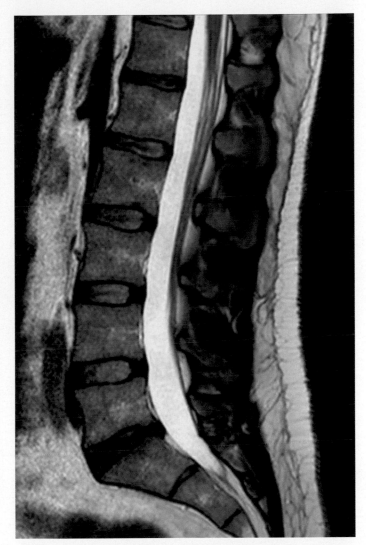

FIGURE 30–4. Midsagittal T2-weighted image. Note that the anatomic structures, such as the spinal cord, cerebrospinal fluid, conus medullaris, cauda equina, vertebral bodies, intervertebral discs, and spinous processes, are very well seen due to patient positioning and slice overlay. Also, notice that the area where the saturation band was placed is dark and motion artifact is greatly reduced. Also, notice the decreased signal shown in the L5-S1 intervertebral disc space.

Axial Sequence Acquisition

Option One: Slice Alignment for Intervertebral Disc Acquisition Only

- On a sagittal scout, align the slice overlay parallel to the intervertebral discs (Figure 30–5).
- An odd number of slices should be used to allow for a mid-intervertebral disc slice.
- Place the mid-intervertebral disc slice in the center of the intervertebral disc.
- Slices should include lower one third of superior vertebral body through to the upper third of the inferior vertebral body.
- Several stacks of slices may be used, but avoid cross-talk artifact in useful anatomy.
- On a coronal scout image, align the slice overlay to be perpendicular to the spinal cord (Figure 30–6).
- The superior-to-inferior FOV only covers the intervertebral disc spaces from the level T12 through the lumbosacral intervertebral disc (L5/S1). If imaging the lumbosacral spine, then extend the inferior FOV to include the sacrum.
- The left-to-right FOV must include the transverse processes.
- The anteroposterior FOV should extend from the vertebral bodies to the muscle posterior to the spinous processes.
- An axial image of the lumbar spine is shown in Figure 30–7.

Option Two: Slice Alignment for One Field of View

- Slices are perpendicular to the spinal cord of the superior portion of the lumbar spine (Figure 30–8).
- Slices are parallel to the intervertebral discs of the superior portion of the lumbar spine.
- The superior-to-inferior FOV should extend from the level of T12 to the level of S2. If imaging the lumbosacral spine, then extend the inferior FOV to include the sacrum.
- The left-to-right FOV must include the transverse processes.
- The anteroposterior FOV should extend from the vertebral bodies to the muscle posterior to the spinous processes.

Phase and Frequency Orientation

- Phase: Anteroposterior
- Frequency: Right to left
- Phase and frequency orientations may be swapped to reduce motion artifact.

Saturation Band Placement

- A saturation band may be used to eliminate or reduce motion artifact from the abdomen.
- If used, the saturation band should be placed anterior to the FOV.

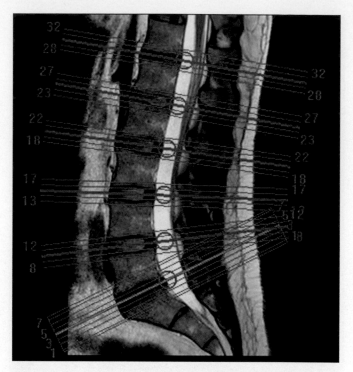

FIGURE 30–5. Midline sagittal scout image showing image slice overlay for an axial sequence of the lumbar spine intervertebral discs. Note the six sets of slice overlays, which are perpendicular to the spine and parallel to the intervertebral discs space. Alternatively, your imaging facility may request a large scan range to include the entire lumbar spine, as opposed to only the intervertebral discs. (See Option 2 in the text and Figure 30–8.) If you use more than one set of slice overlays that overlap, then you must take steps to avoid cross-talk artifact. You may have to split the sets into separate series or, in other words, perform each set of slice overlays separately. Another remedy is to interleave the slices. A saturation band may be placed anterior of the lumbar spine to reduce motion and flow artifacts.

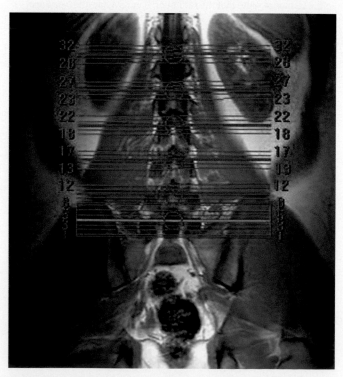

FIGURE 30–6. Coronal scout image showing image slice overlay for an axial sequence of the lumbar spine intervertebral discs.

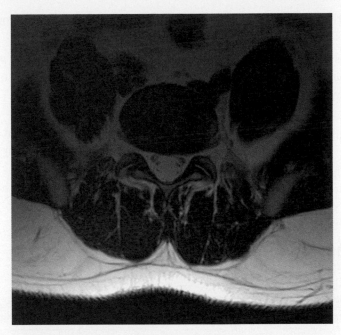

FIGURE 30–7. Axial T2-weighted image of the L5/S1 intervertebral discs. Note the the anatomic structures such as the cauda equina, cerebrospinal fluid, intervertebral discs, and articular facets/processes.

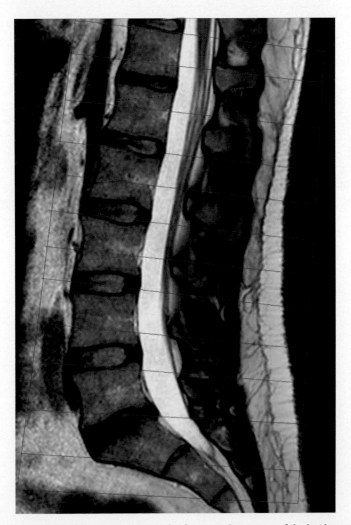

FIGURE 30–8. Sagittal scout image showing image slice overlay for an axial sequence of the lumbar spine in one FOV. Slices will be parallel to the red lines and extend from T12 to S2. Note that the slice thickness and gap of your acquired images will be smaller than in Figure 30–7.

Coronal Sequence Acquisition (if Requested)

Slice Alignment

- Slices are parallel to the transverse processes of the superior portion of the lumbar spine.
- The superior-to-inferior FOV should extend from the level of T12 to the level of S2.
- The left-to-right FOV must include the vertebral bodies.
- The anteroposterior FOV should extend from the vertebral bodies to the muscle posterior to the spinous processes.

Phase and Frequency Orientation

- Phase: Right to left
- Frequency: Superior to inferior
- Phase and frequency orientations may be swapped to reduce motion artifact.

Saturation Band Placement

- A saturation band may be used to eliminate or reduce motion artifact from the abdomen.
- If used, the saturation band should be placed anterior to the FOV.

IMAGING APPLICATION

TABLE 30–1 • General Sequences

General Sequences	TR		TE		TI		FA (degrees)		NEX		SLT/GAP (in millimeters)	
	1.5 T	3.0 T	1.5 T	3.0 T	1.5 T	3.0 T	1.5 T	3.0 T	1.5 T	3.0 T	1.5 T	3.0 T
T1 SE	500	500	8	8	N/A	N/A	90	90	6	2	3/0.3	3/0.3
T2 SE	4000	2000	120	80	N/A	N/A	90	90	6	2	3/0.3	3/0.3
STIR	2500	3000	70	70	170	200	90	90	4	3	3/0.3	3/0.3
T1 SE post C+	500	500	8	8	N/A	N/A	90	90	6	2	3/0.3	3/0.3

Abbreviations: N/A, not applicable; SE, spin echo; STIR, short tau inversion recovery.

SUGGESTED IMAGING APPLICATION VARIATIONS

Trauma

The attending radiologist and/or the requesting physician may ask for additional sequences or orthogonal planes depending on the traumatic injury (Table 30–2).

Scoliosis

A scoliosis protocol may require additional sequences in the coronal plane. Coronal sequences will allow for the evaluation of abnormal left curvature (levoscoliosis) and/or right curvature (dextroscoliosis) of the spine.

Tumor

A tumor protocol may require sequences in addition to the routine spine protocol and a larger FOV to include the lesion. Additional pre- and postcontrast sequences may be included. Three-orthogonal-plane postcontrast sequences may be of benefit to the radiologist. The technologist should follow the protocol provided at their facility.

TABLE 30–2 • Trauma Sequences

Trauma Sequences	TR		TE		TI		FA (degrees)		NEX		SLT/GAP (in millimeters)	
	1.5 T	3.0 T	1.5 T	3.0 T	1.5 T	3.0 T	1.5 T	3.0 T	1.5 T	3.0 T	1.5 T	3.0 T
T2 GRE out-of-phase (fat suppression)	350	150	16	6	N/A	N/A	25	25	4	4	3/0.3	3/0.3

Abbreviations: GRF, gradient echo; N/A, not applicable.

31

Sacrum

COIL SELECTION

- Primary coil: Spine coil

PATIENT/PART POSITIONING AND CENTERING

- The patient is positioned supine and headfirst on the MRI table or patient couch.
- Make the patient comfortable.
- Position the patient so that the spine is parallel to the z-axis of the MRI unit. The spine should be as flat and straight on the coil as possible.
- The pelvis should not be rotated.
- Support the patient's feet and lower legs.
- Center approximately 2 inches inferior to the level of the anterior superior iliac spine (ASIS) so that the pelvis is at isocenter.
- Instruct the patient to lie still and not move any part of their body.
- Instruct the patient to not cross their arms and legs.

SLICE ALIGNMENT AND SCAN RANGE

Sagittal Sequence Acquisition

Slice Alignment

- On the coronal scout image, align the slice overlay to be parallel to the spinal cord and spinous process (Figure 31–1).
- On the axial scout image, align the slice overlay vertical (Figure 31–2).
- Use an odd number of slices to allow for a midline sagittal slice. Extend the slice overlay to include the entire bony vertebra.
- Place the midsagittal slice on a line extending from the middle of the median sacral crest to the middle of the sacral promontory.
- The superior-to-inferior field of view (FOV) should extend from the level of lumbar vertebrae 5 (L5) through the coccyx (Figure 31–3).
- The left-to-right FOV should include the sacroiliac joints.
- The anteroposterior FOV should extend from the sacral promontory to the muscle posterior of the sacral crest.
- A sagittal image of the sacrum is shown in Figure 31–4.

Phase and Frequency Orientation

- Phase: Anteroposterior
- Frequency: Superior to inferior
- Phase and frequency orientations may be swapped to reduce motion artifact.

Saturation Band Placement

- A saturation band may be used to eliminate or reduce motion artifact from the abdomen.
- If used, the saturation band should be placed anterior to the FOV.

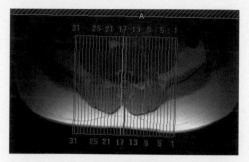

FIGURE 31–2. Axial scout image showing slice overlay for a sagittal sequence.

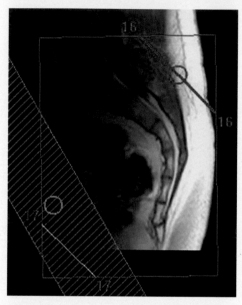

FIGURE 31–3. Sagittal scout image demonstrating the FOV, which is shown as a red perimeter box. Note that the saturation band overlay (blue band) is anterior to the sacrum so that motion artifact from the bowel and bladder will be reduced.

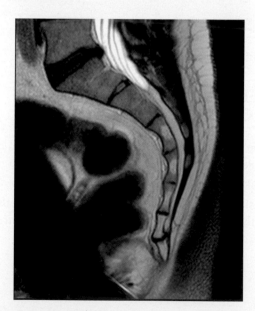

FIGURE 31–4. Midline sagittal T2-weighted image. Note that the anatomic structures, such as the spinal cord, cerebrospinal fluid, cauda equina, L5/S1, sacral canal, transverse ridges (lines of vertebral fusion), and the coccyx, are very well seen due to patient positioning and slice overlay. Also, notice that the area where the saturation band was placed is dark and motion artifact is greatly reduced.

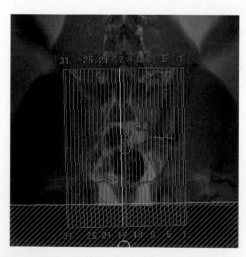

FIGURE 31–1. Coronal scout image showing slice overlay for a sagittal sequence. Note that there is an odd number of slices in this example, so the middle slice would be a midsagittal image.

Axial Sequence Acquisition

Option 1: Slice Alignment for One Field of View

- On a sagittal scout image, align the slice overlay to be perpendicular to the sacral canal of the superior portion of the sacrum (Figure 31–5).
- The superior-to-inferior FOV should extend from the level of L5 through the coccyx.
- The left-to-right FOV should include the sacral foramina (Figure 31–6).
- The anteroposterior FOV should extend from the sacral promontory to the muscle posterior to the sacral crest.
- An axial image of the sacrum is shown in Figure 31–7.

Option 2: Slice Alignment According to Sacral Curvature

- Slices are perpendicular to the sacral canal.
- Several stacks of slices may be used, but avoid cross-talk artifact in useful anatomy.
- The superior-to-inferior FOV should extend from the level of L5 through the coccyx.
- The left-to-right FOV should include the sacral foramina.
- The anteroposterior FOV should extend from the sacral promontory to the muscle posterior to the sacral crest.

Phase and Frequency Orientation

- Phase: Anteroposterior
- Frequency: Right to left
- Phase and frequency orientations may be swapped to reduce motion artifact.

Saturation Band Placement

- A saturation band may be used to eliminate or reduce motion artifact from the abdomen.
- If used, the saturation band should be placed anterior to the FOV.

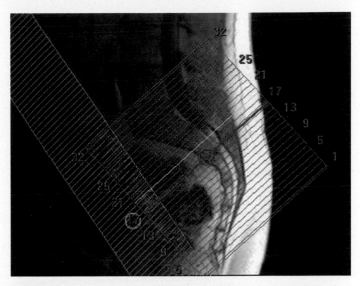

FIGURE 31–5. Midline sagittal scout image showing slice overlay for an axial sequence. Note that the saturation band may be placed anterior of the sacrum to reduce motion and flow artifacts.

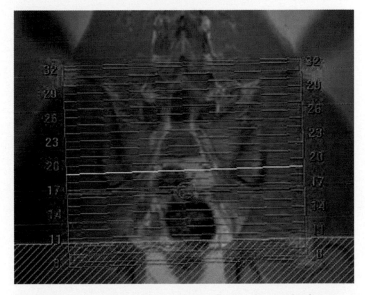

FIGURE 31–6. Coronal scout image showing image slice overlay for an axial sequence.

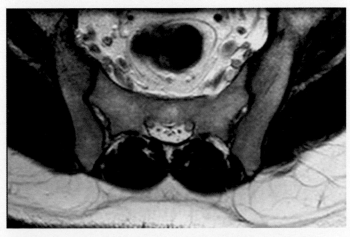

FIGURE 31–7. Axial T2-weighted image. Note the anatomic structures such as the sacroiliac joints and sacral canal.

Coronal Sequence Acquisition

Slice Alignment

- On a sagittal scout image, align the slice overlay to be parallel to the sacral canal (Figure 31–8)
- The superior-to-inferior FOV should extend from the level of L5 through the coccyx.
- The left-to-right FOV should include the sacral foramina (Figure 31–9).
- The anteroposterior FOV should extend from the sacral promontory to the muscle posterior to the sacral crest.
- A coronal image of the sacrum is shown in Figure 31–10.

Phase and Frequency Orientation

- Phase: Right to left
- Frequency: Superior to inferior
- Phase and frequency orientations may be swapped to reduce motion artifact.

Saturation Band Placement

- A saturation band may be used to eliminate or reduce motion artifact from the abdomen.
- If used, the saturation band should be placed anterior to the FOV.

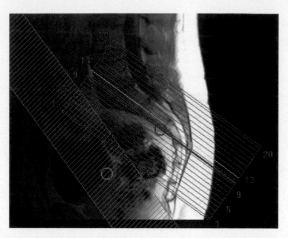

FIGURE 31–8. Sagittal scout image showing slice overlay for a coronal sequence. Note that the saturation band overlay (the *blue band*) is anterior to the sacrum so that motion artifact from blood, bowel, and bladder will be reduced.

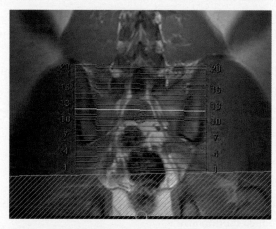

FIGURE 31–9. Coronal scout image showing slice overlay for a coronal sequence. Note that this scout image is included to demonstrate the FOV and is shown as a perimeter box.

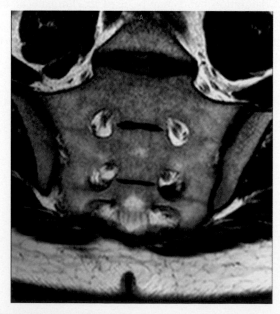

FIGURE 31–10. Coronal T2-weighted image. Note the anatomic structures such as the sacral foramina, nerve roots surrounded by CSF, L5/S1, sacroiliac joints, and transverse ridges.

IMAGING APPLICATION

TABLE 31–1 • General Sequences

General Sequences	TR		TE		TI		FA (degrees)		NEX		SLT/GAP (in millimeters)	
	1.5 T	3.0 T	1.5 T	3.0 T	1.5 T	3.0 T	1.5 T	3.0 T	1.5 T	3.0 T	1.5 T	3.0 T
T1 SE	500	500	8	8	N/A	N/A	90	90	6	2	3/0.3	3/0.3
T2 SE	4000	2000	120	80	N/A	N/A	90	90	6	2	3/0.3	3/0.3
STIR	2500	3000	70	70	170	200	90	90	4	3	3/0.3	3/0.3
T1 SE post C+	500	500	8	8	N/A	N/A	90	90	6	2	3/0.3	3/0.3

Abbreviations: N/A, not applicable; SE, spin echo; STIR, short tau inversion recovery.

SUGGESTED IMAGING APPLICATION VARIATIONS

Trauma

The attending radiologist and/or the requesting physician may ask for additional sequences or orthogonal planes depending on the traumatic injury (Table 31–2).

Tumor

A tumor protocol may require sequences in addition to the routine spine protocol and a larger FOV to include the lesion. Additional pre- and postcontrast sequences may be included. Three-orthogonal-plane postcontrast sequences may be of benefit to the radiologist. The technologist should follow the protocol provided at their facility.

TABLE 31–2 • Trauma Sequences

Trauma Sequences	TR		TE		TI		FA (degrees)		NEX		SLT/GAP (in millimeters)	
	1.5 T	3.0 T	1.5 T	3.0 T	1.5 T	3.0 T	1.5 T	3.0 T	1.5 T	3.0 T	1.5 T	3.0 T
T2 GRE out-of-phase (fat suppression)	350	150	16	6	N/A	N/A	25	25	4	4	3/0.3	3/0.3

Abbreviations: GRE, gradient echo; N/A, not applicable.

32

Neck Angiography (Neck MRA or Carotids)

COIL SELECTION

- Primary coil: Head and neck coil
- Secondary coil: Surface coils

PATIENT/PART POSITIONING AND CENTERING

- The patient is positioned supine and headfirst on the MRI table or patient couch.

- Make the patient comfortable.
- Position the patient so that the spine is parallel to the z-axis of the MRI unit. The neck should be as flat and straight on the coil as possible.
- Center mid-neck so that the neck is at isocenter.
- Instruct the patient to lie still and not move any part of their body.
- Instruct the patient to not cross their arms and legs.

SLICE ALIGNMENT AND SCAN RANGE

Examples of contrast-enhanced angiography (Figures 32–1 to 32–8), phase-contrast angiography (Figures 32–9 to 32–14), and time-of-flight angiography (Figures 32–15 to 32–17) are provided. Please consult the protocol used at your facility to determine which to use.

Coronal Sequence Acquisition

Slice Alignment

- Slices are parallel to the carotid arteries (see Figures 32–1 and 32–9).
- Slices should be aligned according to a line drawn from the left carotid artery to the right carotid artery. Angle the slices so that they enter each carotid artery at the same point (see Figures 32–2 and 32–10).
- The anatomy on each side of the image should correspond to the other side so that it is a mirror image (unless pathology is present).
- The superior-to-inferior field of view (FOV) should extend from the basilar artery to the arch portion of the aortic arch.
- The left-to-right FOV must include the left and right external carotid arteries (see Figures 32–7 and 32–13)
- The anteroposterior FOV must include the carotid arteries and vertebral arteries (see Figures 32–7 and 32–8).
- The 2 examples shown here are contrast enhanced (see Figures 32–7 and 32–8) and phase contrast (see Figures 32–13 and 32–14).

Phase and Frequency Orientation
- Phase: Superior to inferior
- Frequency: Right to left
- Phase and frequency orientations may be swapped to reduce motion artifact.

Saturation Band Placement
- A saturation band is placed superior to the FOV.
- The saturation band will saturate venous flow.

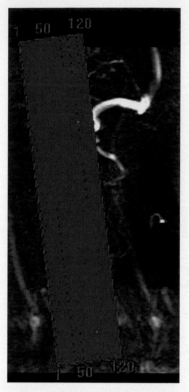

FIGURE 32–1. Sagittal scout image showing slice overlay for a coronal MRA sequence. Note the 120 planned slices and the thin slice thickness and gap.

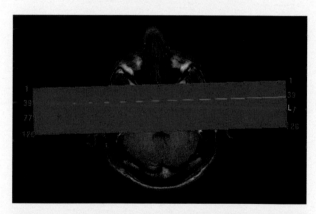

FIGURE 32–2. Axial scout image showing slice overlay for a coronal MRA sequence.

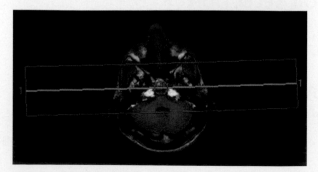

FIGURE 32–3. Axial scout image showing slice overlay for the bolus track. Bolus tracking will provide real-time images of the flow of contrast within the FOV. When sufficient contrast is flowing in the carotid arteries, the MRA sequence planned in Figures 32–1 and 32–2 will begin.

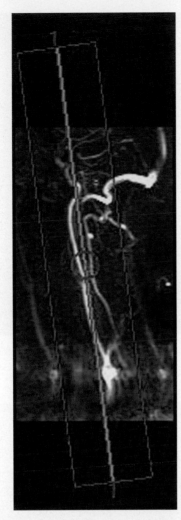

FIGURE 32–4. Sagittal scout image showing slice overlay for the bolus track.

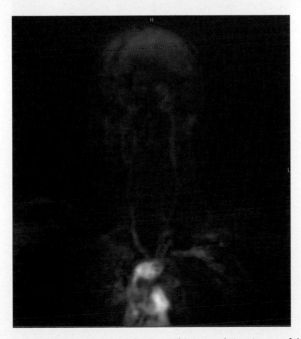

FIGURE 32–5. Coronal bolus track image. This is a real-time image of the flow of contrast within the FOV. Sufficient contrast is flowing in the carotid arteries, so the MRA sequence planned in Figures 32–1 and 32–2 may begin.

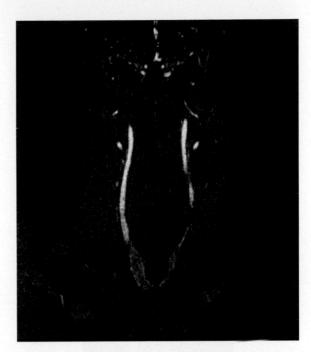

FIGURE 32–6. Coronal image. Note that this is 1 of the 120 planned slices and will be reconstructed to form a maximum intensity projection (MIP) of arterial flow.

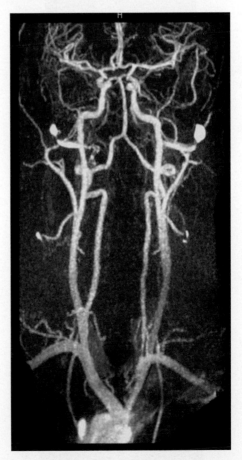

FIGURE 32–7. Coronal maximum intensity projection (MIP) of a contrast-enhanced MRA of the neck. Note the anatomic structures such as the arch portion of the aortic arch, brachiocephalic trunk, common carotid arteries, subclavian artery, internal carotid arteries, external carotid arteries, vertebral arteries, basilar artery, and circle of Willis.

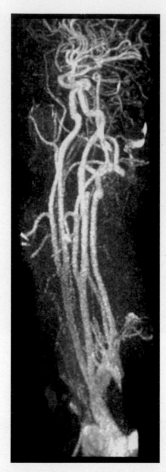

FIGURE 32–8. Sagittal maximum intensity projection (MIP) of a contrast-enhanced MRA of the neck.

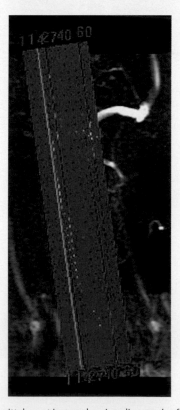

FIGURE 32–9. Sagittal scout image showing slice overlay for a coronal MRA sequence. Note the 60 planned slices and the thin slice thickness and gap.

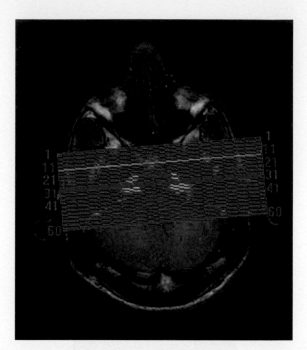

FIGURE 32–10. Axial scout image showing slice overlay for a coronal MRA sequence.

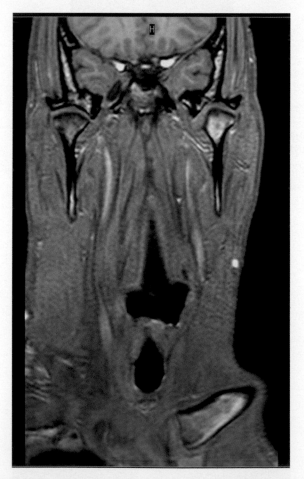

FIGURE 32–11. Coronal image. Note that this is 1 of the 60 planned slices and will be reconstructed to form a maximum intensity projection (MIP) of arterial flow (Figures 32–13 and 32–14).

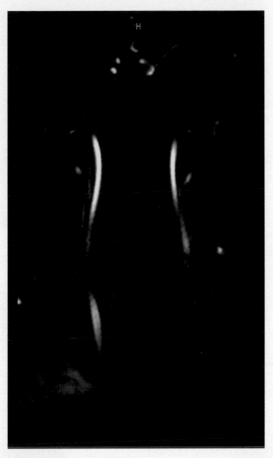

FIGURE 32–12. Coronal reconstructed image. This will be further reformatted to produce Figures 32–13 and 32–14.

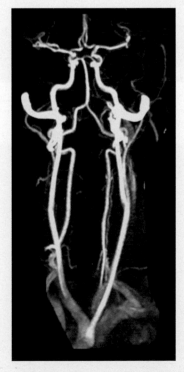

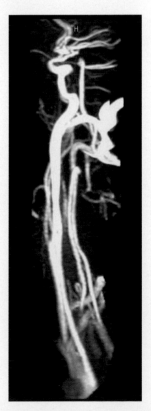

FIGURE 32–13. Coronal maximum intensity projection (MIP) of a phase-contrast MRA of the neck. Note the anatomic structures such as the arch portion of the aortic arch, brachiocephalic trunk, common carotid arteries, subclavian artery, internal carotid arteries, external carotid arteries, vertebral arteries, basilar artery, and circle of Willis.

FIGURE 32–14. Sagittal maximum intensity projection (MIP) of a phase-contrast MRA of the neck.

Axial Sequence Acquisition

Slice Alignment

- Slices are perpendicular to the carotid arteries (see Figure 32–15).

- The superior-to-inferior FOV should extend from the basilar artery to the arch portion of the aortic arch (see Figures 32–15 and 32–16).

- The left-to-right FOV must include the left and right external carotid arteries (see Figure 32–16).

- The anteroposterior FOV must include the carotid arteries and vertebral arteries.

- The example shown here is a time-of-flight magnetic resonance angiography (MRA) of the neck (see Figure 32–17).

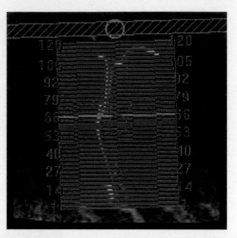

FIGURE 32–15. Sagittal scout image showing slice overlay for an axial MRA sequence. Note that the saturation band overlay (the *blue band*) is superior to the FOV.

Phase and Frequency Orientation

- Phase: Anteroposterior
- Frequency: Right to left
- Phase and frequency orientations may be swapped to reduce motion artifact.

Saturation Band Placement

- Saturation band is placed superior to the FOV (see Figure 32–15).
- The saturation band will saturate venous flow.

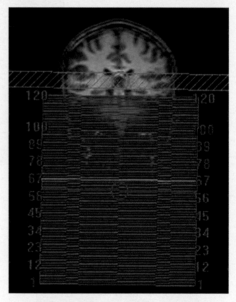

FIGURE 32–16. Coronal scout image showing slice overlay for an axial MRA sequence. Note that the saturation band overlay (the *blue band*) is superior to the FOV.

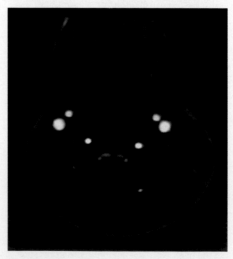

FIGURE 32–17. Axial time-of-flight MRA of the neck. Note the anatomic structures such as the vertebral arteries, internal carotid arteries, and external carotid arteries.

IMAGING APPLICATION

TABLE 32–1 • General Sequences

General Sequences	TR		TE		TI		FA (degrees)		NEX		SLT/GAP (in millimeters)	
	1.5 T	3.0 T	1.5 T	3.0 T	1.5 T	3.0 T	1.5 T	3.0 T	1.5 T	3.0 T	1.5 T	3.0 T
Contrast enhanced (CE)	5	10	2	5	N/A	N/A	40°	40°	1	1	4/0	4/0
Time of flight (TOF)	25	20	7	5	N/A	N/A	20°	20°	1	1	1/0	1/0
Phase contrast (PC)	15	20	5	5	N/A	N/A	15°	15°	2	2	40/0	40/0

Abbreviation: N/A, not applicable.

33

Soft Tissue Neck

COIL SELECTION

- Primary coil: Head and neck coil
- Secondary coil: Surface coils

PATIENT/PART POSITIONING AND CENTERING

- The patient is positioned supine and headfirst on the MRI table or patient couch.

- Make the patient comfortable.
- Position the patient so that the spine is parallel to the z-axis of the MRI unit. The neck should be as flat and straight on the coil as possible.
- Center mid-neck so that the neck is at isocenter.
- Instruct the patient to lie still and not move any part of their body.
- Instruct the patient to not cross their arms and legs.

SLICE ALIGNMENT AND SCAN RANGE

Axial Sequence Acquisition

Slice Alignment

- Slices are parallel to the hard palate (Figure 33–1).
- Slices are perpendicular to the spinal cord (Figures 33–1 and 33–2).
- The superior-to-inferior field of view (FOV) should extend from the hard palate to the arch portion of the aortic arch (see Figures 33–1 and 33–2).
- The left-to-right FOV should extend from the left mid-clavicle to the right mid-clavicle (see Figure 33–2).
- The anteroposterior FOV should extend from the hyoid bone to the cervical spine spinous processes.
- An axial image of the soft tissue neck is shown in Figure 33–3.

Phase and Frequency Orientation

- Phase: Anteroposterior
- Frequency: Right to left
- Phase and frequency orientations may be swapped to reduce motion artifact.

Saturation Band Placement

- A saturation band may be used to eliminate or reduce motion artifact from the thorax.
- If used, the saturation band should be placed inferior to the FOV or may be placed superior and inferior (see Figure 33–1).

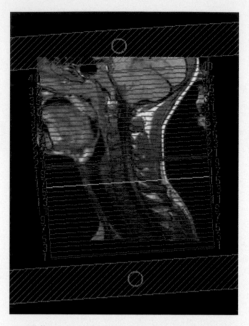

FIGURE 33–1. Midline sagittal scout image showing slice overlay for an axial sequence. Note the two saturation bands (*blue bands*) superior and inferior of the FOV so that vascular flow artifact will be reduced. Also, note that your facility may require additional coverage of the face.

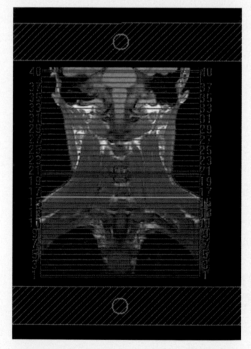

FIGURE 33–2. Coronal scout image showing slice overlay for an axial sequence.

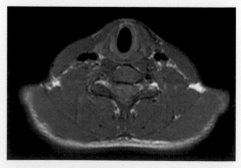

FIGURE 33–3. Axial T1-weighted image.

Sagittal Sequence Acquisition

Slice Alignment

- Slices are parallel to the spinal cord and spinous process (Figure 33–4).
- An odd number of slices should be used to allow for a mid-sagittal slice (see Figures 33–4 and 33–5).
- Place the midsagittal slice on a line extending from the middle of the cervical spine vertebral body through the middle of the cervical spine spinous process. (see Figures 33–47 and 33–5).
- The superior-to-inferior FOV should extend from the hard palate to the arch portion of the aortic arch.
- The left-to-right FOV should extend from the left mid-clavicle to the right mid-clavicle.
- The anteroposterior FOV should extend from the hyoid bone to the cervical spine spinous processes.
- A sagittal image of the soft tissue neck is shown in Figure 33–6.

Phase and Frequency Orientation

- Phase: Superior to inferior
- Frequency: Anteroposterior
- Phase and frequency orientations may be swapped to reduce motion artifact.

Saturation Band Placement

- A saturation band may be used to eliminate or reduce motion artifact from the thorax.
- If used, the saturation band should be placed inferior to the FOV or may be placed superior and inferior.

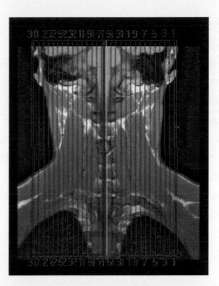

FIGURE 33–4. Coronal scout image showing image slice overlay for a sagittal sequence.

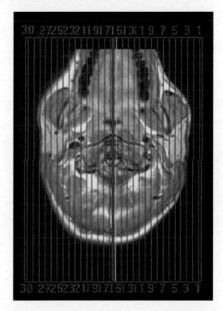

FIGURE 33–5. Axial scout image showing image slice overlay for a sagittal sequence.

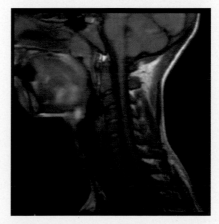

FIGURE 33–6. Midline sagittal T1-weighted image. Note the anatomic structures such as the pharynx, spine, and trachea. As a side note, there is a small amount of motion on this image.

Coronal Sequence Acquisition

Slice Alignment

- Slices are parallel to the spinal cord and spinous process (Figure 33–7).
- Slices are parallel to the transverse processes (Figure 33–8).
- The superior-to-inferior FOV should extend from the hard palate to the arch portion of the aortic arch.
- The left-to-right FOV should extend from the left mid-clavicle to the right mid-clavicle.
- The anteroposterior FOV should extend from the hyoid bone to the cervical spine spinous processes.
- A coronal image of the soft tissue neck is shown in Figure 33–9.

Phase and Frequency Orientation

- Phase: Superior to inferior
- Frequency: Right to left
- Phase and frequency orientations may be swapped to reduce motion artifact.

Saturation Band Placement

- A saturation band may be used to eliminate or reduce motion artifact from the thorax.
- If used, the saturation band should be placed inferior to the FOV.

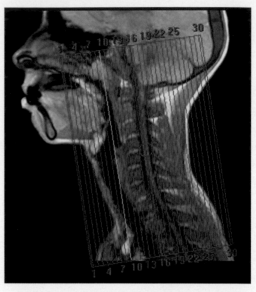

FIGURE 33–7. Midline sagittal scout image showing slice overlay for a coronal sequence.

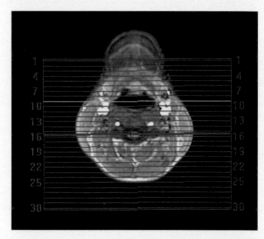

FIGURE 33–8. Axial scout image showing slice overlay for a coronal sequence.

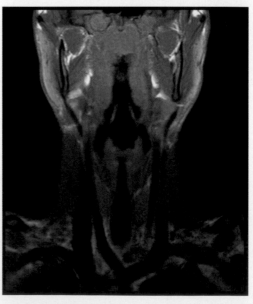

FIGURE 33–9. Coronal T1-weighted fat-saturated image. Note the anatomic structures such as the pharynx, trachea, and carotid arteries.

IMAGING APPLICATION

TABLE 33–1 • General Sequences

General Sequences	TR		TE		TI		FA (degrees)		NEX		SLT/GAP (in millimeters)	
	1.5 T	3.0 T	1.5 T	3.0 T	1.5 T	3.0 T	1.5 T	3.0 T	1.5 T	3.0 T	1.5 T	3.0 T
T1 SE	500	500	15	12	N/A	N/A	90	90	2	2	5/1	5/1
T1 SE FS	500	500	15	12	N/A	N/A	90	90	2	2	5/1	5/1
T2 SE FS	6000	3000	100	70	N/A	N/A	90	90	2	2	5/1	5/1
T1 SE post C+	500	500	15	12	N/A	N/A	90	90	2	2	5/1	5/1

Abbreviations: FS, fat saturated; N/A, not applicable; SE, spin echo.

SUGGESTED IMAGING APPLICATION VARIATIONS

Trauma

The attending radiologist and/or the requesting physician may ask for additional sequences or orthogonal planes depending on the traumatic injury.

Tumor

A tumor protocol may require sequences in addition to the routine soft tissue neck protocol and a larger FOV to include the lesion. Additional pre- and postcontrast sequences may be included. Three-orthogonal-plane postcontrast sequences may be of benefit to the radiologist. The technologist should follow the protocol provided at their facility.

34

Cardiac

COIL SELECTION

- Primary coil: Cardiac coil
- Secondary coil: Body or torso coil

PATIENT/PART POSITIONING AND CENTERING

- The patient is positioned supine and headfirst on the MRI table or patient couch.
- Make the patient comfortable.
- Position the patient so that the spine is parallel to the z-axis of the MRI unit. The patient should be as flat and straight on the coil as possible.

- Center mid-sternum.
- Instruct the patient to lie still and not move any part of their body.
- Instruct the patient to not cross their arms and legs.
- Cardiac gating will most likely be utilized. Place the leads on the patient's chest according to manufacturer guidelines. Alternatively, a peripheral gating system such as a peripheral pulse unit (PPU) may be used. This is helpful if the cardiac gating is difficult due to arrythmia or body habitus.
- Shimming is particularly important for cardiac exams. The examples below use a volume shim placed over the heart and great vessels. The shim is often shown below as a green box. Please consult the protocol used at your facility.

SLICE ALIGNMENT AND SCAN RANGE

Straight Axial Sequence Acquisition

Slice Alignment

- Using the coronal and sagittal scout images, align the slice overlay to be perpendicular to the long axis of the thorax (Figures 34–1 and 34–2).
- The field of view should extend from the apex of the heart through the great vessels.
- Straight axial sequences are show in Figures 31–3 and 31–4.

Phase and Frequency Orientation

- Phase: Superior to inferior
- Frequency: Right to left
- Phase and frequency orientations may be swapped to reduce motion artifact.

Saturation Band Placement

- A saturation band may be used to eliminate or reduce motion artifact.

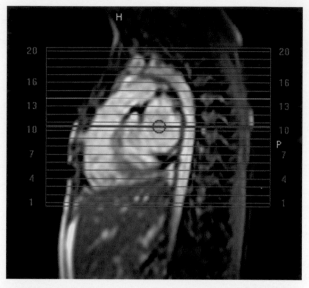

FIGURE 34–2. Sagittal scout image showing image slice overlay for a straight axial sequence.

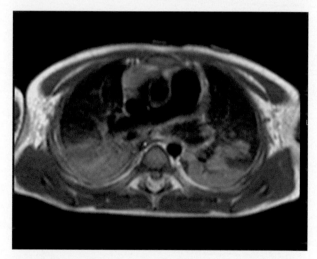

FIGURE 34–3. Axial black blood resultant image.

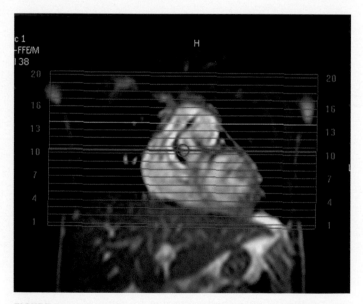

FIGURE 34–1. Coronal scout image showing image slice overlay for a straight axial sequence.

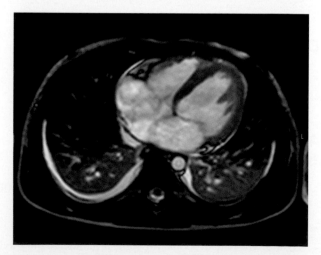

FIGURE 34–4. Axial bright blood image. Note that this is at a lower level than Figure 34–3. Image included to demonstrate the difference between black blood (Figure 34–3) and bright blood (Figure 34–4). Also, note the anatomic structures such as the interventricular septum, mitral valve, tricuspid valve, atria, and ventricles.

Straight Coronal Sequence Acquisition

Slice Alignment

- Using the axial and sagittal scout images, align the slice overlay to be parallel to the long axis of the thorax (Figures 34–5 and 34–6).
- The field of view should extend from the apex of the heart through the great vessels.
- A straight coronal sequence is shown in Figure 34–7.

Phase and Frequency Orientation

- Phase: Superior to inferior
- Frequency: Right to left
- Phase and frequency orientations may be swapped to reduce motion artifact.

Saturation Band Placement

- A saturation band may be used to eliminate or reduce motion artifact.

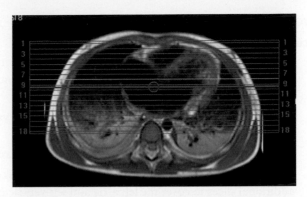

FIGURE 34–5. Axial scout image showing image slice overlay for a straight coronal sequence.

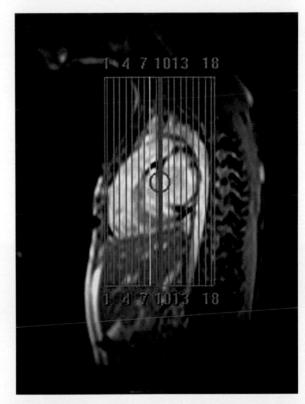

FIGURE 34–6. Sagittal scout image showing image slice overlay for a straight coronal sequence.

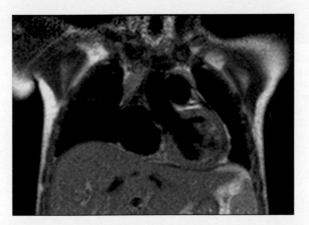

FIGURE 34–7. Coronal black blood image. Note the anatomic structures such as the left ventricle, interventricular septum, and aorta.

Two-Chamber Sequence Acquisition

Slice Alignment

- Using the acquired straight axial and straight coronal images, align the slice overlay to be parallel to the ventricular septum (Figures 34–8 and 34-9).
- Slices should be approximately at mid-mitral valve (see Figure 34–8).
- The field of view must include the heart and great vessels.
- Consult the protocol used at facility as you may ask for additional slices to cover the left atria and left ventricle.
- A 2-chamber (left atrium and left ventricle) sequence is shown in Figure 34–11.

Phase and Frequency Orientation

- Phase: Superior to inferior
- Frequency: Right to left
- Phase and frequency orientations may be swapped to reduce motion artifact.

Saturation Band Placement

- A saturation band may be used to eliminate or reduce motion artifact.

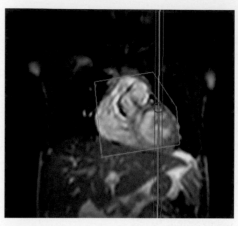

FIGURE 34–9. Coronal scout image showing image slice overlay for a 2-chamber sequence.

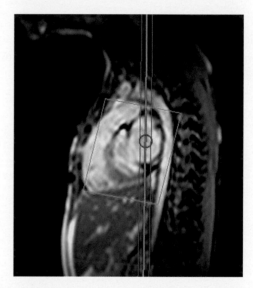

FIGURE 34–10. Sagittal scout image showing image slice overlay for a 2-chamber sequence.

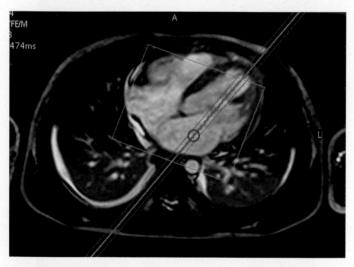

FIGURE 34–8. Acquired straight axial bright blood image (see Figure 34–4) used as a scout for a 2-chamber sequence. Note that the volume shim is shown as a box placed over the heart and great vessels. Shimming is very important in cardiac imaging. Be sure to use the protocol used at your facility.

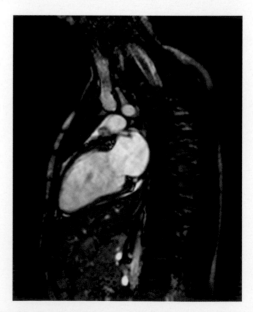

FIGURE 34–11. Two-chamber bright blood image. Note the anatomic structures such as the left ventricle and mitral valve.

Short-Axis Sequence Acquisition

Slice Alignment

- On the straight axial images, align perpendicular to the interventricular septum (Figures 34–12 and 34–15).
- Using the acquired Two-chamber images, align the slice overlay to be perpendicular to the long axis of the heart (Figures 34–13 and 34–16).
- The field of view should extend from the base to apex of the heart. Note that Figures 34–12 and 34–13 demonstrate alignment for a cine sequence and thus do not cover the entire field of view. Figures 34–15 and 34–16 demonstrate the field of view for the full sequence.
- A short-axis (left and right ventricles) sequence is shown in Figures 34–14 and 34–17.

Phase and Frequency Orientation

- Phase: Superior to inferior
- Frequency: Right to left
- Phase and frequency orientations may be swapped to reduce motion artifact.

Saturation Band Placement

- A saturation band may be used to eliminate or reduce motion artifact.

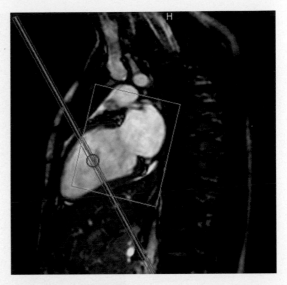

FIGURE 34–13. Acquired 2-chamber bright blood image (see Figure 34–11) used as a scout for a single-slice short-axis sequence. Note that the volume shim is shown as a box placed over the heart and great vessels.

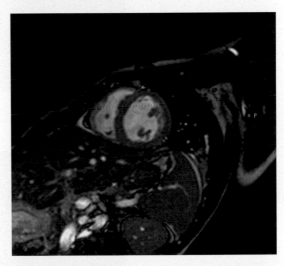

FIGURE 34–14. Short-axis bright blood image. Note that this sequence is used for cine imaging. (See Figures 34–15, 34–16, and 34–17 for full short-axis coverage.)

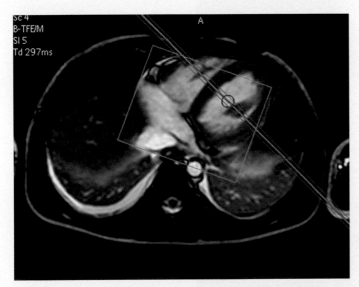

FIGURE 34–12. Acquired straight axial scout image showing image slice overlay for a single-slice short-axis sequence.

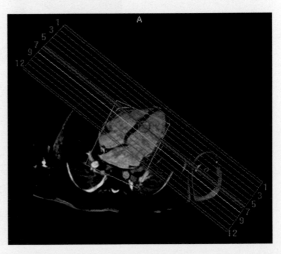

FIGURE 34–15. The straight axial may be used as a scout image, but the 4-chamber may be used as a scout for the short axis.

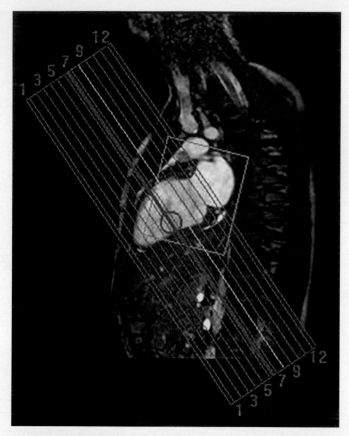

FIGURE 34–16. Acquired 2-chamber bright blood image (see Figure 34–11) used as a scout for a multi-slice short-axis sequence. Note that the volume shim is shown as a box placed over the heart and great vessels.

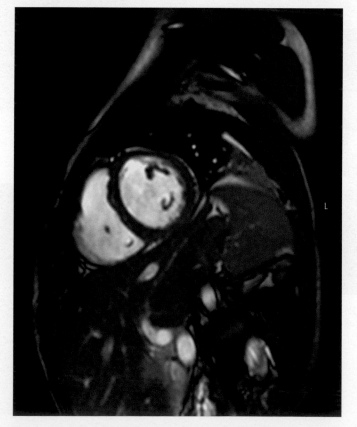

FIGURE 34–17. Short-axis bright blood image. Note the anatomic structures shown such as the ventricles, interventricular septum, and left ventricle wall.

Four-Chamber Sequence Acquisition

Slice Alignment

- Using the acquired 2-chamber images, select an image that depicts the long axis of the heart and align the slice overlay to be parallel (Figures 34–18 and 34–21).
- Using the acquired short-axis images, align the slice overlay through the chamber of the mid-left ventricle (papillary muscles) and apex of the right ventricle (Figures 34–19 and 34–22).
- The field of view must include the heart and great vessels. Note that Figures 34–18 and 34–19 demonstrate alignment for a cine sequence and thus do not cover the entire field of view. Figures 34–20 and 34–21 demonstrate the field of view for the full sequence.
- A 4-chamber (atria and ventricles) sequence is shown in Figures 34–20 and 34–23.

Phase and Frequency Orientation

- Phase: Superior to inferior
- Frequency: Right to left
- Phase and frequency orientations may be swapped to reduce motion artifact.

Saturation Band Placement

- A saturation band may be used to eliminate or reduce motion artifact.

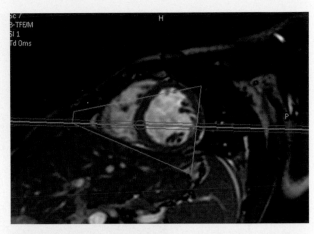

FIGURE 34–19. Acquired short-axis image (see Figure 34–17) used as a scout for a single-slice 4-chamber sequence.

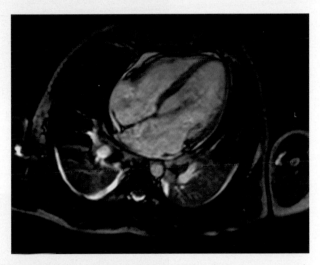

FIGURE 34–20. Four-chamber image. Note that this sequence is used for cine imaging. (See Figures 34–21, 34–22, and 34–23 for full 4-chamber coverage.)

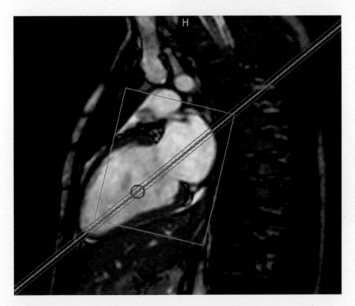

FIGURE 34–18. Acquired 2-chamber image (see Figure 34–11) used as a scout for a 4-chamber sequence. Note that the volume shim is shown as a green box placed over the heart and great vessels.

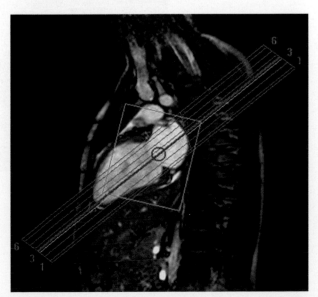

FIGURE 34–21. Acquired 2-chamber image (see Figure 34–11) used as a scout for a 4-chamber sequence. Note that the volume shim is shown as a box placed over the heart and great vessels.

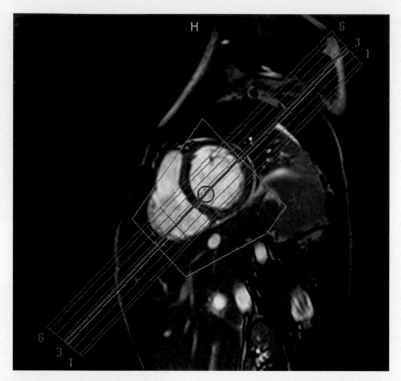

FIGURE 34–22. Acquired short-axis image (see Figure 34–17) used as a scout for a multi-slice 4-chamber sequence.

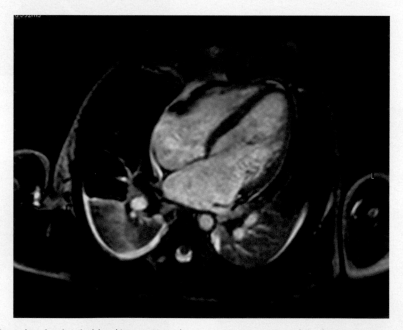

FIGURE 34–23. Four-chamber bright blood image. Note the anatomic structures such as the interventricular septum, mitral valve, tricuspid valve, atria, and ventricles.

Left Ventricular Outflow Tract (LVOT) (3-Chamber) Sequence Acquisition

Slice Alignment

- Using the acquired short-axis images, align the slice overlay to bisect the left ventricle outflow tract (LVOT) (Figure 34–24).
- Using the acquired 2-chamber images, align the slice overlay to be parallel to the long axis (Figure 34–25).
- The field of view must include the heart and great vessels.
- An LVOT (3-chamber) (left atria, left ventricle, right ventricle, and aorta) sequence is shown in Figure 34–26.

Phase and Frequency Orientation

- Phase: Superior to inferior
- Frequency: Right to left
- Phase and frequency orientations may be swapped to reduce motion artifact.

Saturation Band Placement

- A saturation band may be used to eliminate or reduce motion artifact.

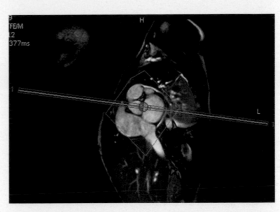

FIGURE 34–24. Acquired short axis image (see Figure 34–17) used as a scout for an LVOT sequence.

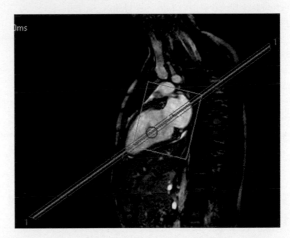

FIGURE 34–25. Acquired 2-chamber bright blood image (see Figure 34–11) used as a scout for an LVOT sequence. Note that the volume shim is shown as a box placed over the heart and great vessels.

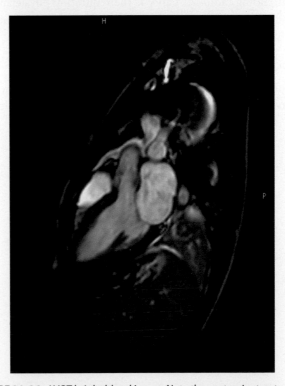

FIGURE 34–26. LVOT bright blood image. Note the anatomic structures such as the left ventricle, mitral valve, aortic valve, and left atrium.

IMAGING APPLICATION

General Sequences	TR		TE		TI		FA (degrees)		NEX		SLT/GAP (in millimeters)	
	1.5 T	3.0 T	1.5 T	3.0 T	1.5 T	3.0 T	1.5 T	3.0 T	1.5 T	3.0 T	1.5 T	3.0 T
Balanced gradient echo	4	4	2	2	N/A	N/A	60	60	1	1	8/0	8/0
Spin echo black blood	Min	Min	50	50	Auto	Auto	40	40	1	1	8/0	8/0
Spin echo black blood fat nulled	Min	Min	50	50	Auto	Auto	40	40	1	1	8/0	8/0
Phase contrast (PC)	15	20	5	5	N/A	N/A	15	15	2	2	8/0	8/0
Contrast enhanced (CE)	5	10	2	5	N/A	N/A	40	40	1	1	8/0	8/0

TABLE 34–1 • General Sequences

Abbreviation: N/A, not applicable.

SUGGESTED IMAGING APPLICATION VARIATIONS

Trauma

The attending radiologist and/or the requesting physician may ask for additional sequences or orthogonal planes depending on the traumatic injury.

Tumor

A tumor protocol may require sequences in addition to the routine liver protocol and a larger field of view to include the lesion.

Additional pre- and postcontrast sequences may be included. Three-orthogonal-plane postcontrast sequences may be of benefit to the radiologist. The technologist should follow the protocol provided at their facility.

Additional Sequences

Additional sequences of the aorta, magnetic resonance angiography of the chest, valves, tagging, and flow quantification may be requested. Please consult the protocol at your facility and requesting physician to determine if any additional sequences are needed.

Great Vessels (Chest MRA)

35

COIL SELECTION

- Primary coil: Body or torso coil
- Secondary coil: Cardiac coil

PATIENT/PART POSITIONING AND CENTERING

- The patient is positioned supine and headfirst on the MRI table or patient couch.
- Make the patient comfortable.
- Position the patient so that the spine is parallel to the z-axis of the MRI unit. The patient should be as flat and straight on the coil as possible.
- Center at mid-sternum.
- Instruct the patient to lie still and not move any part of their body.
- Instruct the patient to not cross their arms and legs.

SLICE ALIGNMENT AND SCAN RANGE

Slice Alignment

- Using the coronal and sagittal scout images, align the slice overlay to be parallel to the long axis of the thorax (Figures 35–1 to 35–4).
- The field of view should extend from mid-neck to the abdomen (see Figures 35–1 to 35–4).

Phase and Frequency Orientation

- Phase: Right to left
- Frequency: Anteroposterior
- Phase and frequency orientations may be swapped.

Saturation Band Placement

- A saturation band is placed superior to and outside the field of view.
- The saturation band will supress (hypointense blood) the venous flow.

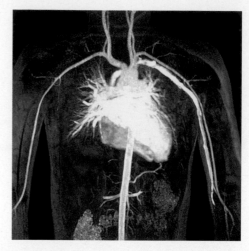

FIGURE 35–2. Coronal maximum intensity projection (MIP). Compare Figures 35–2, 35–3, and 35–4 and note the contrast enhancement. These 3 figures were acquired at different time intervals. By the time Figure 35–4 was acquired, the contrast had dissipated (washed out). The contrast is washing out of the arterial system, thus the arterial system becomes less clearly defined.

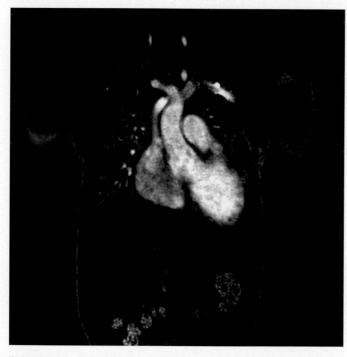

FIGURE 35–1. Contrast-enhanced MRA of the heart and great vessels.

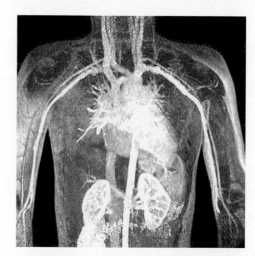

FIGURE 35–3. Coronal maximum intensity projection (MIP). Note the washout of the contrast and increased venous enhancement.

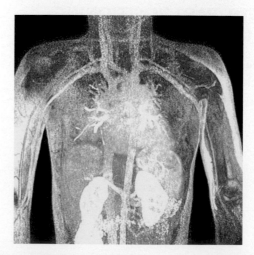

FIGURE 35–4. Coronal maximum intensity projection (MIP). Note the washout of the contrast and increased venous enhancement.

IMAGING APPLICATION

TABLE 35–1 • General Sequences

General Sequences	TR		TE		TI		FA (degrees)		NEX		SLT/GAP (in millimeters)	
	1.5 T	3.0 T	1.5 T	3.0 T	1.5 T	3.0 T	1.5 T	3.0 T	1.5 T	3.0 T	1.5 T	3.0 T
Contrast enhanced (CE)	5	10	2	5	N/A	N/A	40°	40°	1	1	4/1	4/1
Time of flight (TOF)	25	20	7	5	N/A	N/A	20°	20°	1	1	1/0	1/0
Phase contrast (PC)	15	20	5	5	N/A	N/A	15°	15°	2	2	8/0	8/0

Abbreviation: N/A, not applicable.

36

Breast

COIL SELECTION

- Primary coil: Breast coil
- Secondary coil: Surface coil

PATIENT/PART POSITIONING AND CENTERING

- The patient is positioned prone and headfirst on the breast coil.
- The breasts fit into the coil. Depending on the manufacturer, the breasts are often suspended in the coil.

- Make the patient comfortable by supporting the patient's head and legs with pillows and cushions.
- Center on the breasts.
- Instruct the patient to lie still and not move any part of their body.
- Instruct the patient to not cross their arms and legs.
- Place magnetic resonance markers on areas of interest as indicated by the radiologist, such as surgical scars.

SLICE ALIGNMENT AND SCAN RANGE

Axial Sequence Acquisition

Slice Alignment

- As shown on the sagittal and coronal scout images, align the slice overlay perpendicular to the long axis of the sternum (Figures 36–1 and 36–2).
- The superior-to-inferior field of view must include the soft tissue of the breast.
- The left-to-right field of view should extend from the left breast to the right breast and include the soft tissue. Note that this is for bilateral breast imaging. The breasts may also be imaged individually. (see Figure 36–3).
- The anteroposterior field of view should extend from the nipple to the chest wall. Often, the field of view extends to approximately mid-thorax so that the axillary margins are included (Figure 36–4).

Phase and Frequency Orientation

- Phase: Anteroposterior
- Frequency: Right to left
- Phase and frequency orientations may be swapped to reduce motion artifact.

Saturation Band Placement

- A saturation band may be used to eliminate or reduce motion artifact from the thorax.
- If used, the saturation band should be placed medial to the field of view.

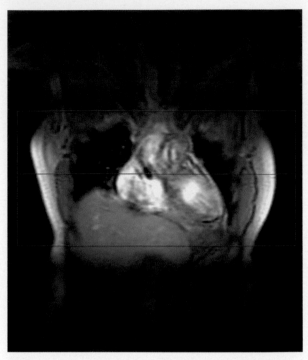

FIGURE 36–2. Coronal scout image showing slice overlay for an axial sequence.

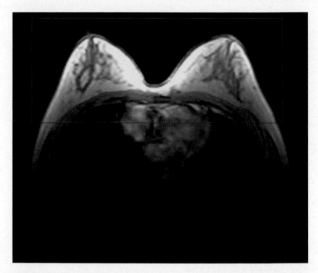

FIGURE 36–3. Axial scout image demonstrating the FOV, which is shown as a red perimeter box.

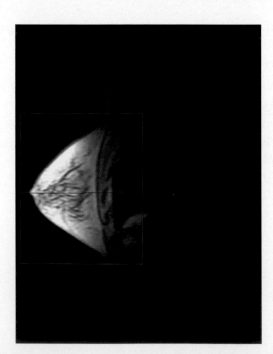

FIGURE 36–1. Sagittal scout image showing slice overlay for an axial sequence. You will align parallel with the red line. The red box demonstrates the field of view.

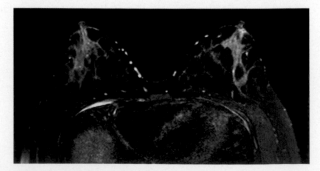

FIGURE 36–4. Axial short tau inversion recovery (STIR).

Sagittal Sequence Acquisition

Slice Alignment

- As shown on the axial and coronal scout images, align the slice overlay parallel to the long axis of the sternum (Figures 36–5 and 36–6).
- The superior-to-inferior field of view must include the soft tissue of the breast.
- The left-to-right field of view must include the soft tissue of the breast.
- The anteroposterior field of view should extend from the nipple to the chest wall. Often, the field of view extends to approximately mid-thorax so that the axillary margins are included (Figure 36–7).
- Note that this is an example of imaging each breast individually; however, both breasts may be imaged in one acquisition. If you decide to acquire the sagittal sequence in one acquisition, make sure to include all the soft tissue of both breasts.

Phase and Frequency Orientation

- Phase: Anteroposterior
- Frequency: Superior to inferior
- Phase and frequency orientations may be swapped to reduce motion artifact.

Saturation Band Placement

- A saturation band may be used to eliminate or reduce motion artifact from the thorax.
- If used, the saturation band should be placed medial to the field of view.

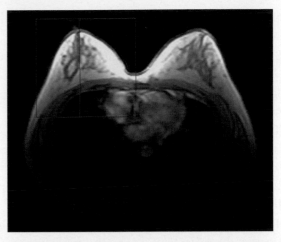

FIGURE 36–5. Axial scout image showing slice overlay for a sagittal sequence. Align parallel with the red line. The red perimeter box demonstrates the field of view.

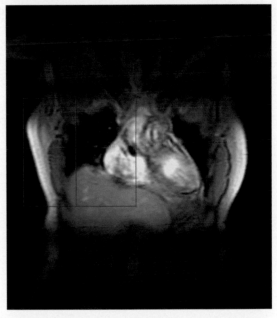

FIGURE 36–6. Coronal scout image showing slice overlay for a sagittal sequence.

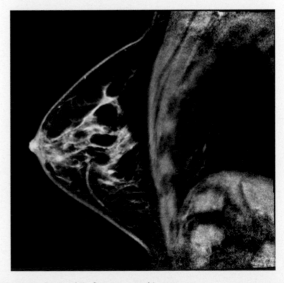

FIGURE 36–7. Sagittal T2 fat-saturated image.

Coronal Sequence Acquisition (if Requested)

Slice Alignment

- Slices are parallel to a line extending from the left breast to the right breast.
- If breasts are symmetric, angle the slices so that they enter each breast at the same point.
- The anatomy on each side of the image should correspond to the other side so that it is a mirror image (unless pathology is present).
- If breasts are asymmetric, angle the slices so that they enter the thoracic cavity at the same point.
- The superior-to-inferior field of view must include the soft tissue of the breast.
- The left-to-right field of view should extend from the left axilla to the right axilla.
- The anteroposterior field of view should include extend from the nipple through the axilla.

Phase and Frequency Orientation

- Phase: Right to left
- Frequency: Superior to inferior
- Phase and frequency orientations may be swapped to reduce motion artifact.

Saturation Band Placement

- A saturation band may be used to eliminate or reduce motion artifact from the thorax.
- If used, the saturation band should be placed medial to the field of view.

SUGGESTED IMAGING APPLICATION VARIATIONS

Tumor

A tumor protocol may require sequences in addition to the routine shoulder protocol and a larger field of view to include the lesion. Additional pre- and postcontrast sequences may be included. Three-orthogonal-plane postcontrast sequences may be of benefit to the radiologist. The technologist should follow the protocol provided at their facility.

Abdomen and Pelvis

37

Liver

COIL SELECTION

- Primary coil: Body or torso coil
- Secondary coil: Cardiac coil

PATIENT/PART POSITIONING AND CENTERING

- The patient is positioned supine and headfirst on the MRI table or patient couch.
- Make the patient comfortable.

- Position the patient so that the spine is parallel to the z-axis of the MRI unit. The patient should be as flat and straight on the coil as possible.
- Center 2 inches inferior the xiphoid process so that the liver is at isocenter.
- Instruct the patient to lie still and not move any part of their body.
- Instruct the patient to not cross their arms and legs.

SLICE ALIGNMENT AND SCAN RANGE

Abdominal imaging, particularly imaging of the liver, will require some sort of respiratory triggering or breath holds due to respiratory motion. The various manufacturers have software and hardware to compensate for respiratory motion. You should consult the protocol used at your facility.

Coronal Sequence Acquisition

Slice Alignment

- Slices are parallel to a line extending from the left lobe of the liver to the right lobe of the liver (Figure 37–1).
- The field of view (FOV) must include the liver (Figures 37–1 to 37–3).
- A coronal image of the liver is shown in Figure 37–4.

Phase and Frequency Orientation

- Phase: Superior to inferior
- Frequency: Right to left
- Phase and frequency orientations may be swapped to reduce motion artifact.

Saturation Band Placement

- A saturation band may be used to eliminate or reduce motion artifact.
- If used, the saturation band should be placed anterior and superior to the FOV.

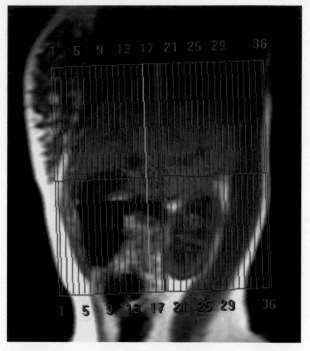

FIGURE 37–2. Sagittal scout image showing slice overlay for a coronal sequence.

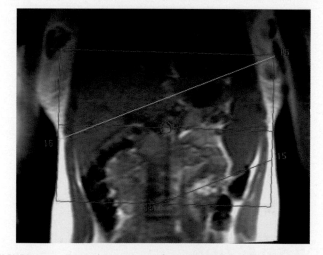

FIGURE 37–3. Coronal scout image demonstrating the FOV, which is shown as a red perimeter box.

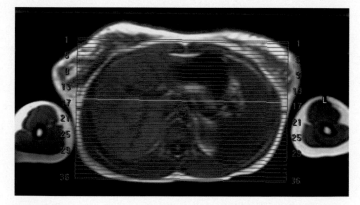

FIGURE 37–1. Axial scout image showing slice overlay for a coronal sequence.

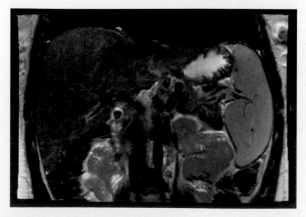

FIGURE 37–4. Coronal T2-weighted image.

Axial Sequence Acquisition

Slice Alignment

- Slices are perpendicular to the abdominal cavity (Figure 37–5).
- The FOV must include the liver (see Figures 37–5 to 37–7).
- An axial image of the liver is shown in Figure 37–8.

Phase and Frequency Orientation

- Phase: Anteroposterior
- Frequency: Right to left
- Phase and frequency orientations may be swapped to reduce motion artifact.

Saturation Band Placement

- A saturation band may be used to eliminate or reduce motion artifact.
- If used, the saturation band should be placed anterior and superior to the FOV.

Sagittal Sequence Acquisition (if Requested)

Slice Alignment

- Slices are perpendicular to a line extending from the left lobe of the liver to the right lobe of the liver.
- The FOV must include the liver.

Phase and Frequency Orientation

- Phase: Superior to inferior
- Frequency: Anteroposterior
- Phase and frequency orientations may be swapped to reduce motion artifact.

Saturation Band Placement

- A saturation band may be used to eliminate or reduce motion artifact.
- If used, the saturation band should be placed anterior and superior to the FOV.

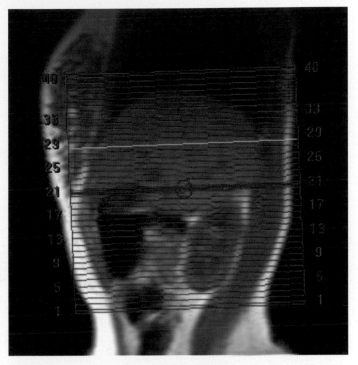

FIGURE 37–6. Sagittal scout image showing slice overlay for an axial sequence.

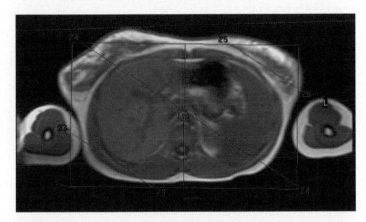

FIGURE 37–7. Axial scout image showing demonstrating the FOV, which is shown as a red perimeter box.

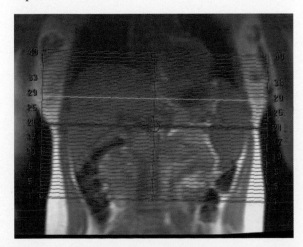

FIGURE 37–5. Coronal scout image showing slice overlay for an axial sequence.

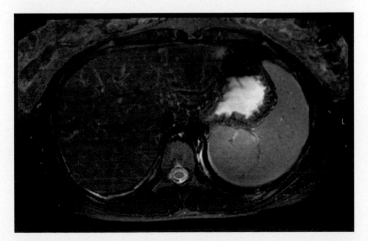

FIGURE 37–8. Axial T2-weighted fat-saturated image.

IMAGING APPLICATION

TABLE 37–1 • General Sequences

General Sequences	TR		TE		TI		FA (degrees)		NEX		SLT/GAP (in millimeters)	
	1.5 T	3.0 T	1.5 T	3.0 T	1.5 T	3.0 T	1.5 T	3.0 T	1.5 T	3.0 T	1.5 T	3.0 T
T2 FS fast spin echo	1600	1800	100	100	N/A	N/A	90°	90°	2	2	5/1	5/1
In phase	10	10	4.6	4.6	N/A	N/A	15°	15°	3	3	5/1	5/1
Out of phase	10	10	2.3	2.3	N/A	N/A	15°	15°	3	3	5/1	5/1
T1 3D with fat suppression post C+	5.8	6	2.9	3	N/A	N/A	10°	10°	1	1		

Abbreviations: 3D, 3-dimensional; FS, fat saturated; N/A, not applicable.

SUGGESTED IMAGING APPLICATION VARIATIONS

Different Contrast Agents (Eovist or Primovist)

The exam may be protocoled with gadoxetate disodium (also known as Eovist and Primovist), instead of the typical contrast gadolinium contrast agents that might be used for other exams. Eovist and Primovist are examples of hepato-specific gadolinium-based contrast agents and are useful in imaging liver lesions. Your protocol may require imaging in several phases of contrast administration or postcontrast delays. Note, however, that the scan alignment and scan range provided earlier would still apply. Please consult your imaging protocol.

Trauma

The attending radiologist and/or the requesting physician may ask for additional sequences or orthogonal planes depending on the traumatic injury.

Tumor

A tumor protocol may require sequences in addition to the routine liver protocol and a larger FOV to include the lesion. Additional pre- and postcontrast sequences may be included. Three-orthogonal-plane postcontrast sequences may be of benefit to the radiologist. The technologist should follow the protocol provided at their facility.

Magnetic Resonance Cholangiopancreatography (MRCP)

COIL SELECTION

- Primary coil: Body or torso coil
- Secondary coil: Cardiac coil

PATIENT/PART POSITIONING AND CENTERING

- The patient is positioned supine and headfirst on the MRI table or patient couch.
- Make the patient comfortable.
- Position the patient so that the spine is parallel to the z-axis of the MRI unit. The patient should be as flat and straight on the coil as possible.

- Center 2 inches inferior the xiphoid process so that the liver is at isocenter.
- Instruct the patient to lie still and not move any part of their body.
- Instruct the patient to not cross their arms and legs.

SLICE ALIGNMENT AND SCAN RANGE

Abdominal imaging, particularly imaging of the liver, will require some sort of respiratory triggering or breath holds due to respiratory motion. The various manufacturers have software and hardware to compensate for respiratory motion. You should consult the protocol used at your facility.

Coronal Sequence Acquisition

Slice Alignment

- Slices are parallel to a line extending from the left lobe of the liver to the right lobe of the liver (Figures 38–1 and 38–3).
- The field of view must include the gallbladder and extra-hepatic bile ducts (see Figures 38–1 to 38–3).
- An axial resultant image is shown in Figure 38–4. Maximum Intensity Projection (MIP) images are demonstrated in Figures 38–5 to 38–7.
- Note: The field of view in the example above includes the entire liver. A smaller field of view may be required by your facility. Please consult your imaging protocol.
- Additional liver imaging will most likely be required per protocol. (See Figures 37–1 to 37–4 for more information.)

Phase and Frequency Orientation

- Phase: Superior to inferior
- Frequency: Right to left
- Phase and frequency orientations may be swapped to reduce motion artifact.

Saturation Band Placement

- A saturation band may be used to eliminate or reduce motion artifact.
- If used, the saturation band should be placed anterior and superior to the field of view.

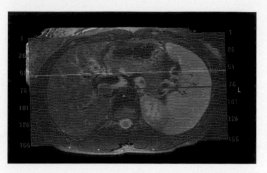

FIGURE 38-1. Axial scout image showing slice overlay for a coronal sequence. Note the 155 planned slices and the thin slice thickness and gap. The field of view may be reduced to only cover the gallbladder and extrahepatic bile ducts; be sure to consult your protocol.

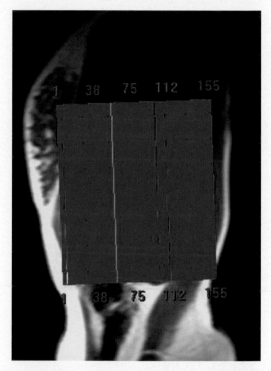

FIGURE 38-2. Sagittal scout image showing slice overlay for a coronal sequence.

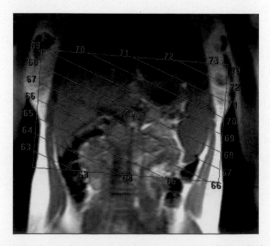

FIGURE 38-3. Coronal scout image demonstrating the FOV, which is shown as a red perimeter box.

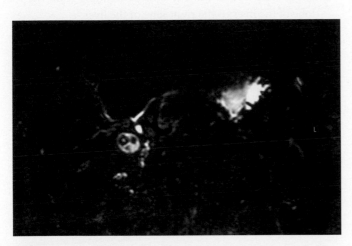

FIGURE 38–4. Coronal MRCP image. Note that it will be reconstructed to form a maximum intensity projection (MIP).

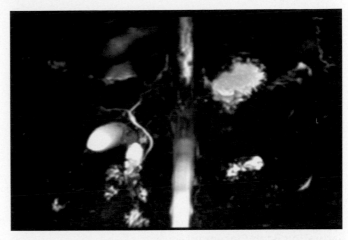

FIGURE 38–5. Maximum intensity projection (MIP) of the MRCP. Note the anatomic structures such as the gallbladder and biliary ducts.

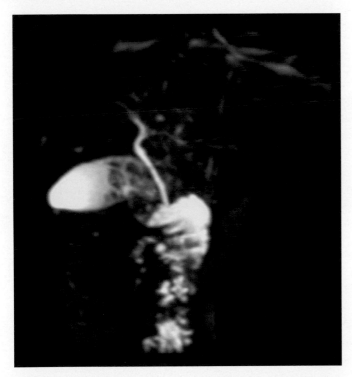

FIGURE 38–6. Maximum intensity projection (MIP) of the MRCP. Note the anatomic structures such as the gallbladder and biliary ducts.

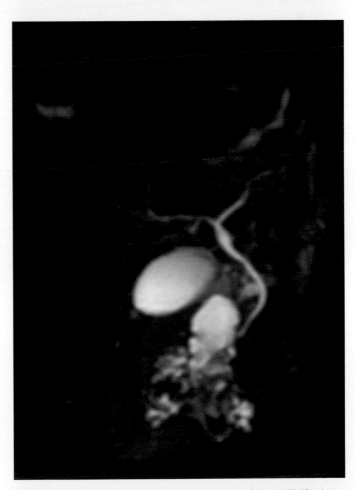

FIGURE 38–7. Maximum intensity projection (MIP) of the MRCP. This is the same MIP reconstruction as Figure 38-6. The only difference is that the projection has been rotated to better visualize the biliary tree and pancreatic ducts.

Axial Sequence Acquisition (if Requested)

Slice Alignment

- Slices are perpendicular to the abdominal cavity.
- The field of view must include the gallbladder and extra-hepatic bile ducts.

Phase and Frequency Orientation

- Phase: Anteroposterior
- Frequency: Right to left
- Phase and frequency orientations may be swapped to reduce motion artifact.

Saturation Band Placement

- A saturation band may be used to eliminate or reduce motion artifact.
- If used, the saturation band should be placed anterior and superior to the field of view.
- Additional liver imaging will most likely be required per protocol. (See Figures 37–5 to 37–8 for more information.)

Sagittal Sequence Acquisition (if Requested)

Slice Alignment

- Slices are perpendicular to a line extending from the left lobe of the liver to the right lobe of the liver.
- The field of view must include the gallbladder and extra-hepatic bile ducts.

Phase and Frequency Orientation

- Phase: Superior to inferior
- Frequency: Anteroposterior
- Phase and frequency orientations may be swapped to reduce motion artifact.

Saturation Band Placement

- A saturation band may be used to eliminate or reduce motion artifact.
- If used, the saturation band should be placed anterior and superior to the field of view.

IMAGING APPLICATION

TABLE 38–1 • General Sequences													
General Sequences	TR		TE		TI		FA (degrees)		NEX		SLT/GAP (in millimeters)		
	1.5T	3.0 T	1.5 T	3.0 T	1.5 T	3.0 T	1.5 T	3.0 T	1.5 T	3.0 T	1.5 T	3.0 T
T2 3D ultra-fast spin echo	2100	2200	650	650	N/A	N/A	N/A	N/A	1	1	40/0	40/0

Abbreviations: 3D, 3-dimensional; N/A, not applicable.

SUGGESTED IMAGING APPLICATION VARIATIONS

Trauma

The attending radiologist and/or the requesting physician may ask for additional sequences or orthogonal planes depending on the traumatic injury.

Tumor

A tumor protocol may require sequences in addition to the routine magnetic resonance cholangiopancreatography (MRCP) protocol and a larger field of view to include the lesion. Additional pre- and postcontrast sequences may be included. Three-orthogonal-plane postcontrast sequences may be of benefit to the radiologist. The technologist should follow the protocol provided at their facility.

Magnetic Resonance Enterography (MRE)

39

COIL SELECTION

- Primary coil: Body or torso coil
- Secondary coil: Cardiac coil

PATIENT/PART POSITIONING AND CENTERING

- The patient is positioned supine and either headfirst or feetfirst on the MRI table or patient couch. If possible, have the patient place their arms up over their head.

- Make the patient comfortable.
- The legs should be extended.
- The pelvis should not be rotated.
- The abdomen should be placed as close to isocenter as possible.
- Center approximately 5 to 6 inches superior of the anterior superior iliac spine (ASIS).
- Support the patient's legs and arms.
- Instruct the patient to lie still and not move any part of their body.
- Instruct the patient to not cross their arms and legs.

SLICE ALIGNMENT AND SCAN RANGE

Please consult the imaging protocol provided by your facility and follow the patient preparation outlined in the protocol. The patient will most likely drink oral contrast such as barium sulfate before imaging. If oral contrast is administered, the patient should slowly drink the contrast over an extended period of time. Many facilities allow the patient to slowly drink the contrast over approximately an hour and a half and then allow approximately 30 minutes before scanning. Also, some facilities administer intravenous drugs to slow down peristalsis for optimal imaging.

Coronal Sequence Acquisition

Slice Alignment

- Slices are parallel to the long axis of the body (Figures 39–1 and 39–2).
- The superior-to-inferior field of view should extend from superior of the liver to inferior of the anus (Figure 39–3).
- The left-to-right field of view should extend from the left side of the abdominal cavity to the right side of the abdominal cavity. The field of view must include the abdominal and pelvic contents (see Figure 39–2).
- The anteroposterior field of view should extend from abdominal body fat to posterior body fat (see Figure 39–1).
- A coronal MRE image is shown in Figure 39–4.

Phase and Frequency Orientation

- Phase: Right to left
- Frequency: Superior to inferior
- Phase and frequency orientations may be swapped to reduce motion artifact.

Saturation Band Placement

- A saturation band may be used to eliminate or reduce motion artifact.
- If used, the saturation band should be placed superior to the field of view.

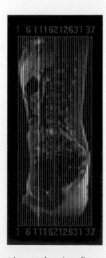

FIGURE 39–1. Sagittal scout image showing slice overlay for a coronal sequence.

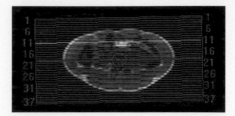

FIGURE 39–2. Axial scout image showing slice overlay for a coronal sequence. Additional slices were added to compensate for an inspiratory breath hold.

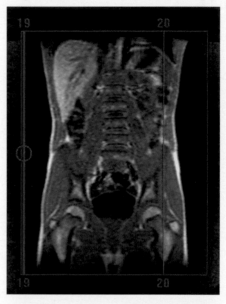

FIGURE 39–3. Coronal scout image demonstrating the FOV, which is shown as a red perimeter box.

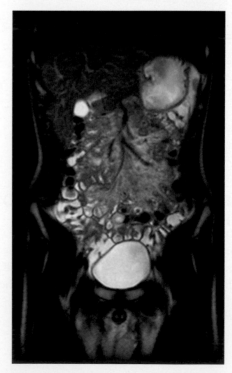

FIGURE 39–4. Coronal T2-weighted fast spin echo image. Note the anatomic structures such as the small bowel, large bowel, mesentery, liver, stomach, and bladder.

Axial Sequence Acquisition

Slice Alignment

- Slices are perpendicular to the long axis of the body (Figures 39–5 and 39–8).
- The superior-to-inferior field of view should extend from superior of the liver to inferior of the anus. Note: In Figures 39–5 and 39–8, axial magnetic resonance enterography (MRE) imaging was split into upper and lower sections so that image acquisition time was short and the patient could hold their breath during image acquisition.
- The left-to-right field of view should extend from the left side of the abdominal cavity to the right side of the abdominal cavity. The field of view must include the abdominal and pelvic contents (see Figures 39–5 and 39–8).
- The anteroposterior field of view should extend from abdominal body fat to posterior body fat (Figures 39–6 and 39–9).

Phase and Frequency Orientation

- Phase: Anteroposterior
- Frequency: Right to left
- Phase and frequency orientations may be swapped to reduce motion artifact.

Saturation Band Placement

- A saturation band may be used to eliminate or reduce motion artifact.
- If used, the saturation band should be placed superior to the field of view.

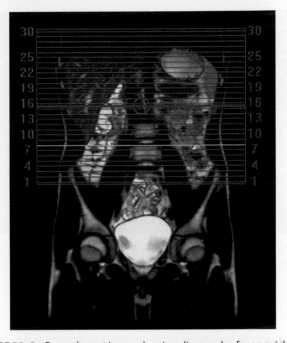

FIGURE 39–5. Coronal scout image showing slice overlay for an axial sequence of the upper abdomen. Note that the axial image acquisition is split between an upper and lower slice overlay (see Figures 39–5 and 39–8), with sufficient overlap of the 2 stacks of overlays. Axial MRE imaging was split into upper and lower sections so that image acquisition time was short and the patient could hold their breath during image acquisition.

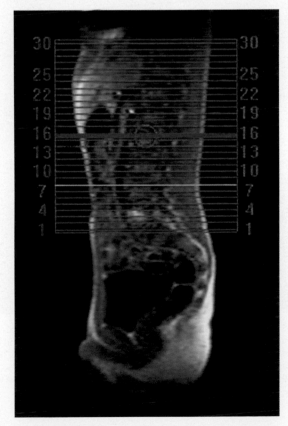

FIGURE 39–6. Sagittal scout image showing slice overlay for an axial sequence of the upper abdomen.

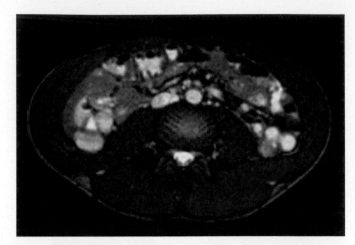

FIGURE 39–7. Axial fast gradient echo T2-weighted image of the upper abdomen. Note the anatomic structures such as the small and large bowel.

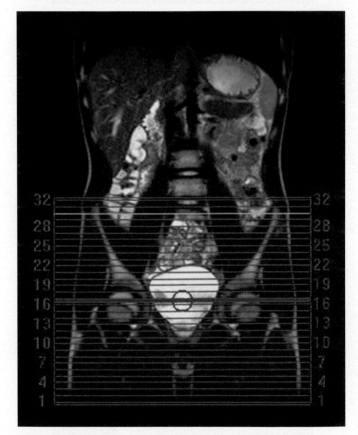

FIGURE 39–8. Coronal scout image showing slice overlay for an axial sequence of the lower abdomen. Note that the axial image acquisition is split between an upper and lower slice overlay (see Figures 39–5 and 39–8), with sufficient overlap of the 2 stacks of overlays. Axial MRE imaging was split into upper and lower sections so that image acquisition time was short and the patient could hold their breath during image acquisition.

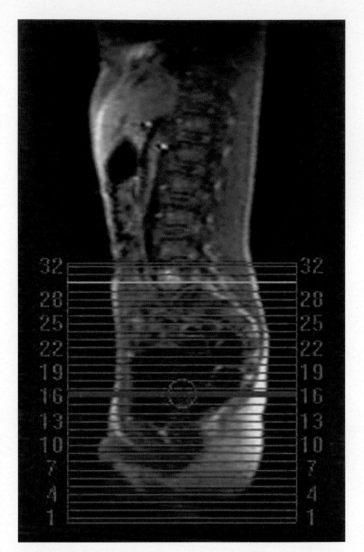

FIGURE 39–9. Sagittal scout image showing slice overlay for an axial sequence of the lower abdomen.

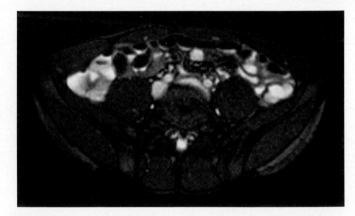

FIGURE 39–10. Axial fast gradient echo T2-weighted image of the lower abdomen/pelvis. Note the anatomic structures such as the small and large bowel.

Sagittal Sequence Acquisition (if Requested)

Slice Alignment

- Slices are perpendicular to a line extending from the left ASIS to the right ASIS.
- The superior-to-inferior field of view should extend from superior of the liver to inferior of the anus.
- The left-to-right field of view should extend from the left side of the abdominal cavity to the right side of the abdominal cavity. The field of view must include the abdominal and pelvic contents.
- The anteroposterior field of view should extend from abdominal body fat to posterior body fat.

Phase and Frequency Orientation

- Phase: Superior to inferior
- Frequency: Anteroposterior
- Phase and frequency orientations may be swapped to reduce motion artifact.

Saturation Band Placement

- A saturation band may be used to eliminate or reduce motion artifact.
- If used, the saturation band should be placed superior to the field of view.

IMAGING APPLICATION

TABLE 39–1 • General Sequences

General Sequences	TR		TE		TI		FA (degrees)		NEX		SLT/GAP (in millimeters)	
	1.5 T	3.0 T	1.5 T	3.0 T	1.5 T	3.0 T	1.5 T	3.0 T	1.5 T	3.0 T	1.5 T	3.0 T
T2 ultra-fast spin echo	440	500	80	80	N/A	N/A	N/A	N/A	2	2	5/1	5/1
Fast balanced gradient echo	4.1	4.1	2.1	2.1	N/A	N/A	90°	90°	1	1	7/1	7/1
T1 3D with fat suppression post C+	5.8	6	2.9	3	N/A	N/A	10	10	1	1		

Abbreviations: 3D, 3-dimensional; N/A, not available.

SUGGESTED IMAGING APPLICATION VARIATIONS

Trauma

The attending radiologist and/or the requesting physician may ask for additional sequences or orthogonal planes depending on the traumatic injury.

Tumor

A tumor protocol may require sequences in addition to the routine MRE protocol and a larger field of view to include the lesion. Additional pre- and postcontrast sequences may be included. Three-orthogonal-plane postcontrast sequences may be of benefit to the radiologist. The technologist should follow the protocol provided at their facility.

Kidneys

40

COIL SELECTION

- Primary coil: Body or torso coil
- Secondary coil: Cardiac coil

PATIENT/PART POSITIONING AND CENTERING

- The patient is positioned supine and either headfirst or feetfirst on the MRI table or patient couch.
- Make the patient comfortable.
- Position the patient so that the spine is parallel to the z-axis of the MRI unit. The patient should be as flat and straight on the coil as possible.
- Center approximately 6 inches superior of the anterior superior iliac spine (ASIS) so that the kidneys are at isocenter.
- Instruct the patient to lie still and not move any part of their body.
- Instruct the patient to not cross their arms and legs.

SLICE ALIGNMENT AND SCAN RANGE

Coronal Sequence Acquisition

Slice Alignment

- Slices are parallel to a line extending from the left kidney to the right kidney (Figure 40–1).

- Angle the slices so that they enter each kidney at the same point.

- On sagittal scout, slices should be aligned according to a line drawn from the superior pole of the kidney to the inferior pole of the kidney (Figure 40–2).

- The anatomy on each side of the image should correspond to the other side so that it is a mirror image (unless pathology is present).

- The field of view must include the kidneys and adrenal glands (Figure 40–3).

- Note: Some radiologists may desire the field of view to include the liver.

Phase and Frequency Orientation

- Phase: Superior to inferior
- Frequency: Right to left
- Phase and frequency orientations may be swapped to reduce motion artifact.

Saturation Band Placement

- A saturation band may be used to eliminate or reduce motion artifact.

- If used, the saturation band should be placed anterior and superior to the field of view.

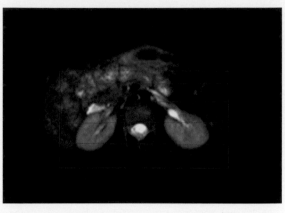

FIGURE 40–1. Axial scout image showing slice overlay for a coronal sequence. Note that you will align parallel with the red lines. The red perimeter box demonstrates the field of view. The slice thickness will be much thinner.

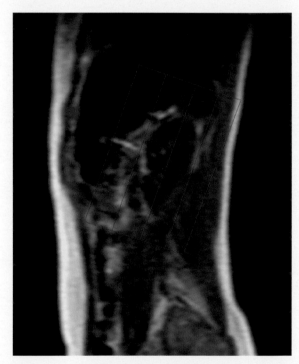

FIGURE 40–2. Sagittal scout image showing slice overlay for a coronal sequence. Note align parallel with the red lines, parallel to the long axis of the kidneys.

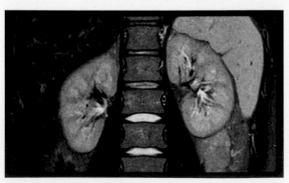

FIGURE 40–3. Coronal short tau inversion recovery (STIR) image of the kidneys. Note the anatomic structures of the kidneys, such as the cortex, medulla, minor calices, major calices, and renal pelvis.

Axial Sequence Acquisition

Slice Alignment

- Angle the slices so that they enter each kidney at the same point.
- On sagittal scout, slices should be aligned perpendicular to a line drawn from the superior pole of the kidney to the inferior pole of the kidney (Figures 40–4 and 40–5).
- The anatomy on each side of the image should correspond to the other side so that it is a mirror image (unless pathology is present).
- The field of view must include the kidneys and adrenal glands (Figure 40–6).
- Note: Radiologists may desire the field of view to include the liver.

Phase and Frequency Orientation

- Phase: Anteroposterior
- Frequency: Right to left
- Phase and frequency orientations may be swapped to reduce motion artifact.

Saturation Band Placement

- A saturation band may be used to eliminate or reduce motion artifact.
- If used, the saturation band should be placed anterior and superior to the field of view.

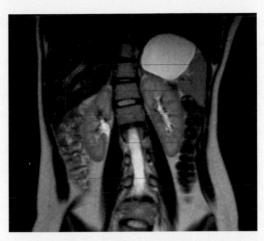

FIGURE 40–4. Coronal scout image showing slice overlay for an axial sequence. Note that you will align parallel with the red lines. The red perimeter box demonstrates the field of view.

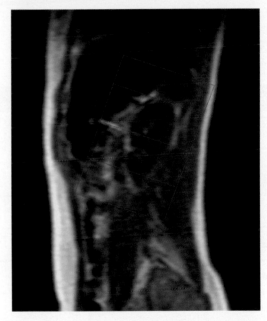

FIGURE 40–5. Sagittal scout image showing slice overlay for an axial sequence. Note that you will align parallel with the red lines. The perimeter box demonstrates the field of view. Note that slices are perpendicular to the long axis of the kidneys.

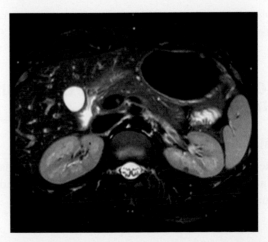

FIGURE 40–6. Axial fat-saturated T2-weighted image of the kidneys. Note the anatomic structures of the kidneys, such as the cortex, medulla, minor calices, major calices, renal artery, and renal vein.

Sagittal Sequence Acquisition (if Requested)

Slice Alignment

- If each kidney will be imaged separately: On coronal and sagittal scout images, slices should be aligned according to a line drawn from the superior pole of the kidney to the inferior pole of the kidney. Use the axial scout images to align with the renal pelvis.
- If a bilateral field of view sagittal image is requested: Use the coronal and axial scout images to align parallel with the spine.
- The field of view must include the kidneys and adrenal glands.
- Note: Radiologists may desire the field of view to include the liver.

Phase and Frequency Orientation

- Phase: Superior to inferior
- Frequency: Anteroposterior
- Phase and frequency orientations may be swapped to reduce motion artifact.

Saturation Band Placement

- A saturation band may be used to eliminate or reduce motion artifact.
- If used, the saturation band should be placed anterior and superior to the field of view.

IMAGING APPLICATION

TABLE 40–1 • General Sequences												
	TR		**TE**		**TI**		**FA (in degrees)**		**NEX**		**SLT/GAP (in millimeters)**	
General Sequences	**1.5 T**	**3.0 T**	**1.5 T**	**3.0 T**	**1.5 T**	**3.0 T**	**1.5 T**	**3.0 T**	**1.5 T**	**3.0 T**	**1.5 T**	**3.0 T**
STIR	3000	3000	60	60	150	150	90°	90°	2	2	4/1	4/1
T2 FS fast spin echo	2000	2000	100	100	N/A	N/A	90°	90°	2	2	4/1	4/1
In phase	10	10	4.6	4.6	N/A	N/A	15°	15°	3	3	5/1	5/1
Out of phase	10	10	2.3	2.3	N/A	N/A	15°	15°	3	3	5/1	5/1
T1 3D with fat suppression post C+	5.8	6	2.9	3	N/A	N/A	10°	10°	1	1		

Abbreviations: 3D, 3-dimensional; FS, fat saturated; N/A, not applicable; STIR, short tau inversion recovery.

SUGGESTED IMAGING APPLICATION VARIATIONS

Trauma

The attending radiologist and/or the requesting physician may ask for additional sequences or orthogonal planes depending on the traumatic injury.

Tumor

A tumor protocol may require sequences in addition to the routine kidney protocol and a larger field of view to include the lesion. Additional pre- and postcontrast sequences may be included. Three-orthogonal-plane postcontrast sequences may be of benefit to the radiologist. The technologist should follow the protocol provided at their facility.

Female Pelvis

COIL SELECTION

- Primary coil: Body or torso coil
- Secondary coil: Cardiac coil

PATIENT/PART POSITIONING AND CENTERING

- The patient is positioned supine and either headfirst or feetfirst on the MRI table or patient couch.
- Make the patient comfortable.

- The legs should be extended with the feet medially rotated 15 to 20 degrees. The feet should be secured in this position with tape and/or sandbags.
- The pelvis should not be rotated.
- Center approximately 2 inches inferior to the anterior superior iliac spine (ASIS) so that the pelvis is at isocenter.
- Instruct the patient to lie still and not move any part of their body.
- Instruct the patient to not cross their arms and legs.

SLICE ALIGNMENT AND SCAN RANGE

Sagittal Sequence Acquisition

Slice Alignment

- On coronal scout images, slices are parallel to the long axis of the body (Figure 41–1).
- On axial scout images, slices are perpendicular to a line extending from the left ASIS to the right ASIS (Figure 41–2).
- An odd number of slices should be used to allow for a mid-sagittal slice.
- Place the midsagittal slice on the pubic symphysis.
- The superior-to-inferior field of view should extend from superior of the iliac crest to inferior of the ramus of ischium (Figure 41–1).
- The left-to-right field of view should extend from the left femoral head to the right femoral head (see Figure 41–1).
- The anteroposterior field of view should extend from abdominal body fat through the rectum (Figure 41–4).
- A sagittal image of the female pelvis is shown in Figure 41–4.

Phase and Frequency Orientation

- Phase: Superior to inferior
- Frequency: Anteroposterior
- Phase and frequency orientations may be swapped to reduce motion artifact.

Saturation Band Placement

- A saturation band may be used to eliminate or reduce motion artifact.
- If used, the saturation band should be placed superior and anterior of the field of view.

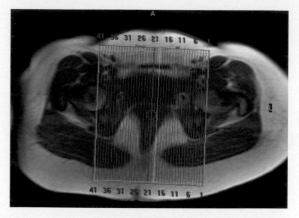

FIGURE 41–2. Axial scout image showing slice overlay for a sagittal sequence.

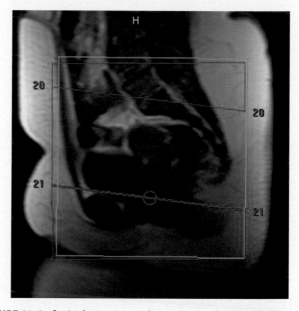

FIGURE 41–3. Sagittal scout image demonstrating the FOV, which is shown as a red perimeter box.

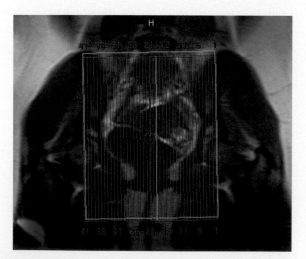

FIGURE 41–1. Coronal scout image showing slice overlay for a sagittal sequence. Note that there is an odd number of slices in this example so the middle slice would be a midsagittal image.

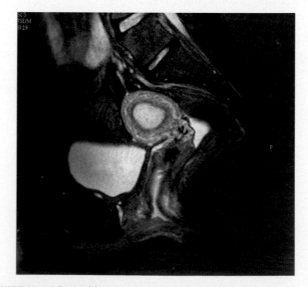

FIGURE 41–4. Sagittal fat-saturated T2-weighted image. Note the anatomic structures such as the uterus, vagina, and bladder.

Coronal Sequence Acquisition

Option 1: Slices Aligned to the Uterus

- On sagittal scout, slices are parallel to the uterus (Figure 41–5).
- The superior-to-inferior field of view should extend from superior of the iliac crest to inferior of the ramus of ischium.
- The left-to-right field of view should extend from the left femoral head to the right femoral head (Figures 41–6 and 41–7).
- The anteroposterior field of view should extend from abdominal body fat through the rectum.
- A coronal image of the female pelvis aligned with the uterus is shown in Figure 41–8.

Option 2: Slices Aligned to the Pelvic Floor (if Requested)

- On axial images, slices are parallel to a line extending from the left ASIS to the right ASIS.
- The superior-to-inferior field of view should extend from superior of the iliac crest to inferior of the ramus of ischium.
- The left-to-right field of view should extend from the left femoral head to the right femoral head.
- The anteroposterior field of view should extend from abdominal body fat through the rectum.

Phase and Frequency Orientation

- Phase: Superior to inferior
- Frequency: Right to left
- Phase and frequency orientations may be swapped to reduce motion artifact.

Saturation Band Placement

- A saturation band may be used to eliminate or reduce motion artifact.
- If used, the saturation band should be placed superior and anterior to the field of view (see Figure 41–5).

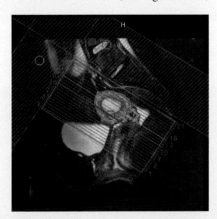

FIGURE 41–5. Midline sagittal scout image showing slice overlay for a coronal sequence aligned with the uterus (option 1). Note that the inferior field of view should extend to the ramus. Also, the saturation bands overlay (the *blue band*) is anterior and superior to the slice overlay so that motion and flow artifacts will be reduced. Note, in this example, the anteroposterior field of view does not extend through the pelvic floor. You may extend the field of view through the pelvic floor.

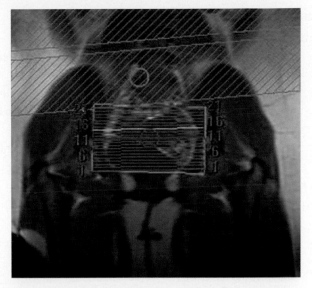

FIGURE 41–6. Coronal scout image demonstrating the FOV, which is shown as a red perimeter box, aligned with the uterus (option 1).

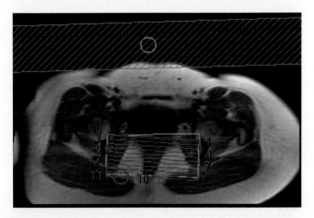

FIGURE 41–7. Axial scout image showing slice overlay for a coronal sequence aligned with the uterus (option 1).

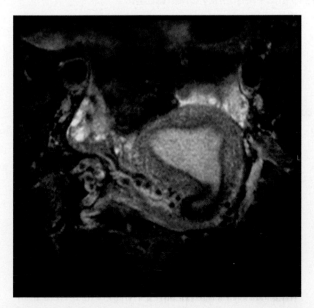

FIGURE 41–8. Coronal fat-saturated T2-weighted image aligned with the uterus (option 1). Note the anatomic structures such as the body of the uterus, uterine cavity, and ovaries.

Axial Sequence Acquisition

Option 1: Slices Aligned to the Uterus

- On sagittal scout, slices are parallel to the uterus (Figure 41–9).
- The superior-to-inferior field of view should extend from superior of the iliac crest to inferior of the ramus of ischium.
- The left-to-right field of view should extend from the left femoral head to the right femoral head (Figures 41–10 and 41–11).
- The anteroposterior field of view should extend from abdominal body fat through the rectum.
- An axial image of the female pelvis aligned with the uterus is shown in Figure 41–12.

Option 2: Slices Aligned to the Pelvic Floor (if Requested)

- On sagittal scout, slices are parallel to the pelvic floor (Figure 41–13).
- Slices are perpendicular to the femoral shafts. (Figure 41–14)
- The superior-to-inferior field of view should extend from superior of the iliac crest to inferior of the ramus of ischium (Figure 41–14).
- The left-to-right field of view should extend from the left femoral head to the right femoral head (see Figure 41–14).
- The anteroposterior field of view should extend from abdominal body fat through the rectum.
- An axial image of the female pelvis aligned with the uterus is shown in Figure 41–15.

Phase and Frequency Orientation

- Phase: Anteroposterior
- Frequency: Right to left
- Phase and frequency orientations may be swapped to reduce motion artifact.

Saturation Band Placement

- A saturation band may be used to eliminate or reduce motion artifact.
- If used, the saturation band should be placed superior and anterior to the field of view.

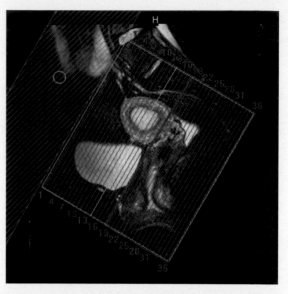

FIGURE 41–9. Midline sagittal scout image showing islice overlay for an axial sequence aligned with the uterus (option 1). Note that the saturation band overlay (the *blue band*) is superior to the slice overlay so that motion and flow artifacts will be reduced.

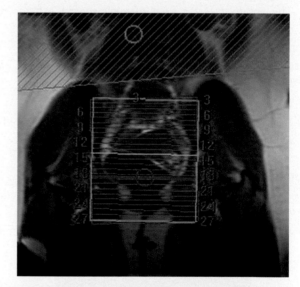

FIGURE 41–10. Coronal scout image showing slice overlay for an axial sequence aligned with the uterus (option 1).

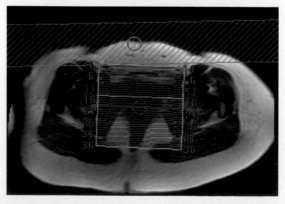

FIGURE 41–11. Axial scout image demonstrating the FOV, which is shown as a red perimeter box, aligned with the uterus (option 1).

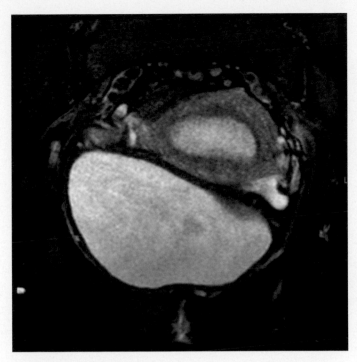

FIGURE 41–12. Axial fat-saturated T2-weighted image that was aligned with the uterus. Note the anatomic structures such as the body of the uterus, uterine cavity, and large urine filled bladder.

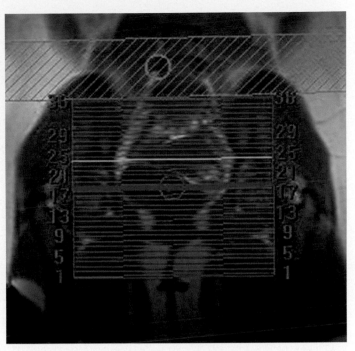

FIGURE 41–14. Coronal scout image showing slice overlay for an axial sequence aligned with the pelvic floor (option 2).

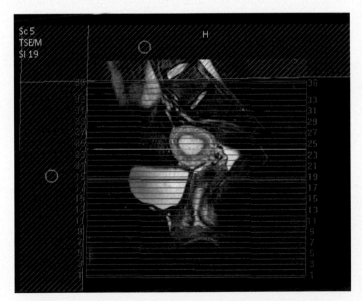

FIGURE 41–13. Midline sagittal scout image showing slice overlay for an axial sequence aligned with the pelvic floor (option 2). Note that the saturation band overlay (the *blue band*) is anterior and superior to the slice overlay so that motion and flow artifacts will be reduced.

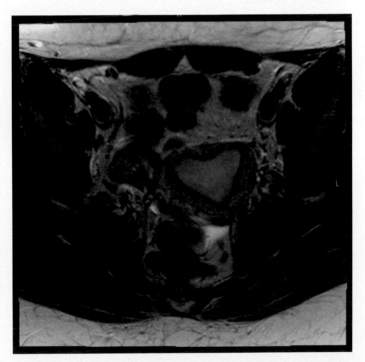

FIGURE 41–15. Axial T2-weighted image that was aligned with the pelvic floor.

IMAGING APPLICATION

TABLE 41–1 • General Sequences

General Sequences	TR		TE		TI		FA (degrees)		NEX		SLT/GAP (in millimeters)	
	1.5 T	3.0 T	1.5 T	3.0 T	1.5 T	3.0 T	1.5 T	3.0 T	1.5 T	3.0 T	1.5 T	3.0 T
T1 SE	500	500	15	20	N/A	N/A	90	90	3	3	3/0.3	3/0.3
T2 SE	4500	4000	70	70	N/A	N/A	90	90	3	3	3/0.3	3/0.3
PD	5000	6500	30	30	N/A	N/A	90	90	3	3	3/0.3	3/0.3
STIR	3000	6000	60	60	150	200	90	90	3	3	3/0.3	3/0.3
T1 SE post C+	500	500	15	20	N/A	N/A	90	90	3	3	3/0.3	3/0.3

Abbreviations: N/A, not applicable; PD, proton density; SE, spin echo; STIR, short tau inversion recovery.

SUGGESTED IMAGING APPLICATION VARIATIONS

Trauma

The attending radiologist and/or the requesting physician may ask for additional sequences or orthogonal planes depending on the traumatic injury.

Tumor

A tumor protocol may require sequences in addition to the routine pelvis protocol and a larger field of view to include the lesion. Additional pre- and postcontrast sequences may be included. Three-orthogonal-plane postcontrast sequences may be of benefit to the radiologist. The technologist should follow the protocol provided at their facility.

42

Male Pelvis

COIL SELECTION

- Primary coil: Body or torso coil
- Secondary coil: Cardiac coil
- Note: Endorectal coils may be used at some facilities but may not be necessary due to good image quality while using a body or torso coil. If an endorectal coil is used, make sure to follow the protocol used at your imaging facility.

PATIENT/PART POSITIONING AND CENTERING

- The patient is positioned supine and either headfirst or feetfirst on the MRI table or patient couch.
- Make the patient comfortable.
- The legs should be extended with the feet medially rotated 15 to 20 degrees. The feet should be secured in this position with tape and/or sandbags.
- The pelvis should not be rotated.
- Center approximately 2 inches inferior of the anterior superior iliac spine (ASIS) so that the pelvis is at isocenter.
- Instruct the patient to lie still and not move any part of their body.
- Instruct the patient to not cross their arms and legs.

SLICE ALIGNMENT AND SCAN RANGE

Sagittal Sequence Acquisition

Slice Alignment

- On coronal scout images, slices are parallel to the long axis of the body (Figure 42–1).
- On axial scout images, slices are perpendicular to a line extending from the left ASIS to the right ASIS (Figure 42–2).
- An odd number of slices should be used to allow for a mid-sagittal slice.
- Place the midsagittal slice on the pubic symphysis.
- The superior-to-inferior field of view should extend from superior of the iliac crest to inferior of the ramus of ischium (Figure 42–3).
- The left-to-right field of view should extend from the left femoral head to the right femoral head, to fully cover the area of the prostate gland (Figure 42–2).
- The anteroposterior field of view should extend from abdominal body fat through the rectum (see Figure 42–3).
- The field of view must include not only the prostate but also the seminal vesicles.
- A sagittal image of the male pelvis is shown in Figure 42–4.

Phase and Frequency Orientation

- Phase: Superior to inferior
- Frequency: Anteroposterior
- Phase and frequency orientations may be swapped to reduce motion artifact.

Saturation Band Placement

- A saturation band may be used to eliminate or reduce motion artifact.
- If used, the saturation band should be placed superior and anterior to the field of view (see Figure 42–3).

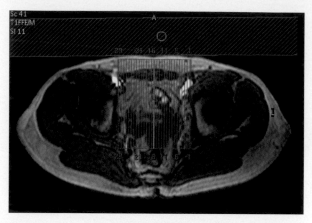

FIGURE 42–2. Axial scout image showing slice overlay for a sagittal sequence.

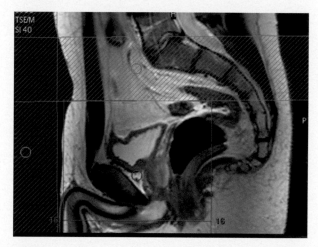

FIGURE 42–3. Sagittal scout image demonstrating the FOV, which is shown as a red perimeter box. Note that the saturation band overlay (the *blue band*) is anterior and superior to the slice overlay so that motion and flow artifacts will be reduced.

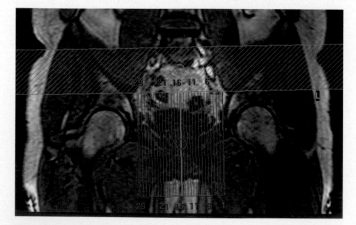

FIGURE 42–1. Coronal scout image showing slice overlay for a sagittal sequence. Note that there is an odd number of slices in this example so the middle slice would be a midsagittal image.

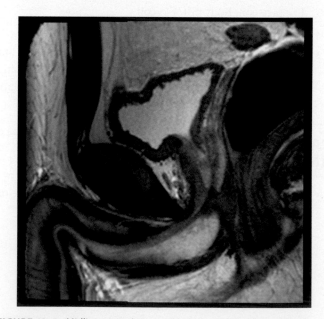

FIGURE 42–4. Midline sagittal T2-weighted image. Note the anatomic structures such as the bladder, prostate, a portion of the penis, and rectum.

Coronal Sequence Acquisition

Option 1: Slices Aligned to the Prostate

- On sagittal scout, slices are parallel to the long axis of the prostate (Figure 42–5).
- The superior-to-inferior field of view should extend from superior of the iliac crest to inferior of the ramus of ischium.
- The left-to-right field of view should extend from the left femoral head to the right femoral head (Figures 42–6 and 42–7).
- The anteroposterior field of view should extend from abdominal body fat through the rectum (see Figure 42–5).
- The field of view must include not only the prostate but also the seminal vesicles.
- A coronal image of the male pelvis aligned with the prostate is shown in Figure 42–8.

Option 2: Slices Aligned to the Pelvic Floor (if Requested)

- On axial images, slices are parallel to a line extending from the left ASIS to the right ASIS.
- The superior-to-inferior field of view should extend from superior of the iliac crest to inferior of the ramus of ischium.
- The left-to-right field of view should extend from the left femoral head to the right femoral head.
- The anteroposterior field of view should extend from abdominal body fat through the rectum.
- The field of view must include not only the prostate but also the seminal vesicles.

Phase and Frequency Orientation

- Phase: Superior to inferior
- Frequency: Right to left
- Phase and frequency orientations may be swapped to reduce motion artifact.

Saturation Band Placement

- A saturation band may be used to eliminate or reduce motion artifact.
- If used, the saturation band should be placed superior and anterior to the field of view.

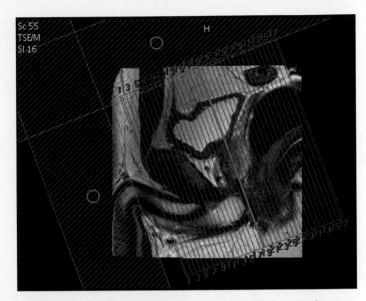

FIGURE 42–5. Midline sagittal scout image showing slice overlay for a coronal sequence aligned with the prostate (option 1). Note that the saturation band overlay (the *blue band*) is anterior and superior to the slice overlay so that motion and flow artifacts will be reduced.

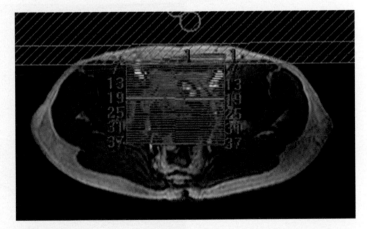

FIGURE 42–6. Axial scout image showing slice overlay for a coronal sequence aligned with the prostate (option 1).

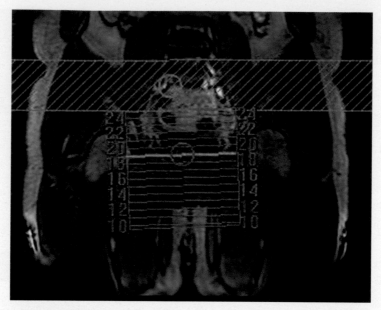

FIGURE 42–7. Coronal scout image showing slice overlay for a coronal sequence aligned with the prostate (option 1).

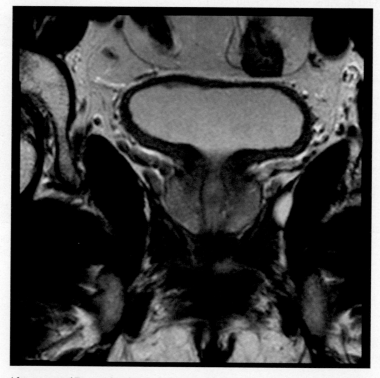

FIGURE 42–8. Coronal fat-saturated T2-weighted image aligned with the prostate (option 1). Note the anatomic structures such as the bladder, prostate, and prostatic urethra.

Axial Sequence Acquisition

Option 1: Slices Aligned to the Prostate

- On sagittal scout, slices are perpendicular to the long axis of the prostate (Figure 42–9).
- The superior-to-inferior field of view should extend from superior of the iliac crest to inferior of the ramus of ischium.
- The left-to-right field of view should extend from the left femoral head to the right femoral head (Figures 42–10 and 42–11).
- The anteroposterior field of view should extend from abdominal body fat through the rectum (see Figure 42–9)
- The field of view must include not only the prostate but also the seminal vesicles.
- An axial image of the male pelvis aligned with the prostate is shown in Figure 41–12.

Option 2: Slices Aligned by Pelvic Floor (if Requested)

- Slices are perpendicular to the femoral shafts.
- The superior-to-inferior field of view should extend from superior of the iliac crest to inferior of the ramus of ischium.
- The left-to-right field of view should extend from the left femoral head to the right femoral head.
- The anteroposterior field of view should extend from abdominal body fat through the rectum.
- The field of view must include not only the prostate but also the seminal vesicles.

Phase and Frequency Orientation

- Phase: Anteroposterior
- Frequency: Right to left
- Phase and frequency orientations may be swapped to reduce motion artifact.

Saturation Band Placement

- A saturation band may be used to eliminate or reduce motion artifact.
- If used, the saturation band should be placed superior and anterior to the field of view (see Figure 42–9).

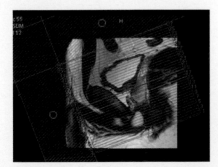

FIGURE 42–9. Midline sagittal scout image showing slice overlay for an axial sequence aligned with the prostate (option 1). Note that the saturation band overlay (the *blue band*) is superior and anterior to the slice overlay so that motion and flow artifacts will be reduced.

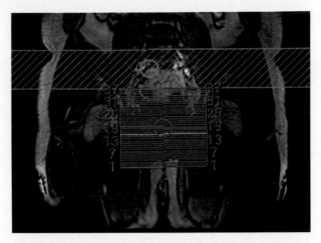

FIGURE 42–10. Coronal scout image showing slice overlay for an axial sequence aligned with the prostate (option 1).

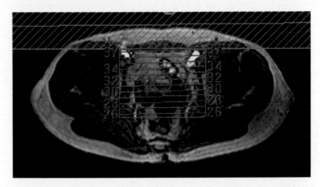

FIGURE 42–11. Axial scout image showing slice overlay for an axial sequence aligned with the prostate (option 1).

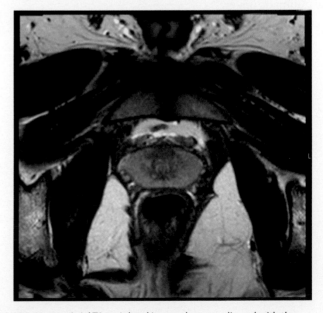

FIGURE 42–12. Axial T2-weighted image that was aligned with the prostate.

IMAGING APPLICATION

TABLE 42–1 • General Sequences

General Sequences	TR		TE		TI		FA (degrees)		NEX		SLT/GAP (in millimeters)	
	1.5 T	3.0 T	1.5 T	3.0 T	1.5 T	3.0 T	1.5 T	3.0 T	1.5 T	3.0 T	1.5 T	3.0 T
T1 SE	500	500	15	20	N/A	N/A	90	90	3	3	3/0.3	3/0.3
T2 SE	4500	4000	70	70	N/A	N/A	90	90	3	3	3/0.3	3/0.3
PD	5000	6500	30	30	N/A	N/A	90	90	3	3	3/0.3	3/0.3
STIR	3000	6000	60	60	150	200	90	90	3	3	3/0.3	3/0.3
T1 SE post C+	500	500	15	20	N/A	N/A	90	90	3	3	3/0.3	3/0.3

Abbreviations: N/A, not applicable; PD, proton density; SE, spin echo; STIR, short tau inversion recovery.

SUGGESTED IMAGING APPLICATION VARIATIONS

Trauma

The attending radiologist and/or the requesting physician may ask for additional sequences or orthogonal planes depending on the traumatic injury.

Tumor

A tumor protocol may require sequences in addition to the routine pelvis protocol and a larger field of view to include the lesion. Additional pre- and postcontrast sequences may be included. Three-orthogonal-plane postcontrast sequences may be of benefit to the radiologist. The technologist should follow the protocol provided at their facility.

43

Shoulder

COIL SELECTION

- Primary coil: Extremity coil
- Secondary coil: Surface coil

PATIENT/PART POSITIONING AND CENTERING

- The patient is positioned supine and headfirst on the MRI table or patient couch.
- Make the patient comfortable.
- Two options for positioning:
  - Option 1: External rotation of the humerus: Supinate the hand and extend the elbow. Adjust the humeral epicondyles parallel to the MRI table. This will place the elbow in true anteroposterior (AP) position.
  - Option 2: Neutral rotation of the humerus: Extend the elbow and place the palm of the hand on the patient's hip. The humeral epicondyles should be at an approximate 45-degree angle to the MRI table.
- Support the patient's hand and shoulder. A sandbag supporting the hand and/or forearm will help keep the elbow in true AP position and aid in patient comfort.
- Center on the coracoid process so that the shoulder is at isocenter.
- Instruct the patient to lie still and not move any part of their body.
- Instruct the patient to not cross their arms and legs.

SLICE ALIGNMENT AND SCAN RANGE

Axial Sequence Acquisition

Slice Alignment

- As shown on Figures 43–1 and 43–2, slices are perpendicular to the shaft of the humerus.
- The superior-to-inferior field of view should extend from superior to the acromioclavicular joint to the surgical neck of the humerus (see Figures 43–1 and 43–2).
- The left-to-right field of view should extend from the deltoid muscle to the scapular notch (Figure 43–3).
- The AP field of view should include the musculature of the rotator cuff.
- An axial image of the shoulder is shown in Figure 43–4.

Phase and Frequency Orientation

- Phase: AP
- Frequency: Right to left
- Phase and frequency orientations may be swapped to reduce motion artifact.

Saturation Band Placement

- A saturation band may be used to eliminate or reduce motion artifact from the thorax.
- If used, the saturation band should be placed medial to the field of view.

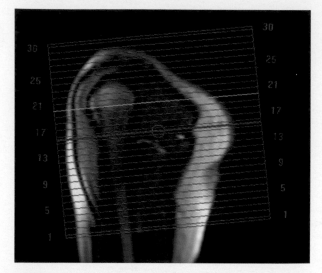

FIGURE 43–2. Sagittal scout image showing slice overlay for an axial sequence.

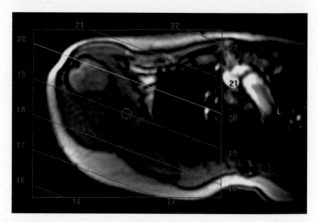

FIGURE 43–3. Axial scout image demonstrating the FOV, which is shown as a red perimeter box.

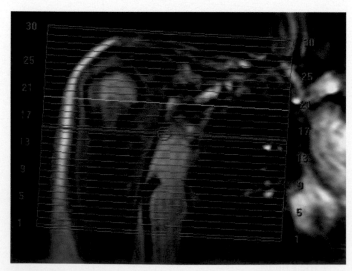

FIGURE 43–1. Coronal scout image showing slice overlay for an axial sequence.

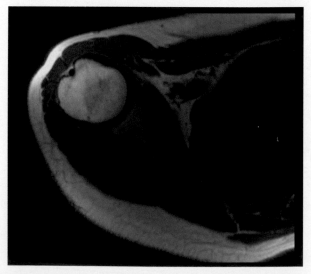

FIGURE 43–4. Axial T1-weighted image. Note that the field of view may be reduced, so be sure to consult your protocol. Also, notice the anatomic structures such as the head of the humerus, glenoid, and labrum.

Coronal Oblique Sequence Acquisition

Slice Alignment

- On axial scout, slices are perpendicular to a line extending from the anterior surface of the glenoid to the posterior surface of the glenoid (Figures 43–5 and 43–6).
- As shown in Figures 43–7 and 43–8, slices are parallel to the shaft of the humerus.
- The superior-to-inferior field of view should extend from superior to the acromioclavicular joint to the surgical neck of the humerus.
- The left-to-right field of view should extend from the deltoid muscle to the scapular notch.
- The AP field-of-view should include the musculature of the rotator cuff.
- A coronal oblique image of the shoulder is shown in Figure 43–9.

Phase and Frequency Orientation

- Phase: Right to left
- Frequency: Superior to inferior
- Phase and frequency orientations may be swapped to reduce motion artifact.

Saturation Band Placement

- A saturation band may be used to eliminate or reduce motion artifact from the thorax.
- If used, the saturation band should be placed medial to the field of view (Figures 43–5 and 43–8).

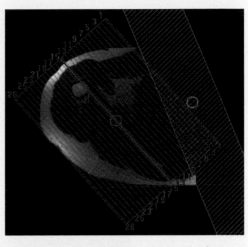

FIGURE 43–5. Axial scout image showing slice overlay for a coronal oblique sequence. Note that the saturation band overlay (the *blue band*) is medial to the field of view so that motion and flow artifacts, such as the subclavian artery, will be reduced.

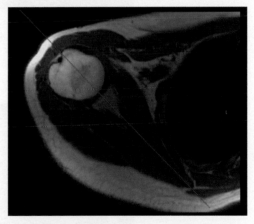

FIGURE 43–6. Additional axial scout image showing slice orientation for a coronal oblique sequence. Note align parallel with the red line and extend to cover entire joint area. The joint is better visualized at this level than in Figure 43–5. Also, your field of view should include the entire joint and pertinent soft tissue.

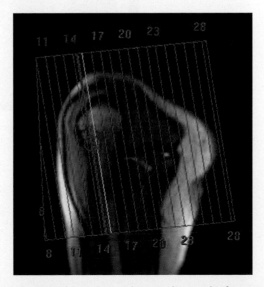

FIGURE 43–7. Sagittal scout image showing slice overlay for a coronal oblique sequence.

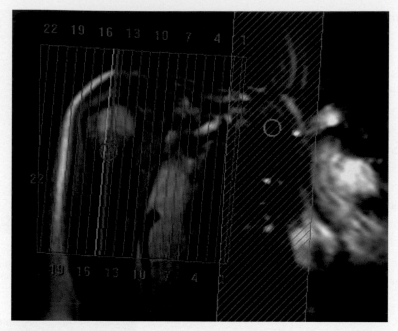

FIGURE 43–8. Coronal scout image demonstrating the FOV, which is shown as a red perimeter box. Note that this image is included to demonstrate the field of view and placement of the saturation band.

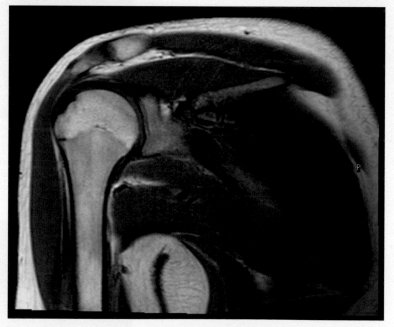

FIGURE 43–9. Coronal oblique T1-weighted image. Note that the field of view may be reduced, so be sure to consult your protocol. Also, notice the anatomic structures such as the head of the humerus, glenoid, labrum, and acromion.

Sagittal Oblique Sequence Acquisition

Slice Alignment

- On axial scout, slices are parallel to a line extending from the anterior surface of the glenoid to the posterior surface of the glenoid (Figures 43–10 and 43–11).
- Slices are parallel to the shaft of the humerus (Figure 43–12).
- The superior-to-inferior field of view should extend from superior to the acromioclavicular joint to the surgical neck of the humerus.
- The left-to-right field of view should extend from the deltoid muscle to the scapular notch.
- The AP field of view should include the musculature of the rotator cuff.
- A sagittal oblique image is shown in Figure 43–13.

Phase and Frequency Orientation

- Phase: AP
- Frequency: Superior to inferior
- Phase and frequency orientations may be swapped to reduce motion artifact.

Saturation Band Placement

- A saturation band may be used to eliminate or reduce motion artifact from the thorax.
- If used, the saturation band should be placed medial to the field of view (Figure 43–10).

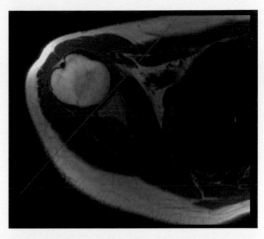

FIGURE 43–11. Additional axial scout image showing slice orientation for a sagittal oblique sequence. Note align parallel with the red line and extend to cover entire joint area. The joint is better visualized at this level than in Figure 43–10. Also, your field of view should include the entire joint and pertinent soft tissue.

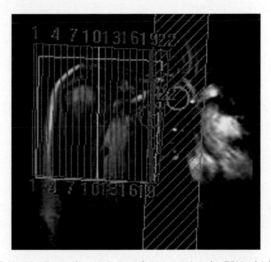

FIGURE 43–12. Coronal scout image demonstrating the FOV, which is shown as a red perimeter box. Note that the saturation band overlay (the *blue band*) is medial to the field of view.

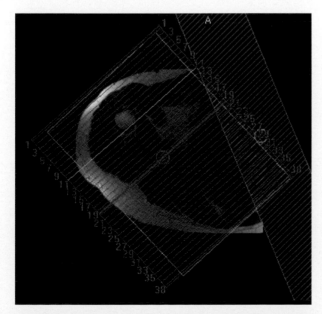

FIGURE 43–10. Axial scout image showing slice overlay for a sagittal oblique sequence. Note that the saturation band overlay (the *blue band*) is medial to the field of view so that motion and flow artifacts will be reduced.

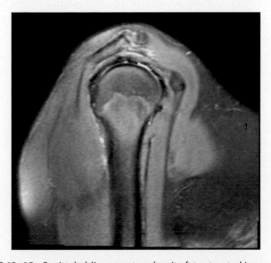

FIGURE 43–13. Sagittal oblique proton density fat-saturated image. Note that the field of view may be reduced, so be sure to consult your protocol. Also, notice the anatomic structures such as the head of the humerus, acromion, and acromioclavicular joint.

IMAGING APPLICATION

General Sequences	TR		TE		TI		FA (degrees)		NEX		SLT/GAP (in millimeters)	
	1.5 T	3.0 T	1.5 T	3.0 T	1.5 T	3.0 T	1.5 T	3.0 T	1.5 T	3.0 T	1.5 T	3.0 T
T1 SE	500	500	15	20	N/A	N/A	90	90	3	3	3/1	3/1
T2 SE	4500	4000	70	70	N/A	N/A	90	90	3	3	3/1	3/1
PD	2500	3500	30	30	N/A	N/A	90	90	3	3	3/1	3/1
STIR	3000	4000	60	15	150	220	90	90	3	3	3/1	3/1
T1 SE post C+	500	500	15	20	N/A	N/A	90	90	3	3	3/1	3/1

TABLE 43–1 • General Sequences

Abbreviations: N/A, not applicable; PD, proton density; SE, spin echo; STIR, short tau inversion recovery.

SUGGESTED IMAGING APPLICATION VARIATIONS

Arthrogram

The injection of contrast media and/or gas in the capsular space may be requested. The requested media will be injected, usually under the guidance of fluoroscopy. The patient will then be imaged in MRI. Additional sequences to the routine protocol may be requested by the radiologist. (See Chapter 50.)

Trauma

The attending radiologist and/or the requesting physician may ask for additional sequences or orthogonal planes depending on the traumatic injury.

Tumor

A tumor protocol may require sequences in addition to the routine shoulder protocol and a larger field of view to include the lesion. Additional pre- and postcontrast sequences may be included. Three-orthogonal-plane postcontrast sequences may be of benefit to the radiologist. The technologist should follow the protocol provided at their facility.

44

Humerus

COIL SELECTION

- Primary coil: Extremity coil
- Secondary coil: Surface coil

PATIENT/PART POSITIONING AND CENTERING

- The patient is positioned supine and headfirst on the MRI table or patient couch.
- Make the patient comfortable.
- Two options for positioning:
  - Option 1: External rotation of the humerus: Supinate the hand and extend the elbow. Adjust the humeral epicondyles parallel to the MRI table. This will place the elbow in true anteroposterior (AP) position.
  - Option 2: Neutral rotation of the humerus: Extend the elbow and place the palm of the hand on the patient's hip. The humeral epicondyles should be at an approximate 45-degree angle to the MRI table.
- Support the patient's hand and shoulder. A sandbag supporting the hand and/or forearm will help keep the elbow in true AP position and aid in patient comfort.
- Center midshaft so that the humerus is at isocenter.
- Instruct the patient to lie still and not move any part of their body.
- Instruct the patient to not cross their arms and legs.

SLICE ALIGNMENT AND SCAN RANGE

Coronal Oblique Sequence Acquisition

Slice Alignment

- As shown on Figures 44–1 and 44–2, slices are parallel to the shaft of the humerus.
- Slices are parallel to the humeral condyle.
- Resultant images should demonstrate the full shaft of the humerus (Figure 44–3).
- The superior-to-inferior field of view should extend from the acromion to the neck of the radius (Figure 44–3).
- The left-to-right field of view must include the shoulder joint and musculature of the humerus.
- The anteroposterior field of view should include the musculature of the humerus.
- A coronal oblique image of the humerus is shown in Figure 44–4.

Phase and Frequency Orientation

- Phase: Right to left
- Frequency: Superior to inferior
- Phase and frequency orientations may be swapped to reduce motion artifact.

Saturation Band Placement

- A saturation band may be used to eliminate or reduce motion artifact from the thorax.
- If used, the saturation band should be placed medial to the field of view.

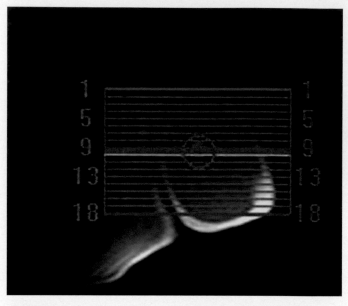

FIGURE 44–2. Axial scout image showing slice overlay for a coronal sequence.

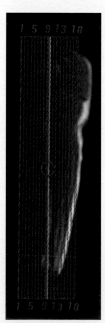

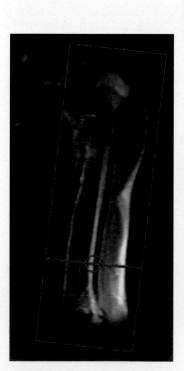

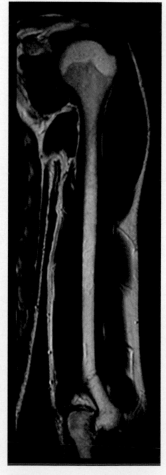

FIGURE 44–1. Sagittal scout image showing slice overlay for a coronal sequence. Note that the slice overlay is aligned parallel with the long axis of the humerus and the resulting image should display the full shaft of the humerus (see Figure 44–4).

FIGURE 44–3. Coronal scout image demonstrating the FOV, which is shown as a red perimeter box

FIGURE 44–4. Coronal oblique T2-weighted image. Note the anatomic structures such as the head of the humerus, greater tubercle, lateral condyle of the humerus.

Sagittal Oblique Sequence Acquisition

Slice Alignment

- As shown in Figures 44–5 and 44–6, slices are parallel to the shaft of the humerus.
- Slices are perpendicular to the humeral condyle.
- Resultant images should demonstrate the full shaft of the humerus (Figure 44–8).
- The superior-to-inferior field of view should extend from the acromion to the neck of the radius.
- The left-to-right field of view must include the shoulder joint and musculature of the humerus (Figure 44–7).
- The anteroposterior field of view should include the musculature of the humerus.
- A sagittal oblique image of the humerus is shown in Figure 44–8.

Phase and Frequency Orientation

- Phase: AP
- Frequency: Superior to inferior
- Phase and frequency orientations may be swapped to reduce motion artifact.

Saturation Band Placement

- A saturation band may be used to eliminate or reduce motion artifact from the thorax.
- If used, the saturation band should be placed medial to the field of view.

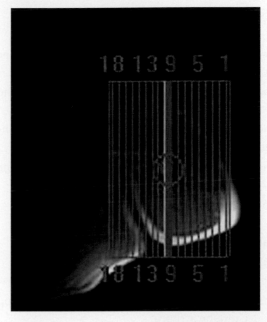

FIGURE 44–6. Axial scout image showing slice overlay for a sagittal oblique sequence.

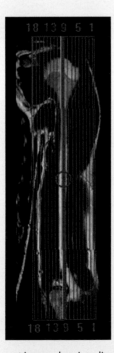

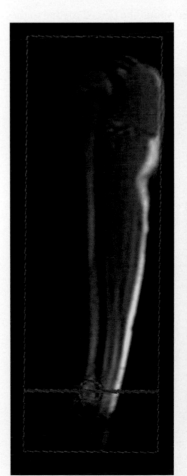

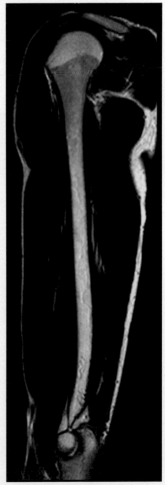

FIGURE 44–5. Coronal scout image showing slice overlay for a sagittal oblique sequence. Note that the slice overlay is aligned parallel with the long axis of the humerus and the resulting image should display the full shaft of the humerus.

FIGURE 44–7. Sagittal scout image demonstrating the FOV, which is shown as a red perimeter box.

FIGURE 44–8. Sagittal oblique T2-weighted image. Note the anatomic structures such as the head of the humerus, greater tubercle, trochlea of the humerus, and the olecranon process of the ulna.

Axial Sequence Acquisition

Slice Alignment

- As shown in Figures 44–9 and 44–10, slices are perpendicular to the shaft of the humerus.
- The superior-to-inferior field of view should extend from the acromion to the neck of the radius.
- The left-to-right field of view must include the shoulder joint and musculature of the humerus (Figure 44–11).
- The anteroposterior field of view should include the musculature of the humerus.
- An axial image of the humerus is shown in Figure 44–12.

Phase and Frequency Orientation

- Phase: AP
- Frequency: Right to left
- Phase and frequency orientations may be swapped to reduce motion artifact.

Saturation Band Placement

- A saturation band may be used to eliminate or reduce motion artifact from the thorax.
- If used, the saturation band should be placed medial to the field of view.

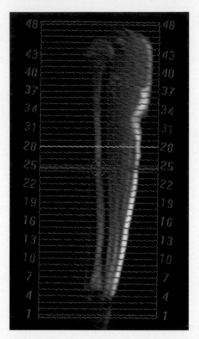

FIGURE 44–10. Sagittal scout image showing slice overlay for an axial sequence.

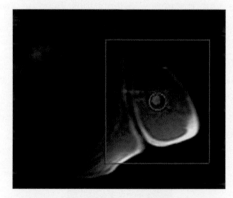

FIGURE 44–11. Axial scout image demonstrating the FOV, which is shown as a red perimeter box.

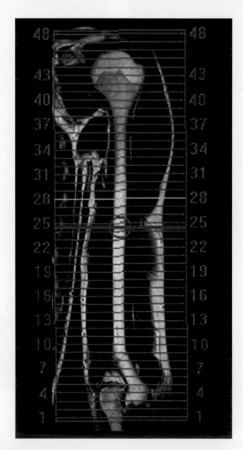

FIGURE 44–9. Coronal scout image showing slice overlay for an axial sequence.

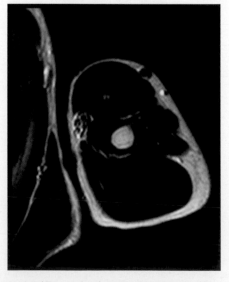

FIGURE 44–12. Axial T2-weighted image. Note that this slice is at the midshaft level.

IMAGING APPLICATION

TABLE 44–1 • General Sequences

General Sequences	TR		TE		TI		FA (degrees)		NEX		SLT/GAP (in millimeters)	
	1.5 T	3.0 T	1.5 T	3.0 T	1.5 T	3.0 T	1.5 T	3.0 T	1.5 T	3.0 T	1.5 T	3.0 T
T1 SE	500	500	15	20	N/A	N/A	90	90	3	3	3/1	3/1
T2 SE	4500	4000	70	70	N/A	N/A	90	90	3	3	3/1	3/1
PD	3000	2500	30	30	N/A	N/A	90	90	3	3	3/1	3/1
STIR	3000	4000	60	15	150	220	90	90	3	3	3/1	3/1
T1 SE post C+	500	500	15	20	N/A	N/A	90	90	3	3	3/1	3/1

Abbreviations: N/A, not applicable; PD, proton density; SE, spin echo; STIR, short tau inversion recovery.

SUGGESTED IMAGING APPLICATION VARIATIONS

Trauma

The attending radiologist and/or the requesting physician may ask for additional sequences or orthogonal planes depending on the traumatic injury.

Tumor

A tumor protocol may require sequences in addition to the routine humerus protocol and a larger field of view to include the lesion. Additional pre- and postcontrast sequences may be included. Three-orthogonal-plane postcontrast sequences may be of benefit to the radiologist. The technologist should follow the protocol provided at their facility.

Elbow

45

COIL SELECTION

- Primary coil: Extremity coil
- Secondary coil: Surface coil

PATIENT/PART POSITIONING AND CENTERING

There are 2 options for positioning the patient and part.

Option 1: Patient Supine

- The patient is positioned supine and headfirst on the MRI table or patient couch.
- Make the patient comfortable.
- Supinate the hand and extend the elbow. This will place the elbow in true anteroposterior (AP) position.
- The elbow should be placed as close to isocenter of the magnet as possible, so the patient may need to slide on the table as far as possible to the opposite side.
- Support the patient's hand and shoulder. A sandbag supporting the hand and/or forearm will help keep the elbow in true AP position and aid in patient comfort.

- Center on the humeral epicondyles.
- Instruct the patient to lie still and not move any part of their body.
- Instruct the patient to not cross their legs.

Option 2: Patient Prone

- The patient is positioned prone and headfirst on the MRI table or patient couch.
- Make the patient comfortable.
- Extend the patient's arm and supinate the hand. This will place the elbow in true AP position.
- The elbow should be placed as close to isocenter of the magnet as possible, so the patient may need to slide on the table as far as possible to the opposite side.
- Support the patient's hand and shoulder. A sandbag supporting the hand and/or forearm will help keep the elbow in true AP position and aid in patient comfort.
- Center on the humeral epicondyles.
- Instruct the patient to lie still and not move any part of their body.
- Instruct the patient to not cross their legs.

SLICE ALIGNMENT AND SCAN RANGE

Axial Sequence Acquisition

Slice Alignment

- As shown in Figures 45–1 and 45–2, slices are parallel to the elbow joint capsule.
- Slices are perpendicular to the shafts of the humerus, radius, and ulna (see Figures 45–1 and 45–2).
- Slices are parallel to a line extending from the trochlea to the capitulum (see Figure 45–1).
- The superior-to-inferior field of view should extend from the distal humerus to the radial tuberosity.
- The left-to-right field of view must include the musculature of the elbow (Figure 45–3).
- The AP field of view should include the musculature of the elbow.
- An axial image of the elbow is shown in Figure 45–4.

Phase and Frequency Orientation

- Phase: AP
- Frequency: Right to left
- Phase and frequency orientations may be swapped to reduce motion artifact.

Saturation Band Placement

- A saturation band may be used to eliminate or reduce motion artifact from the abdomen or blood flow motion artifact in the upper extremity.
- If used, the saturation band should be placed medial and/or superior and inferior to the field of view.

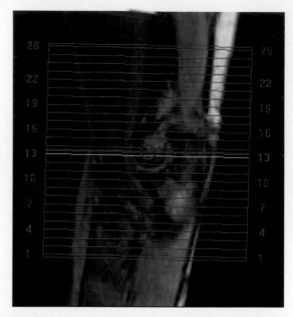

FIGURE 45–2. Sagittal scout image showing slice overlay for an axial sequence.

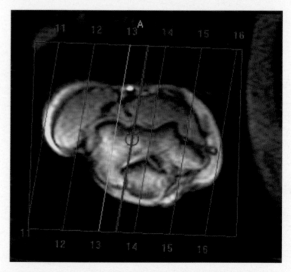

FIGURE 45–3. Axial scout image demonstrating the FOV, which is shown as a red perimeter box.

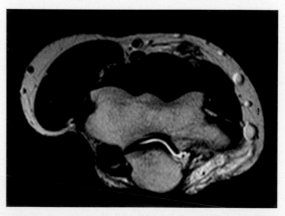

FIGURE 45–4. Axial T2-weighted image. Note the anatomic structures such as the olecranon process of the ulna, olecranon fossa of the humerus, and medial epicondyle.

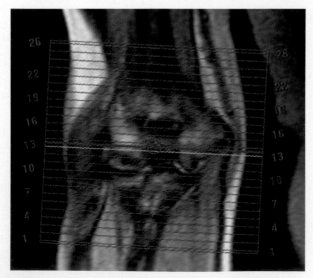

FIGURE 45–1. Coronal scout image showing slice overlay for an axial sequence.

Coronal Oblique Sequence Acquisition

Slice Alignment

- On axial scout, slices are parallel to a line extending from the anterior surface of the trochlea to the anterior surface of the capitulum (Figure 45–5).
- Slices are parallel to the shafts of the humerus, radius, and ulna (Figure 45–6).
- The superior-to-inferior field of view should extend from the distal humerus to the radial tuberosity.
- The left-to-right field of view must include the musculature of the elbow (Figure 45–7).
- The AP field of view should include the musculature of the elbow.
- A coronal oblique image of the elbow is shown in Figure 45–8.

Phase and Frequency Orientation

- Phase: Right to left
- Frequency: Superior to inferior
- Phase and frequency orientations may be swapped to reduce motion artifact.

Saturation Band Placement

- A saturation band may be used to eliminate or reduce motion artifact from the abdomen or blood flow motion artifact in the upper extremity.
- If used, the saturation band should be placed medial and/or superior and inferior to the field of view.

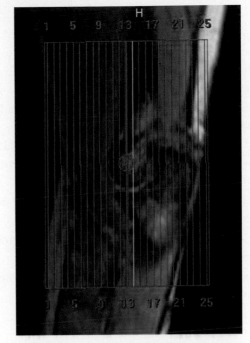

FIGURE 45–6. Sagittal scout image showing slice overlay for a coronal oblique sequence.

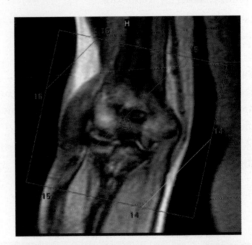

FIGURE 45–7. Coronal scout image demonstrating the FOV, which is shown as a red perimeter box.

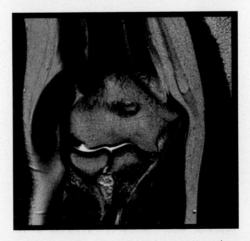

FIGURE 45–8. Coronal oblique T2-weighted image. Note the anatomic structures such as the head of the radius, ulna, trochlea, capitulum, medial condyle, and lateral condyle.

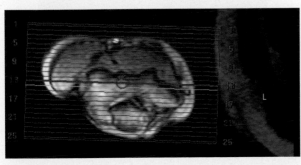

FIGURE 45–5. Axial scout image showing slice overlay for a coronal oblique sequence.

Sagittal Oblique Sequence Acquisition

Slice Alignment

- On axial scout, slices are perpendicular to a line extending from the anterior surface of the trochlea to the anterior surface of the capitulum.
- Slices are parallel to the shafts of the humerus, radius, and ulna (Figures 45–9 and 45–10).
- The superior-to-inferior field of view should extend from the distal humerus to the radial tuberosity (see Figure 45–11).
- The left-to-right field of view must include the musculature of the elbow.
- The AP field of view should include the musculature of the elbow.
- A sagittal oblique image of the elbow is shown in Figure 45–12.

Phase and Frequency Orientation

- Phase: AP
- Frequency: Superior to inferior
- Phase and frequency orientations may be swapped to reduce motion artifact.

Saturation Band Placement

- A saturation band may be used to eliminate or reduce motion artifact from the abdomen or blood flow motion artifact in the upper extremity.
- If used, the saturation band should be placed medial and/ or superior and inferior to the field of view.

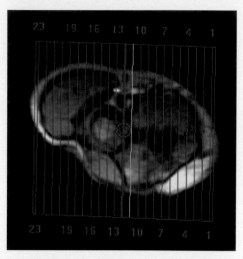

FIGURE 45–10. Axial scout image showing slice overlay for a sagittal sequence.

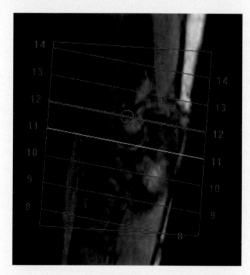

FIGURE 45–11. Sagittal scout image demonstrating the FOV, which is shown as a red perimeter box.

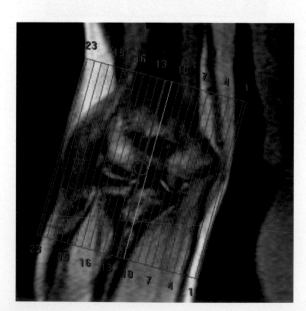

FIGURE 45–9. Coronal scout image showing slice overlay for a sagittal oblique sequence.

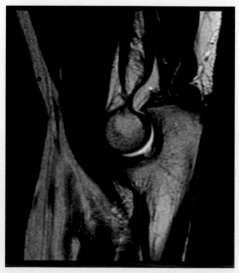

FIGURE 45–12. Midline sagittal oblique T2-weighted image. Note the anatomic structures such as the olecranon process of the ulna, trochlea of the humerus, And coronoid process.

IMAGING APPLICATION

TABLE 45–1 • General Sequences

General Sequences	TR		TE		TI		FA (degrees)		NEX		SLT/GAP (in millimeters)	
	1.5 T	3.0 T	1.5 T	3.0 T	1.5 T	3.0 T	1.5 T	3.0 T	1.5 T	3.0 T	1.5 T	3.0 T
T1 SE	500	500	15	20	N/A	N/A	90	90	3	3	3/0.3	3/0.3
T2 SE	4500	4000	70	70	N/A	N/A	90	90	3	3	3/0.3	3/0.3
PD	2500	3500	30	30	N/A	N/A	90	90	3	3	3/0.3	3/0.3
STIR	3000	4000	60	15	150	220	90	90	3	3	3/0.3	3/0.3
T1 SE post C+	500	500	15	20	N/A	N/A	90	90	3	3	3/0.3	3/0.3

Abbreviations: N/A, not applicable; PD, proton density; SE, spin echo; STIR, short tau inversion recovery.

SUGGESTED IMAGING APPLICATION VARIATIONS

Arthrogram

The injection of contrast media and/or gas in the capsular space may be requested. The requested media will be injected, usually under the guidance of fluoroscopy. The patient will then be imaged in MRI. Additional sequences to the routine protocol may be requested by the radiologist.

Trauma

The attending radiologist and/or the requesting physician may ask for additional sequences or orthogonal planes depending on the traumatic injury.

Tumor

A tumor protocol may require sequences in addition to the routine elbow protocol and a larger field of view to include the lesion. Additional pre- and postcontrast sequences may be included. Three-orthogonal-plane postcontrast sequences may be of benefit to the radiologist. The technologist should follow the protocol provided at their facility.

46

Forearm

COIL SELECTION

- Primary coil: Extremity coil
- Secondary coil: Surface coil

PATIENT/PART POSITIONING AND CENTERING

There are 2 options for positioning the patient and part.

Option 1: Patient Supine

- The patient is positioned supine and headfirst on the MRI table or patient couch.
- Make the patient comfortable.
- Supinate the hand and extend the elbow. Adjust the humeral epicondyles parallel to the MRI table. This will place the elbow in true anteroposterior (AP) position.
- The forearm should be placed as close to isocenter as possible, so the patient may need to slide on the table as far as possible to the opposite side.
- Support the patient's hand and shoulder. A sandbag supporting the hand and/or forearm will help keep the elbow in true AP position and aid in patient comfort.

- Center mid-forearm.
- Instruct the patient to lie still and not move any part of their body.
- Instruct the patient to not cross their legs.

Option 2: Patient Prone

- The patient is positioned prone and headfirst on the MRI table or patient couch.
- Make the patient comfortable.
- Extend the patient's arm and supinate the hand. This will place the elbow in true AP position.
- The forearm should be placed as close to isocenter as possible, so the patient may need to slide on the table as far as possible to the opposite side.
- Support the patient's hand and shoulder. A sandbag supporting the hand and/or forearm will help keep the elbow in true AP position and aid in patient comfort.
- Center mid-forearm.
- Instruct the patient to lie still and not move any part of their body.
- Instruct the patient to not cross their legs.

SLICE ALIGNMENT AND SCAN RANGE

Coronal Sequence Acquisition

Slice Alignment

- Slices are parallel to a line extending from the radial head to the radial styloid process (Figure 46–1).

- Slices are also parallel to the humeral condyles.

- Resultant images should demonstrate the full shafts of the ulna and radius (Figure 46–3).

- The superior-to-inferior field of view should extend from the humeral epicondyle to the metacarpals (see Figure 46–1).

- The left-to-right field of view must include the musculature of the forearm (Figure 46–2).

- The AP field of view must include the musculature of the forearm.

- A coronal image of the forearm is shown in Figure 46–1.

Phase and Frequency Orientation

- Phase: Right to left
- Frequency: Superior to inferior
- Phase and frequency orientations may be swapped to reduce motion artifact.

Saturation Band Placement

- A saturation band may be used to eliminate or reduce motion artifact from the abdomen or blood flow motion artifact in the upper extremity.

- If used, the saturation band should be placed medial and/ or superior and inferior to the field of view.

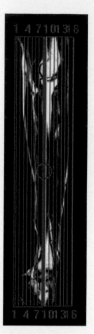

FIGURE 46–1. Sagittal scout image showing slice overlay for a coronal sequence.

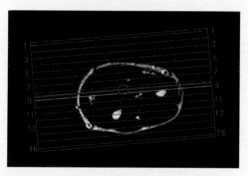

FIGURE 46–2. Axial scout image showing slice overlay for a coronal sequence. As a side note, a more proximal scout showing the humeral condyles should be used.

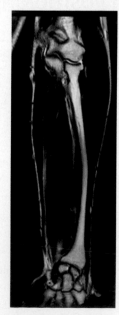

FIGURE 46–3. Coronal T2-weighted image.

Sagittal Sequence Acquisition

Slice Alignment

- Slices are parallel to a line extending from the radial notch of the ulna to the ulnar notch of the radius.
- Slices are perpendicular to the humeral condyle (Figures 46–4 and 46–5).
- Resultant images should demonstrate the full shafts of the ulna and radius (Figure 46–7).
- The superior-to-inferior field of view should extend from the humeral epicondyle to the metacarpals (see Figure 46–4).
- The left-to-right field of view must include the musculature of the forearm (see Figure 46–5).
- The AP field of view must include the musculature of the forearm (Figure 46–6).
- A sagittal image of the forearm is shown in Figure 46–7.

Phase and Frequency Orientation

- Phase: AP
- Frequency: Superior to inferior
- Phase and frequency orientations may be swapped to reduce motion artifact.

Saturation Band Placement

- A saturation band may be used to eliminate or reduce motion artifact from the abdomen or blood flow motion artifact in the upper extremity.
- If used, the saturation band should be placed medial and/ or superior and inferior to the field of view.

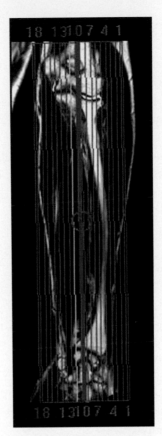

FIGURE 46–4. Coronal scout image showing slice overlay for a sagittal sequence.

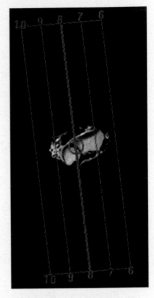

FIGURE 46–5. Axial scout image showing slice overlay for a sagittal sequence.

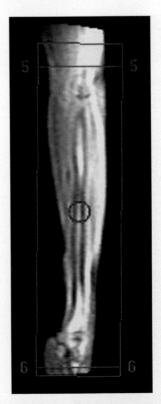

FIGURE 46–6. Sagittal scout image demonstrating the FOV, which is shown as a red perimeter box.

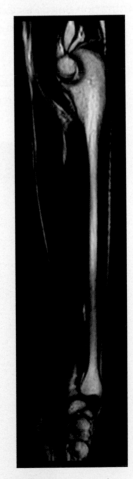

FIGURE 46–7. Sagittal T2-weighted image. Note the anatomic structures such as the ulna, olecranon process of the ulna, trochlea of the humerus, and the styloid process of the ulna.

Axial Sequence Acquisition

Slice Alignment

- As shown in Figures 46–8 and 46–9, slices are perpendicular to the shafts of the ulna and radius.
- The superior-to-inferior field of view should extend from the humeral epicondyle to the metacarpals (see Figure 46–8).
- The left-to-right field of view must include the musculature of the forearm (Figures 46–9 and 46–10).
- The AP field of view must include the musculature of the forearm.
- An axial image of the forearm is shown in Figure 46–11.

Phase and Frequency Orientation

- Phase: AP
- Frequency: Right to left
- Phase and frequency orientations may be swapped to reduce motion artifact.

Saturation Band Placement

- A saturation band may be used to eliminate or reduce motion artifact from the abdomen or blood flow motion artifact in the upper extremity.
- If used, the saturation band should be placed medial and/or superior and inferior to the field of view.

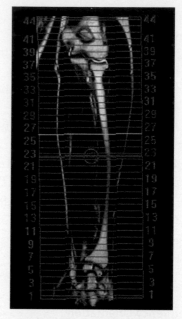

FIGURE 46–9. Coronal scout image showing slice overlay for an axial sequence.

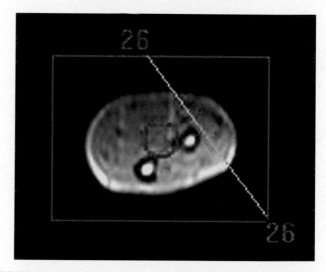

FIGURE 46–10. Axial scout image demonstrating the FOV, which is shown as a red perimeter box.

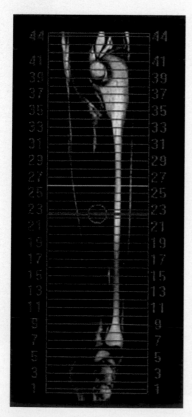

FIGURE 46–8. Sagittal scout image showing slice overlay for an axial sequence.

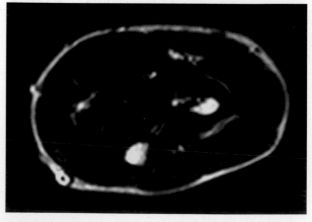

FIGURE 46–11. Axial T2-weighted image. Note that this slice is at the midshaft of the forearm showing the radius and ulna.

IMAGING APPLICATION

TABLE 46–1 • General Sequences												
General Sequences	TR		TE		TI		FA (degrees)		NEX		SLT/GAP (in millimeters)	
	1.5 T	3.0 T	1.5 T	3.0 T	1.5 T	3.0 T	1.5 T	3.0 T	1.5 T	3.0 T	1.5 T	3.0 T
T1 SE	500	500	15	20	N/A	N/A	90	90	3	3	3/0.3	3/0.3
T2 SE	4500	4000	70	70	N/A	N/A	90	90	3	3	3/0.3	3/0.3
PD	3000	2500	30	30	N/A	N/A	90	90	3	3	3/0.3	3/0.3
STIR	4000	5000	15	15	150	220	90	90	3	3	3/0.3	3/0.3
T1 SE post C+	500	500	15	20	N/A	N/A	90	90	3	3	3/0.3	3/0.3

Abbreviations: N/A, not applicable; PD, proton density; SE, spin echo; STIR, short tau inversion recovery.

SUGGESTED IMAGING APPLICATION VARIATIONS

Trauma

The attending radiologist and/or the requesting physician may ask for additional sequences or orthogonal planes depending on the traumatic injury.

Tumor

A tumor protocol may require sequences in addition to the routine forearm protocol and a larger field of view to include the lesion. Additional pre- and postcontrast sequences may be included. Three-orthogonal-plane postcontrast sequences may be of benefit to the radiologist. The technologist should follow the protocol provided at their facility.

Wrist

47

COIL SELECTION

- Primary coil: Extremity coil
- Secondary coil: Surface coil

PATIENT/PART POSITIONING AND CENTERING

There are 2 options for positioning the patient and part.

Option 1: Patient Supine

- The patient is positioned supine and headfirst on the MRI table or patient couch.
- Make the patient comfortable.
- Extend the elbow and place the palm of the hand next to the patient's hip. This will place the hand perpendicular to the MRI table.
- The wrist should be placed as close to isocenter as possible, so the patient may need to slide on the table as far as possible to the opposite side.
- Support the patient's hand and shoulder. A sandbag supporting the forearm will help keep the hand in position and aid in patient comfort.

- Center mid-carpal.
- Instruct the patient to lie still and not move any part of their body.
- Instruct the patient to not cross their legs.

Option 2: Patient Prone

- The patient is positioned prone and headfirst on the MRI table or patient couch.
- Make the patient comfortable.
- Extend the patient's arm and pronate the hand. If permissible, the hand should be perpendicular to the MRI table.
- The wrist should be placed as close to isocenter as possible, so the patient may need to slide on the table as far as possible to the opposite side.
- Support the patient's hand and shoulder. A sandbag supporting the forearm will help keep the hand in position and aid in patient comfort.
- Center mid-carpal.
- Instruct the patient to lie still and not move any part of their body.
- Instruct the patient to not cross their legs.

SLICE ALIGNMENT AND SCAN RANGE

Axial Sequence Acquisition

Slice Alignment

- As shown in Figures 47–1 and 47–2, slices are perpendicular to the shafts of the radius and ulna.
- The superior-to-inferior field of view should extend from the distal radius and ulna to the proximal metacarpals.
- The left-to-right field of view must include the musculature of the wrist.
- The anteroposterior field of view should include the musculature of the wrist.
- An axial image of the wrist is shown in Figure 47–3.

Phase and Frequency Orientation

- Phase: Anteroposterior
- Frequency: Right to left
- Phase and frequency orientations may be swapped to reduce motion artifact.

Saturation Band Placement

- A saturation band may be used to eliminate or reduce motion artifact from the abdomen or blood flow motion artifact in the upper extremity.
- If used, the saturation band should be placed medial and/or superior and inferior to the field of view.

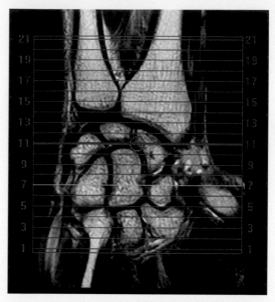

FIGURE 47–1. Coronal scout image showing slice overlay for an axial sequence.

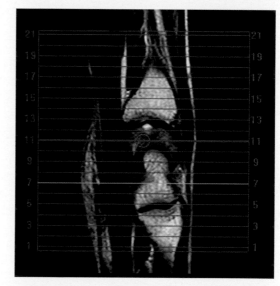

FIGURE 47–2. Sagittal scout image showing slice overlay for an axial sequence.

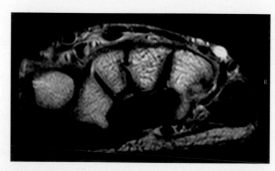

FIGURE 47–3. Axial T2-weighted image. Note the anatomic structures such as the hook of the hamate, hamate, capitate, trapezoid, tubercle of the trapezium, and trapezium. Also note the hypointense area between the hook of the hamate and tubercle of the trapezium, which is the carpal tunnel. The carpal tunnel consists of the transverse carpel ligament (flexor retinaculum), 9 tendons, and the median nerve.

Coronal Sequence Acquisition

Slice Alignment

- On the sagittal scout, slices are parallel to the shaft of the radius and ulna (Figure 47–4).
- On axial scout, slices are parallel to a line extending from the hook of the hamate to the tubercle of the trapezium (Figure 47–5).
- The superior-to-inferior field of view should extend from the distal radius and ulna to the proximal metacarpals.
- The left-to-right field of view must include the musculature of the wrist. (Figure 47–6).
- The anteroposterior field of view should include the musculature of the wrist.
- A coronal image of the wrist is shown in Figure 47–7.

Phase and Frequency Orientation

- Phase: Right to left
- Frequency: Superior to inferior
- Phase and frequency orientations may be swapped to reduce motion artifact.

Saturation Band Placement

- A saturation band may be used to eliminate or reduce motion artifact from the abdomen or blood flow motion artifact in the upper extremity.
- If used, the saturation band should be placed medial and/or superior and inferior to the field of view.

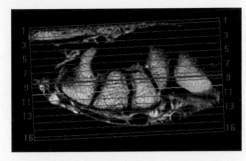

FIGURE 47–5. Axial scout image showing slice overlay for a coronal sequence.

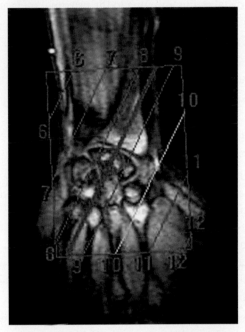

FIGURE 47–6. Coronal scout image demonstrating the FOV, which is shown as a red perimeter box.

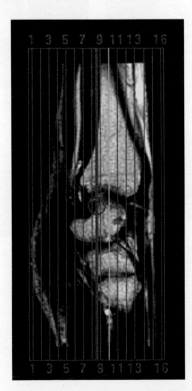

FIGURE 47–4. Sagittal scout image showing slice overlay for a coronal sequence.

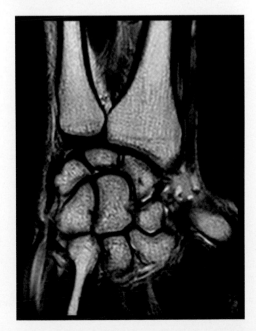

FIGURE 47–7. Coronal T2-weighted image. Note the anatomic structures such as the radius, ulna, scaphoid, lunate, triquetrum, hamate, capitate, trapezoid, trapezium, and proximal metacarpals.

Sagittal Sequence Acquisition

Slice Alignment

- On the coronal scout, slices are parallel to the shaft of the radius and ulna (Figure 47–8).
- On axial scout, slices are perpendicular to a line extending from the hook of the hamate to the tubercle of the trapezium (Figure 47–9).
- Slices are parallel to the shaft of the radius and ulna (Figure 47–8).
- The superior-to-inferior field of view should extend from the distal radius and ulna to the proximal metacarpals.
- The left-to-right field of view must include the musculature of the wrist.
- The anteroposterior field of view should include the musculature of the wrist. (Figure 47–10).
- A sagittal image of the wrist is shown in Figure 47–11.

Phase and Frequency Orientation

- Phase: Anteroposterior
- Frequency: Superior to inferior
- Phase and frequency orientations may be swapped to reduce motion artifact.

Saturation Band Placement

- A saturation band may be used to eliminate or reduce motion artifact from the abdomen or blood flow motion artifact in the upper extremity.
- If used, the saturation band should be placed medial and/or superior and inferior to the field of view.

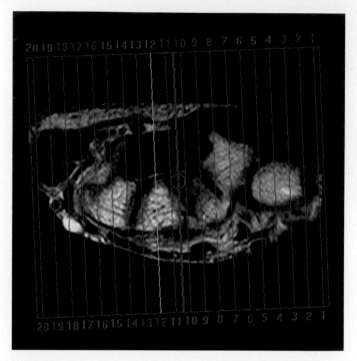

FIGURE 47–9. Axial scout image showing slice overlay for a sagittal sequence.

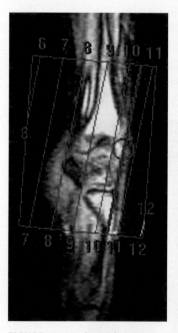

FIGURE 47–10. Sagittal scout image demonstrating the FOV, which is shown as a red perimeter box.

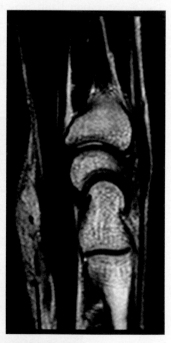

FIGURE 47–11. Sagittal T2-weighted image.

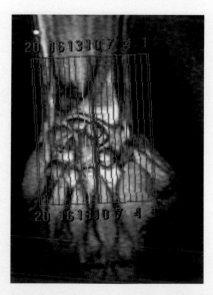

FIGURE 47–8. Coronal scout image showing slice overlay for a sagittal sequence.

IMAGING APPLICATION

TABLE 47–1 • General Sequences											
General Sequences	**TR**		**TE**		**TI**		**FA (degrees)**		**NEX**		**SLT/GAP (in millimeters)**	
	1.5 T	3.0 T	1.5 T	3.0 T	1.5 T	3.0 T	1.5 T	3.0 T	1.5 T	3.0 T	1.5 T	3.0 T
T1 SE	500	500	15	20	N/A	N/A	90	90	3	3	3/0.3	3/0.3
T2 SE	4500	4000	70	70	N/A	N/A	90	90	3	3	3/0.3	3/0.3
PD	2500	3500	30	30	N/A	N/A	90	90	3	3	3/0.3	3/0.3
STIR	3000	4000	60	15	150	220	90	90	3	3	3/0.3	3/0.3
T1 SE post C+	500	500	15	20	N/A	N/A	90	90	3	3	3/0.3	3/0.3

Abbreviations: N/A, not applicable; PD, proton density; SE, spin echo; STIR, short tau inversion recovery.

SUGGESTED IMAGING APPLICATION VARIATIONS

Arthrogram

The injection of contrast media and/or gas in the capsular space may be requested. The requested media will be injected, usually under the guidance of fluoroscopy. The patient will then be imaged in MRI. Additional sequences to the routine protocol may be requested by the radiologist.

Trauma

The attending radiologist and/or the requesting physician may ask for additional sequences or orthogonal planes depending on the traumatic injury.

Tumor

A tumor protocol may require sequences in addition to the routine wrist protocol and a larger field of view to include the lesion. Additional pre- and postcontrast sequences may be included. Three-orthogonal-plane postcontrast sequences may be of benefit to the radiologist. The technologist should follow the protocol provided at their facility.

48

Hand

COIL SELECTION

- Primary coil: Extremity coil
- Secondary coil: Surface coil

PATIENT/PART POSITIONING AND CENTERING

There are 2 options for positioning the patient and part.

Option 1: Patient Supine

- The patient is positioned supine and headfirst on the MRI table or patient couch.
- Make the patient comfortable.
- Extend the elbow and place the palm of the hand next to the patient's hip. This will place the hand perpendicular to the MRI table.
- The fingers should be extended, straight, close together, and immobilized.
- The hand should be placed as close to isocenter as possible, so the patient may need to slide on the table as far as possible to the opposite side.
- Support the patient's hand and shoulder. A sandbag supporting the forearm will help keep the hand in position and aid in patient comfort.

- Center on the metacarpophalangeal (MCP) joints.
- Instruct the patient to lie still and not move any part of their body.
- Instruct the patient to not cross their legs.

Option 2: Patient Prone

- The patient is positioned prone and headfirst on the MRI table or patient couch.
- Make the patient comfortable.
- Extend the patient's arm and pronate the hand. If permissible, the hand should be perpendicular to the MRI table.
- The fingers should be extended, straight, close together, and immobilized.
- The hand should be placed as close to isocenter as possible, so the patient may need to slide on the table as far as possible to the opposite side.
- Support the patient's hand and shoulder. A sandbag supporting the forearm will help keep the hand in position and aid in patient comfort.
- Center on the MCP joints.
- Instruct the patient to lie still and not move any part of their body.
- Instruct the patient to not cross their legs.

SLICE ALIGNMENT AND SCAN RANGE

Axial Sequence Acquisition

Slice Alignment

- As shown in Figures 48–1 and 48–2, slices are perpendicular to the shafts of the radius and ulna.
- Slices are also perpendicular to the long axis of the hand.
- The superior-to-inferior field of view should extend from the distal radius and ulna through the distal phalanges (see Figure 48–1).
- The left-to-right field of view must include the digits (see Figure 48–3).
- The anteroposterior field of view should include the musculature of the hand.
- An axial image of the hand is shown in Figure 48–4.

Phase and Frequency Orientation

- Phase: Anteroposterior
- Frequency: Right to left
- Phase and frequency orientations may be swapped to reduce motion artifact.

Saturation Band Placement

- A saturation band may be used to eliminate or reduce motion artifact from the abdomen or blood flow motion artifact in the upper extremity.
- If used, the saturation band should be placed medial and/or inferior to the field of view.

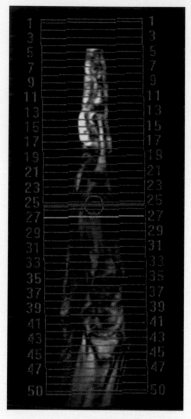

FIGURE 48–2. Sagittal scout image showing slice overlay for an axial sequence.

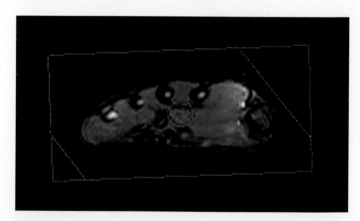

FIGURE 48–3. Axial scout image demonstrating the FOV, which is shown as a red perimeter box.

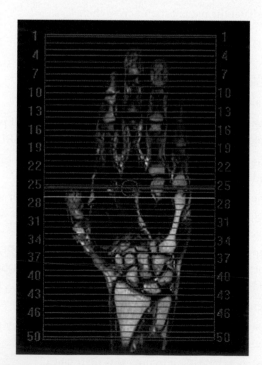

FIGURE 48–1. Coronal scout image showing slice overlay for an axial sequence.

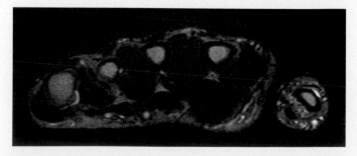

FIGURE 48–4. Axial T2-weighted image.

Coronal Sequence Acquisition

Slice Alignment

- On the sagittal scout, slices are parallel to the long axis of the hand and also the shafts of the radius and ulna (Figure 48–5).
- On axial scout, slices are parallel to a line extending from the first metacarpal to the fifth metacarpal (see Figure 48–6).
- The superior-to-inferior field of view should extend from the distal radius and ulna through the distal phalanges (Figure 48–7).
- The left-to-right field of view must include the digits.
- The anteroposterior field of view should include the musculature of the hand.
- A coronal image of the hand is shown in Figure 48–8.

Phase and Frequency Orientation

- Phase: Right to left
- Frequency: Superior to inferior
- Phase and frequency orientations may be swapped to reduce motion artifact.

Saturation Band Placement

- A saturation band may be used to eliminate or reduce motion artifact from the abdomen or blood flow motion artifact in the upper extremity.
- If used, the saturation band should be placed medial and/or inferior to the field of view.

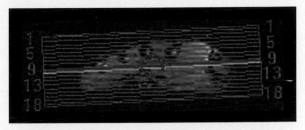

FIGURE 48–6. Axial scout image showing slice overlay for a coronal sequence.

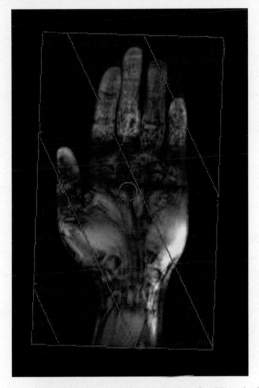

FIGURE 48–7. Coronal scout image demonstrating the FOV, which is shown as a red perimeter box.

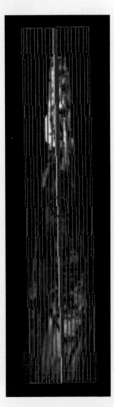

FIGURE 48–5. Sagittal scout image showing slice overlay for a coronal sequence.

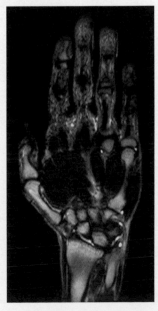

FIGURE 48–8. Coronal T2-weighted image. Note that the fingers are fully extended and are tight together (ie, not spread out).

Sagittal Sequence Acquisition

Slice Alignment

- On the coronal scout, slices are parallel to the long axis of the hand and also the shafts of the radius and ulna (Figure 48–9).
- On axial scout, slices are perpendicular to a line extending from the first metacarpal to the fifth metacarpal (see Figure 48–10).
- The superior-to-inferior field of view should extend from the distal radius and ulna through the distal phalanges (see Figures 48–9 and 48–11).
- The left-to-right field of view must include the digits.
- The anteroposterior field of view should include the musculature of the hand.
- A sagittal image of the hand is shown in Figure 48–12.

Phase and Frequency Orientation

- Phase: Anteroposterior
- Frequency: Superior to inferior
- Phase and frequency orientations may be swapped to reduce motion artifact.

Saturation Band Placement

- A saturation band may be used to eliminate or reduce motion artifact from the abdomen or blood flow motion artifact in the upper extremity.
- If used, the saturation band should be placed medial and/ or inferior to the field of view.

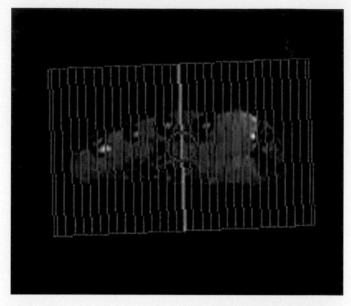

FIGURE 48–10. Axial scout image showing slice overlay for a sagittal sequence.

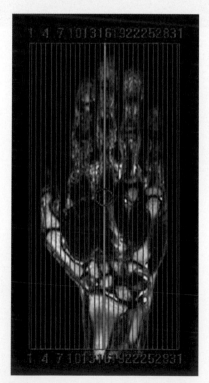

FIGURE 48–9. Coronal scout image showing slice overlay for a sagittal sequence.

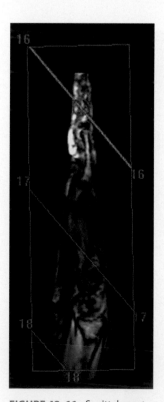

FIGURE 48–11. Sagittal scout image demonstrating the FOV, which is shown as a red perimeter box.

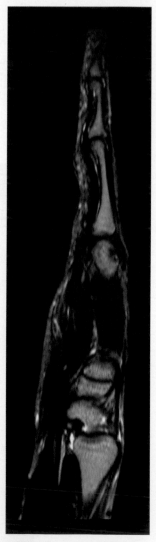

FIGURE 48–12. Sagittal T2-weighted image. Note that the fingers are fully extended.

IMAGING APPLICATION

TABLE 48–1 • General Sequences

General Sequences	TR		TE		TI		FA (degrees)		NEX		SLT/GAP (in millimeters)	
	1.5 T	3.0 T	1.5 T	3.0 T	1.5 T	3.0 T	1.5 T	3.0 T	1.5 T	3.0 T	1.5 T	3.0 T
T1 SE	500	500	15	20	N/A	N/A	90	90	3	3	3/0.3	3/0.3
T2 SE	4500	4000	70	70	N/A	N/A	90	90	3	3	3/0.3	3/0.3
PD	2500	3500	30	30	N/A	N/A	90	90	3	3	3/0.3	3/0.3
STIR	3000	4000	60	15	150	220	90	90	3	3	3/0.3	3/0.3
T1 SE post C+	500	500	15	20	N/A	N/A	90	90	3	3	3/0.3	3/0.3

Abbreviations: N/A, not applicable; PD, proton density; SE, spin echo; STIR, short tau inversion recovery.

SUGGESTED IMAGING APPLICATION VARIATIONS

Arthrogram

The injection of contrast media and/or gas in the capsular space may be requested. The requested media will be injected, usually under the guidance of fluoroscopy. The patient will then be imaged in MRI. Additional sequences to the routine protocol may be requested by the radiologist.

Trauma

The attending radiologist and/or the requesting physician may ask for additional sequences or orthogonal planes depending on the traumatic injury.

Tumor

A tumor protocol may require sequences in addition to the routine hand protocol and a larger field of view to include the lesion. Additional pre- and postcontrast sequences may be included. Three-orthogonal-plane postcontrast sequences may be of benefit to the radiologist. The technologist should follow the protocol provided at their facility.

49

Thumb

COIL SELECTION

- Primary coil: Extremity coil
- Secondary coil: Surface coil

PATIENT/PART POSITIONING AND CENTERING

There are 2 options for positioning the patient and part.

Option 1: Patient Supine

- The patient is positioned supine and headfirst on the MRI table or patient couch.
- Make the patient comfortable.
- First, extend the elbow and place the hand next to the patient's hip. Next, close the second, third, fourth, and fifth digits, creating a fist. Finally, lay the thumb on the medial side of the second digit. This position will be similar to giving a closed "thumbs up."
- The thumb should be placed as close to isocenter as possible, so the patient may need to slide on the table as far as possible to the opposite side.
- Support the patient's hand and shoulder. A sandbag supporting the forearm will help keep the hand in position and aid in patient comfort.
- Center on the metacarpophalangeal (MCP) joint.

- Instruct the patient to lie still and not move any part of their body.
- Instruct the patient to not cross their legs.

Option 2: Patient Prone

- The patient is positioned prone and headfirst on the MRI table or patient couch.
- Make the patient comfortable.
- Extend the patient's arm and pronate the hand. First, extend the elbow and place the hand next to the patient's hip. Next, close the second, third, fourth, and fifth digits, creating a fist. Finally, lay the thumb on the medial side of the second digit. This position will be similar to giving a closed "thumbs up." If permissible, the wrist should be perpendicular to the MRI table.
- The thumb should be placed as close to isocenter as possible, so the patient may need to slide on the table as far as possible to the opposite side.
- Support the patient's hand and shoulder. A sandbag supporting the forearm will help keep the hand in position and aid in patient comfort.
- Center on the MCP joint.
- Instruct the patient to lie still and not move any part of their body.
- Instruct the patient to not cross their legs.

SLICE ALIGNMENT AND SCAN RANGE

Note that the slice alignment and scan range described here demonstrate how to acquire a thumb exam, but the concepts may be applied to the other digits.

Axial Sequence Acquisition

Slice Alignment

- As shown in Figures 49–1 and 49–2, slices are perpendicular to the shafts of the first metacarpal, proximal phalanx, and distal phalanx.
- The superior-to-inferior field of view should extend from the distal phalanx through the trapezium.
- The left-to-right field of view must include the first digit.
- The anteroposterior field of view should include the first digit.
- An axial image of the thumb is shown in Figure 49–3.

Phase and Frequency Orientation

- Phase: Anteroposterior
- Frequency: Right to left
- Phase and frequency orientations may be swapped to reduce motion artifact.

Saturation Band Placement

- A saturation band may be used to eliminate or reduce motion artifact from the abdomen or blood flow motion artifact in the upper extremity.
- If used, the saturation band should be placed medial and/or inferior to the field of view.

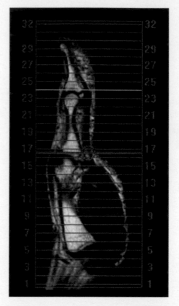

FIGURE 49–1. Sagittal scout image showing slice overlay for an axial sequence.

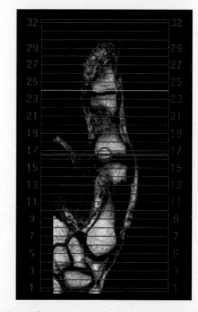

FIGURE 49–2. Coronal scout image showing slice overlay for an axial sequence.

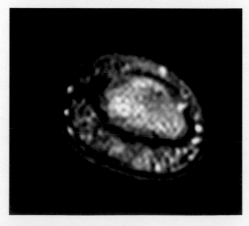

FIGURE 49–3. Axial T2-weighted image.

Coronal Sequence Acquisition

Slice Alignment

- On sagittal scout, slices are parallel to the shafts of the first metacarpal, proximal phalanx, and distal phalanx (Figure 49-4).
- On axial scout, slices are parallel to a line extending from the left side of the first metacarpal to the right side of the first metacarpal (Figure 49-5).
- The superior-to-inferior field of view should extend from the distal phalanx through the trapezium.
- The left-to-right field of view must include the first digit (Figure 49-6).
- The anteroposterior field of view should include the first digit.
- A coronal image of the thumb is shown in Figure 49-7).

Phase and Frequency Orientation

- Phase: Right to left
- Frequency: Superior to inferior
- Phase and frequency orientations may be swapped to reduce motion artifact.

Saturation Band Placement

- A saturation band may be used to eliminate or reduce motion artifact from the abdomen or blood flow motion artifact in the upper extremity.
- If used, the saturation band should be placed medial and/or inferior to the field of view.

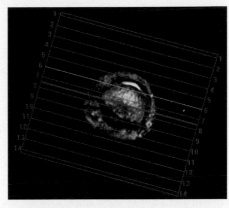

FIGURE 49-5. Axial scout image showing slice overlay for a coronal sequence.

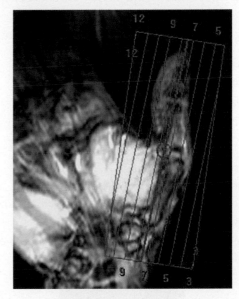

FIGURE 49-6. Coronal scout image demonstrating the FOV, which is shown as a red perimeter box.

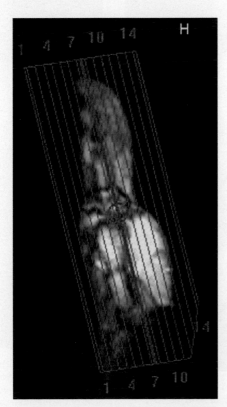

FIGURE 49-4. Sagittal scout image showing slice overlay for a coronal sequence.

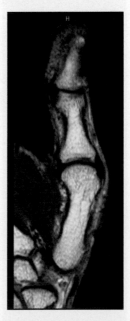

FIGURE 49-7. Coronal T2-weighted image. Note the anatomic structures such as the head of the first metacarpal, proximal phalanx of the thumb, and distal phalanx of the thumb.

Sagittal Sequence Acquisition

Slice Alignment

- On coronal scout, slices are parallel to the shafts of the first metacarpal, proximal phalanx, and distal phalanx (Figure 49–8).
- On axial scout, slices are perpendicular to a line extending from the left side of the first metacarpal to the right side of the first metacarpal (Figure 49–9).
- The superior-to-inferior field of view should extend from the distal phalanx through the trapezium (see Figure 49–10).
- The left-to-right field of view must include the first digit (Figure 49–10).
- The anteroposterior field of view should include the first digit.
- A sagittal image of the thumb is shown in Figure 49–11.

Phase and Frequency Orientation

- Phase: Anteroposterior
- Frequency: Superior to inferior
- Phase and frequency orientations may be swapped to reduce motion artifact.

Saturation Band Placement

- A saturation band may be used to eliminate or reduce motion artifact from the abdomen or blood flow motion artifact in the upper extremity.
- If used, the saturation band should be placed medial and/or inferior to the field of view.

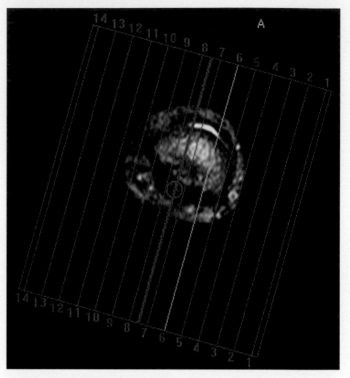

FIGURE 49–9. Axial scout image showing slice overlay for a sagittal sequence.

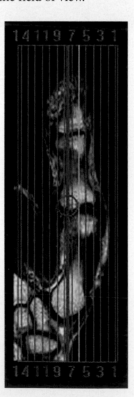

FIGURE 49–8. Coronal scout image showing slice overlay for a sagittal sequence.

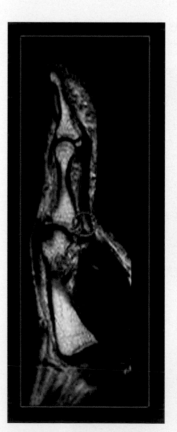

FIGURE 49–10. Sagittal scout image demonstrating the FOV, which is shown as a red perimeter box.

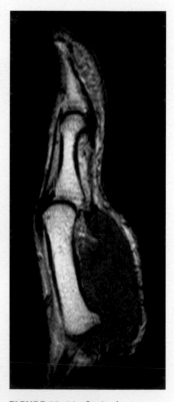

FIGURE 49–11. Sagittal T2-weighted image. Note the anatomic structures such as the head of the first metacarpal, proximal phalanx of the thumb, and distal phalanx of the thumb.

IMAGING APPLICATION

TABLE 49–1 • General Sequences												
General Sequences	TR		TE		TI		FA (degrees)		NEX		SLT/GAP (in millimeters)	
	1.5 T	3.0 T	1.5 T	3.0 T	1.5 T	3.0 T	1.5 T	3.0 T	1.5 T	3.0 T	1.5 T	3.0 T
T1 SE	500	500	15	20	N/A	N/A	90	90	3	3	3/0.3	3/0.3
T2 SE	4500	4000	70	70	N/A	N/A	90	90	3	3	3/0.3	3/0.3
PD	2500	3500	30	30	N/A	N/A	90	90	3	3	3/0.3	3/0.3
STIR	3000	4000	60	15	150	220	90	90	3	3	3/0.3	3/0.3
T1 SE post C+	500	500	15	20	N/A	N/A	90	90	3	3	3/0.3	3/0.3

Abbreviations: N/A, not applicable; PD, proton density; SE, spin echo; STIR, short tau inversion recovery.

SUGGESTED IMAGING APPLICATION VARIATIONS

Arthrogram

The injection of contrast media and/or gas in the capsular space may be requested. The requested media will be injected, usually under the guidance of fluoroscopy. The patient will then be scanned in MRI. Additional sequences to the routine protocol may be requested by the radiologist.

Trauma

The attending radiologist and/or the requesting physician may ask for additional sequences or orthogonal planes depending on the traumatic injury.

Tumor

A tumor protocol may require sequences in addition to the routine thumb protocol and a larger field of view to include the lesion. Additional pre- and postcontrast sequences may be included. Three-orthogonal-plane postcontrast sequences may be of benefit to the radiologist. The technologist should follow the protocol provided at their facility.

Upper Extremity Arthrogram

50

Injection of contrast media into the capsular space (direct method) may be requested. The requested media will be injected, usually under the guidance of fluoroscopy. The patient will then be imaged in MRI. Additional sequences to the routine protocol may be requested by the radiologist. As the arthrogram may be performed on a variety of joints, use the guidelines for the specific joint of interest.

This is an example of a shoulder arthrogram (Figures 50–1 to 50–4).

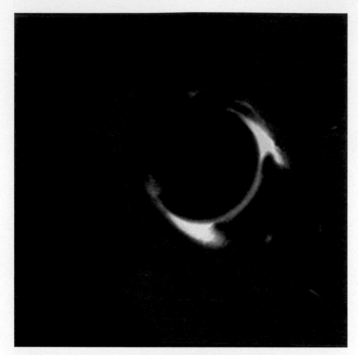

FIGURE 50–1. Axial image of a shoulder arthrogram. Note the hyperintense contrast injected into the joint space.

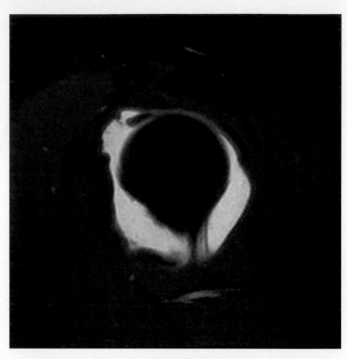

FIGURE 50–3. Sagittal image of a shoulder arthrogram. Note the hyperintense contrast injected into the joint space.

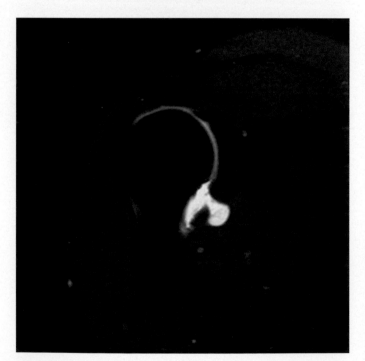

FIGURE 50–2. Coronal image of a shoulder arthrogram. Note the hyperintense contrast injected into the joint space.

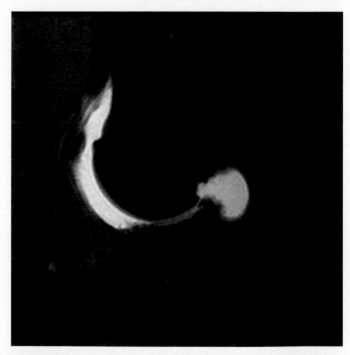

FIGURE 50–4. Image of a shoulder arthrogram in the ABER (abducted and externally rotated) position. A true ABER position requires a 90-degree abduction and 90-degree flexion of the arm; however, this may be very difficult to position in a closed-bore magnet. The patient may need to abduct the arm greater than 90 degrees to fit into the bore of the magnet. This may be accomplished by having the patient place their hand on top of their head and position the coil over/around the shoulder. Sandbags and pads may be required to assist the patient in holding this position.

51

Musculoskeletal Pelvis

COIL SELECTION

- Primary coil: Body coil
- Secondary coil: Surface coil

PATIENT/PART POSITIONING AND CENTERING

- The patient is positioned supine and either headfirst or feetfirst on the MRI table or patient couch.
- Make the patient comfortable.

- The legs should be extended with the feet medially rotated 15 to 20 degrees. The feet should be secured in this position with tape and/or sandbags.
- The pelvis should not be rotated.
- Center approximately 2 inches inferior of the anterior superior iliac spine (ASIS) so that the pelvis is at isocenter.
- Instruct the patient to lie still and not move any part of their body.
- Instruct the patient to not cross their arms and legs.

SLICE ALIGNMENT AND SCAN RANGE

Coronal Sequence Acquisition

Slice Alignment

- On the axial scout, slices are parallel to a line extending from the left ASIS to the right ASIS (Figure 51–1).
- Slices are parallel to the long axis of the body and pelvis (Figure 51–2).
- The superior-to-inferior field of view should extend from superior to the iliac crest to inferior to the ramus of ischium (Figure 51–3).
- The left-to-right field of view should extend from the lateral musculature of the left greater trochanter to the lateral musculature of the right greater trochanter (see Figure 51–3).
- The anteroposterior field of view should extend from abdominal body fat to posterior body fat.
- A coronal image of the pelvis is shown in Figure 51–4.

Phase and Frequency Orientation

- Phase: Superior to inferior
- Frequency: Right to left
- Phase and frequency orientations may be swapped to reduce motion artifact.

Saturation Band Placement

- A saturation band may be used to eliminate or reduce motion artifact.
- If used, the saturation band should be placed superior to the field of view.

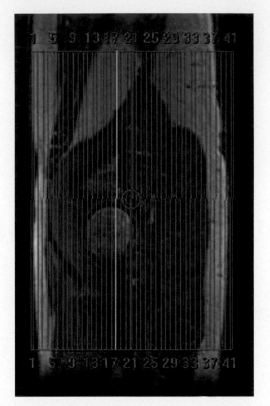

FIGURE 51–2. Sagittal scout image showing slice overlay for a coronal sequence.

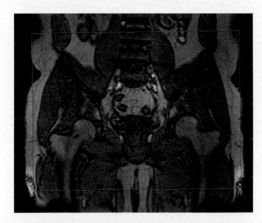

FIGURE 51–3. Coronal scout image demonstrating the FOV, which is shown as a red perimeter box.

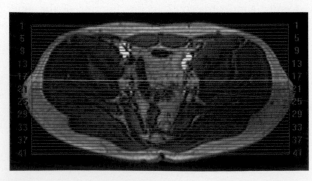

FIGURE 51–1. Axial scout image showing slice overlay for a coronal sequence.

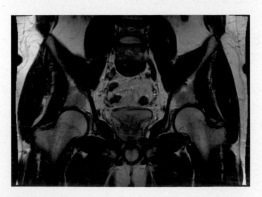

FIGURE 51–4. Coronal T2-weighted image. Note the anatomic structures such as the femoral head, femoral neck, acetabulum, and ilium.

Sagittal Sequence Acquisition

Slice Alignment

- On the coronal scout, slices are perpendicular to a line extending from the left ASIS to the right ASIS (see Figure 51–5).

- As shown in Figure 51–5, slices are perpendicular to the long axis of the body.

- The superior-to-inferior field of view should extend from superior to the iliac crest to inferior to the ramus of ischium (see Figure 51–5).

- The left-to-right field of view should extend from the lateral musculature of the left greater trochanter to the lateral musculature of the right greater trochanter (Figures 51–5 and 51–6).

- The anteroposterior field of view should extend from abdominal body fat to posterior body fat (see Figure 51–6).

- A sagittal image of the pelvis is shown in Figure 51–7.

Phase and Frequency Orientation

- Phase: Superior to inferior
- Frequency: Anteroposterior
- Phase and frequency orientations may be swapped to reduce motion artifact.

Saturation Band Placement

- A saturation band may be used to eliminate or reduce motion artifact.

- If used, the saturation band should be placed superior to the field of view.

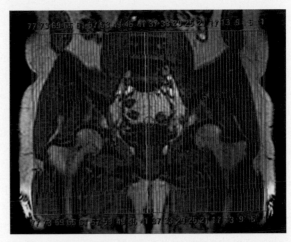

FIGURE 51–5. Coronal scout image showing slice overlay for a sagittal sequence.

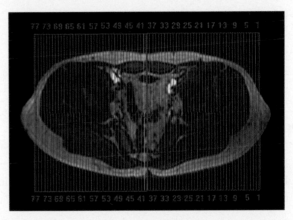

FIGURE 51–6. Axial scout image showing slice overlay for a sagittal sequence.

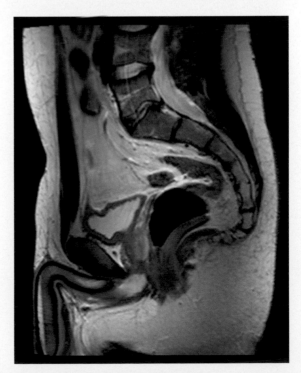

FIGURE 51–7. Midline sagittal T2-weighted image.

Axial Sequence Acquisition

Slice Alignment

- On the coronal scout, slices are parallel to a line extending from the left ASIS to the right ASIS (see Figure 51–8).
- As shown in Figures 51–8 and 51–9, slices are perpendicular to the long axis of the body.
- The superior-to-inferior field of view should extend from the ASIS to inferior to the lesser trochanter (see Figure 51–8).
- The left-to-right field of view should extend from the pubis through the musculature around the greater trochanter.
- The anteroposterior field of view should include the musculature of the hip.
- An axial image of the pelvis is shown in Figure 51–10.

Phase and Frequency Orientation

- Phase: Anteroposterior
- Frequency: Right to left
- Phase and frequency orientations may be swapped to reduce motion artifact.

Saturation Band Placement

- A saturation band may be used to eliminate or reduce motion artifact.
- If used, the saturation band should be placed superior to the field of view.

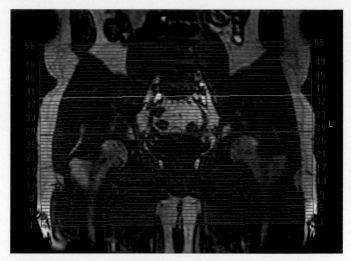

FIGURE 51–8. Coronal scout image showing slice overlay for an axial sequence.

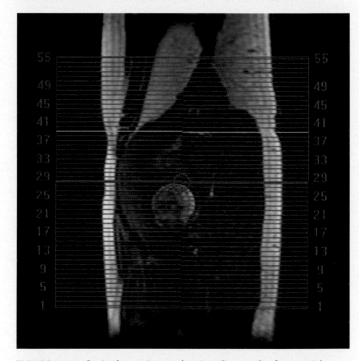

FIGURE 51–9. Sagittal scout image showing slice overlay for an axial sequence.

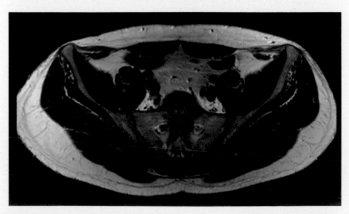

FIGURE 51–10. Axial T2-weighted image. Note the anatomic structures such as the sacrum, sacroiliac joints, and ilium.

IMAGING APPLICATION

	TABLE 51–1 • General Sequences												

General Sequences	TR		TE		TI		FA (degrees)		NEX		SLT/GAP (in millimeters)	
	1.5 T	3.0 T	1.5 T	3.0 T	1.5 T	3.0 T	1.5 T	3.0 T	1.5 T	3.0 T	1.5 T	3.0 T
T1 SE	500	500	15	20	N/A	N/A	90	90	3	3	3/0.3	3/0.3
T2 SE	4500	4000	70	70	N/A	N/A	90	90	3	3	3/0.3	3/0.3
PD	5000	6500	30	30	N/A	N/A	90	90	3	3	3/0.3	3/0.3
STIR	3000	6000	60	60	150	200	90	90	3	3	3/0.3	3/0.3
T1 SE post C+	500	500	15	20	N/A	N/A	90	90	3	3	3/0.3	3/0.3

Abbreviations: N/A, not applicable; PD, proton density; SE, spin echo; STIR, short tau inversion recovery.

SUGGESTED IMAGING APPLICATION VARIATIONS

Arthrogram

The injection of contrast media and/or gas in the capsular space may be requested. The requested media will be injected, usually under the guidance of fluoroscopy. The patient will then be scanned in MRI. Additional sequences to the routine protocol may be requested by the radiologist.

Trauma

The attending radiologist and/or the requesting physician may ask for additional sequences or orthogonal planes depending on the traumatic injury.

Tumor

A tumor protocol may require sequences in addition to the routine pelvis protocol and a larger field of view to include the lesion. Additional pre- and postcontrast sequences may be included. Three-orthogonal-plane postcontrast sequences may be of benefit to the radiologist. The technologist should follow the protocol provided at their facility.

Sacroiliac Joints (SI Joints)

COIL SELECTION

- Primary coil: Body coil
- Secondary coil: Surface coil

PATIENT/PART POSITIONING AND CENTERING

- The patient is positioned supine and either headfirst or feetfirst on the MRI table or patient couch.

- Make the patient comfortable.
- Support the patient's feet and lower legs.
- The pelvis should not be rotated.
- Center approximately 2 inches inferior of the anterior superior iliac spine so that the pelvis is at isocenter.
- Instruct the patient to lie still and not move any part of their body.
- Instruct the patient to not cross their arms and legs.

SLICE ALIGNMENT AND SCAN RANGE

Axial Sequence Acquisition

Slice Alignment

- As shown in Figures 52–1 and 52–2, slices are perpendicular to the body of the sacrum.
- The superior-to-inferior field of view should extend from the level of the fifth lumbar vertebrae (L5) through the coccyx (see Figure 52–1).
- The left-to-right field of view should extend from the left ilium to the right ilium (see Figure 52–2).
- The anteroposterior field of view should extend from the sacral promontory to the muscle posterior of the sacral crest.
- An axial image of the SI Joints is shown in Figure 52–3.

Phase and Frequency Orientation

- Phase: Right to left
- Frequency: Superior to inferior
- Phase and frequency orientations may be swapped to reduce motion artifact.

Saturation Band Placement

- A saturation band may be used to eliminate or reduce motion artifact from the abdomen.
- If used, the saturation band should be placed anterior to the field of view (see Figure 52–1).

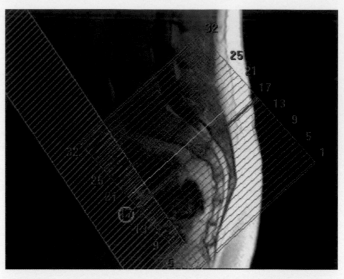

FIGURE 52–1. Midline sagittal scout image showing islice overlay (red box) for an axial sequence. Note that the saturation band (*blue box*) may be placed anterior of the sacrum to reduce motion and flow artifacts.

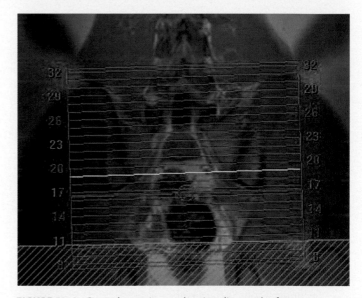

FIGURE 52–2. Coronal scout image showing slice overlay for an axial sequence. The slice overlay is slightly tilted so that the slices are perpendicular to the SI Joints.

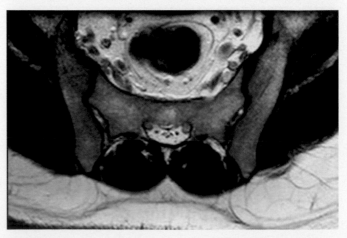

FIGURE 52–3. Axial T2-weighted image. Note the anatomic structures such as the sacral alum, sacroiliac joints, and ilium.

Coronal Sequence Acquisition

Slice Alignment

- As shown in Figure 52–4, slices are parallel to the body of the sacrum.
- The superior-to-inferior field of view should extend from the level of L5 through the coccyx.
- The left-to-right field of view should extend from the left ilium to the right ilium (Figure 52–5).
- The anteroposterior field of view should extend from the sacral promontory to the muscle posterior of the sacral crest.
- A coronal image of the SI Joints is shown in Figure 52–6.

Phase and Frequency Orientation

- Phase: Right to left
- Frequency: Superior to inferior
- Phase and frequency orientations may be swapped to reduce motion artifact.

Saturation Band Placement

- A saturation band may be used to eliminate or reduce motion artifact from the abdomen.
- If used, the saturation band should be placed anterior to the field of view (see Figure 52–4).

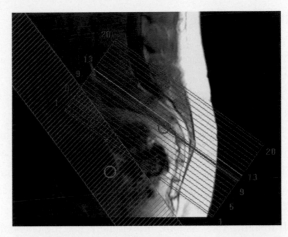

FIGURE 52–4. Sagittal scout image showing slice overlay for a coronal sequence. Note that the saturation band overlay (the *blue band*) is anterior of the sacrum so that motion artifact will be reduced.

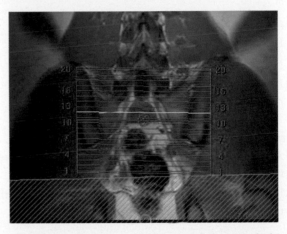

FIGURE 52–5. Coronal scout image demonstrating the FOV, which is shown as a red perimeter box.

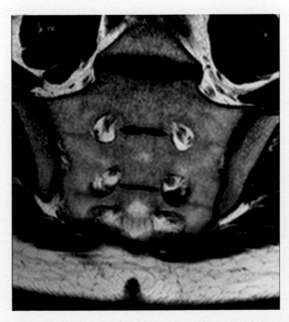

FIGURE 52–6. Coronal T2-weighted image. Note the anatomic structures such as the sacral foramina (showing CSF as hyperintense and nerve roots as hypointense), sacroiliac joints, and transverse ridges.

Sagittal Sequence Acquisition

Slice Alignment

- As shown in Figure 52–7, slices are parallel to the body of the sacrum.
- The superior-to-inferior field of view should extend from the level of L5 through the coccyx (Figure 52–9).
- The left-to-right field of view should extend from the left ilium to the right ilium (see Figures 52–7 and 52–8).
- The anteroposterior field of view should extend from the sacral promontory to the muscle posterior of the sacral crest.
- If imaging each SI joint individually, use the coronal and axial scout images to align parallel with the joint space.
- A midline sagittal image of the sacrum is shown in Figure 52–10.

Phase and Frequency Orientation

- Phase: Anteroposterior
- Frequency: Superior to inferior
- Phase and frequency orientations may be swapped to reduce motion artifact.

Saturation Band Placement

- A saturation band may be used to eliminate or reduce motion artifact from the abdomen.
- If used, the saturation band should be placed anterior to the field of view (see Figure 52–9).

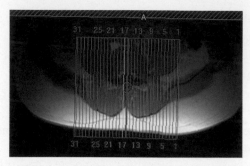

FIGURE 52–8. Axial scout image showing slice overlay for a sagittal sequence.

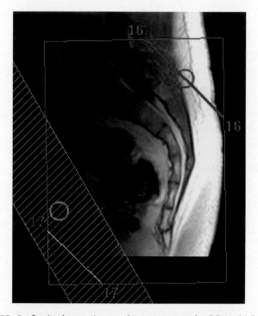

FIGURE 52–9. Sagittal scout image demonstrating the FOV, which is shown as a red perimeter box. Note that the saturation band overlay (the *blue band*) is anterior of the sacrum so that motion artifact will be reduced.

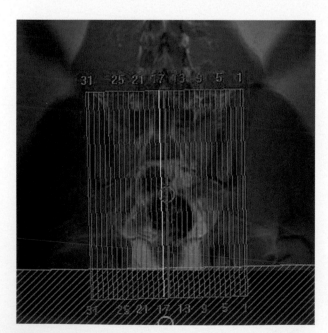

FIGURE 52–7. Coronal scout image showing slice overlay for a sagittal sequence. The slice overlay is slightly tilted so that the slices are parallel to the spinous processes and midsacrum.

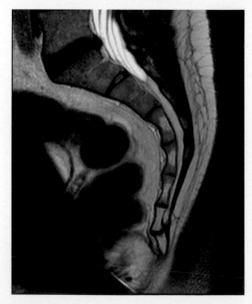

FIGURE 52–10. Sagittal T2-weighted image. Notice the area where the saturation band was placed is dark and motion artifact is greatly reduced. Note, if imaging each SI joint individually, use the coronal and axial scout images to align parallel with the joint space.

IMAGING APPLICATION

TABLE 52–1 • General Sequences

General Sequences	TR		TE		TI		FA (degrees)		NEX		SLT/GAP (in millimeters)	
	1.5 T	3.0 T	1.5 T	3.0 T	1.5 T	3.0 T	1.5 T	3.0 T	1.5 T	3.0 T	1.5 T	3.0 T
T1 SE	500	500	15	20	N/A	N/A	90	90	3	3	3/0.3	3/0.3
T2 SE	4500	4000	70	70	N/A	N/A	90	90	3	3	3/0.3	3/0.3
PD	5000	6500	30	30	N/A	N/A	90	90	3	3	3/0.3	3/0.3
STIR	3000	6000	60	60	150	200	90	90	3	3	3/0.3	3/0.3
T1 SE post C+	500	500	15	20	N/A	N/A	90	90	3	3	3/0.3	3/0.3

Abbreviations: N/A, not applicable; PD, proton density; SE, spin echo; STIR, short tau inversion recovery.

SUGGESTED IMAGING APPLICATION VARIATIONS

Trauma

The attending radiologist and/or the requesting physician may ask for additional sequences or orthogonal planes depending on the traumatic injury.

53

Hip

COIL SELECTION

- Primary coil: Body coil
- Secondary coil: Surface coil

PATIENT/PART POSITIONING AND CENTERING

- The patient is positioned supine and either headfirst or feetfirst on the MRI table or patient couch.
- Make the patient comfortable.

- The legs should be extended with the feet medially rotated 15 to 20 degrees. The feet should be secured in this position with tape and/or sandbags.
- The pelvis should not be rotated.
- Center approximately 2 inches inferior to the anterior superior iliac spine (ASIS) so that the pelvis is at isocenter.
- Instruct the patient to lie still and not move any part of their body.
- Instruct the patient to not cross their arms and legs.

SLICE ALIGNMENT AND SCAN RANGE

Coronal Sequence Acquisition

Slice Alignment

- Slices are parallel to the femoral shaft and femoral neck (Figures 53–1 and 53–2).
- The superior-to-inferior field of view should extend from the ASIS to inferior to the lesser trochanter (Figure 53–3).
- The left-to-right field of view should extend from the pubis through the musculature around the greater trochanter (Figure 53–3).
- The anteroposterior field of view should include the musculature of the hip.
- A coronal image of the hip is shown in Figure 53–4.

Phase and Frequency Orientation

- Phase: Superior to inferior
- Frequency: Right to left
- Phase and frequency orientations may be swapped to reduce motion artifact.

Saturation Band Placement

- A saturation band may be used to eliminate or reduce motion artifact.
- If used, the saturation band should be placed medial to the field of view.

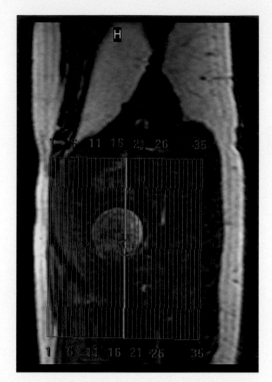

FIGURE 53–2. Sagittal scout image showing slice overlay for a coronal sequence.

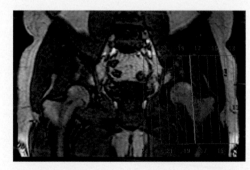

FIGURE 53–3. Coronal scout image demonstrating the FOV, which is shown as a red perimeter box.

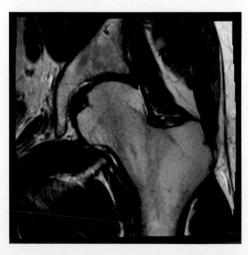

FIGURE 53–4. Coronal T2-weighted image of the left hip. Note the anatomic structures such as the head of the femur, fovea capitis, ligament of the head of the femur connecting the fovea capitis to the acetabulum, femoral neck, greater trochanter, acetabulum, and labrum.

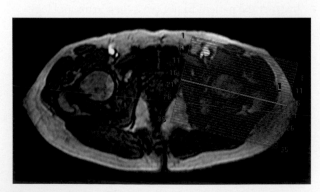

FIGURE 53–1. Axial scout image showing slice overlay for a coronal sequence of the left hip. Note the alignment with the femoral neck.

Sagittal Sequence Acquisition

Option 1: Slices Aligned Parallel with the Femoral Shaft

- On coronal scout images, slices are parallel to the femoral shaft (Figure 53–5).
- On axial scout images, slices are perpendicular to the femoral neck (Figure 53–6).
- The superior-to-inferior field of view should extend from the ASIS to inferior to the lesser trochanter (see Figure 53–5).
- The left-to-right field of view should extend from the pubis through the musculature around the greater trochanter.
- The anteroposterior field of view should include the musculature of the hip.
- A sagittal image of the hip aligned parallel with the femoral shaft is shown in Figure 53–7.

Option 2: Slices Aligned Perpendicular to the Acetabulum

- The sagittal sequence may also be aligned (perpendicular) with the acetabulum so that it is a true acetabular view (ie, sagittal oblique) (Figure 53–8). Using the coronal scout, slices would be parallel with the femoral neck so that it is perpendicular to the acetabulum. Further, using the axial scout images, align parallel to a line extending from the anterior acetabular labrum to the posterior acetabular labrum.

Phase and Frequency Orientation

- Phase: Superior to inferior
- Frequency: Anteroposterior
- Phase and frequency orientations may be swapped to reduce motion artifact.

Saturation Band Placement

- A saturation band may be used to eliminate or reduce motion artifact.
- If used, the saturation band should be placed medial to the field of view.

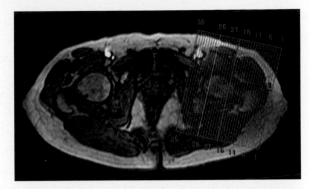

FIGURE 53–6. Axial scout image showing slice overlay for a sagittal sequence of the left hip.

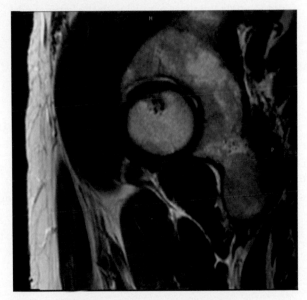

FIGURE 53–7. Sagittal T2-weighted image of the left hip. Note the anatomic structures such as the head of the femur and acetabulum.

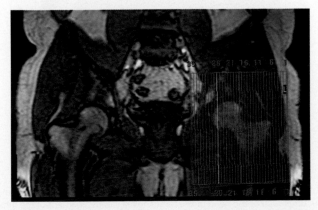

FIGURE 53–5. Coronal scout image showing slice overlay for a sagittal sequence of the left hip.

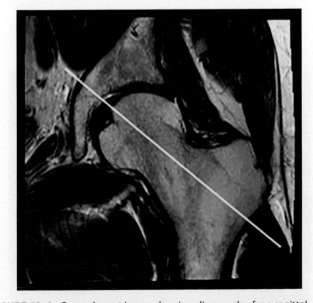

FIGURE 53–8. Coronal scout image showing slice overlay for a sagittal oblique sequence of the left hip for Option 2. Note that slices would be parallel with the white line. The field of view would extend just beyond the edge of the acetabulum.

Axial Sequence Acquisition

Slice Alignment

- As shown in Figures 53–9 and 53–10, slices are perpendicular to the femoral shaft.
- The superior-to-inferior field of view should extend from the ASIS to inferior to the lesser trochanter (see Figure 53–9).
- The left-to-right field of view should extend from the pubis through the musculature around the greater trochanter.
- The anteroposterior field of view should include the musculature of the hip (Figure 53–11).
- Note: Your protocol may include an oblique axial that is aligned with the femoral neck. If required, use the coronal scout to angle the slices parallel with the femoral neck.
- An axial image of the hip is shown in Figure 53–12.

Phase and Frequency Orientation

- Phase: Anteroposterior
- Frequency: Right to left
- Phase and frequency orientations may be swapped to reduce motion artifact.

Saturation Band Placement

- A saturation band may be used to eliminate or reduce motion artifact.
- If used, the saturation band should be placed medial to the field of view.

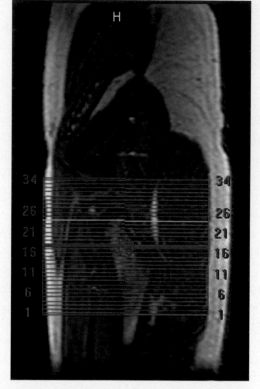

FIGURE 53–10. Sagittal scout image showing slice overlay for an axial sequence.

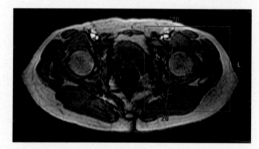

FIGURE 53–11. Axial scout image demonstrating the FOV, which is shown as a red perimeter box.

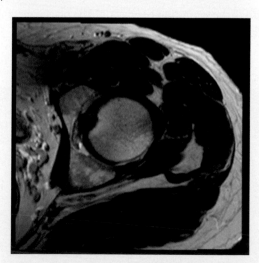

FIGURE 53–12. Axial T2-weighted image of the left hip. Note the anatomic structures such as the head of the femur, fovea capitis, ligament of the head of the femur connecting the fovea capitis to the acetabulum, acetabulum, and labrum.

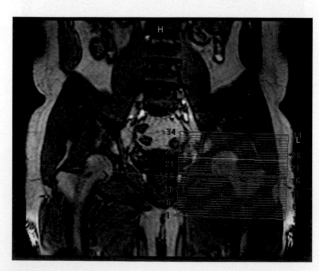

FIGURE 53–9. Coronal scout image showing slice overlay for an axial sequence of the left hip.

IMAGING APPLICATION

TABLE 53–1 • General Sequences												
General Sequences	**TR**		**TE**		**TI**		**FA (degrees)**		**NEX**		**SLT/GAP (in millimeters)**	
	1.5 T	**3.0 T**	**1.5 T**	**3.0 T**	**1.5 T**	**3.0 T**	**1.5 T**	**3.0 T**	**1.5 T**	**3.0 T**	**1.5 T**	**3.0 T**
T1 SE	500	500	15	20	N/A	N/A	90	90	3	3	3/1	3/1
T2 SE	4500	4000	70	70	N/A	N/A	90	90	3	3	3/1	3/1
PD	5000	3000	30	30	N/A	N/A	90	90	3	3	3/1	3/1
STIR	4000	4500	60	15	150	220	90	90	3	3	3/1	3/1
T1 SE post C+	500	500	15	20	N/A	N/A	90	90	3	3	3/1	3/1

Abbreviations: N/A, not applicable; PD, proton density; SE, spin echo; STIR, short tau inversion recovery.

SUGGESTED IMAGING APPLICATION VARIATIONS

Arthrogram

The injection of contrast media and/or gas in the capsular space may be requested. The requested media will be injected, usually under the guidance of fluoroscopy. The patient will then be imaged in MRI. Additional sequences to the routine protocol may be requested by the radiologist. (See Chapter 59.)

Trauma

The attending radiologist and/or the requesting physician may ask for additional sequences or orthogonal planes depending on the traumatic injury.

Tumor

A tumor protocol may require sequences in addition to the routine hip protocol and a larger field of view to include the lesion. Additional pre- and postcontrast sequences may be included. Three-orthogonal-plane postcontrast sequences may be of benefit to the radiologist. The technologist should follow the protocol provided at their facility.

54

Femur

COIL SELECTION

- Primary coil: Body or torso coil
- Secondary coil: Surface coil

PATIENT/PART POSITIONING AND CENTERING

- The patient is positioned supine and either headfirst or feetfirst on the MRI table or patient couch.
- Make the patient comfortable.

- Support the patient's foot and lower leg. A supporting sandbag will help keep the leg in position and aid in patient comfort.
- The legs should be extended with the feet medially rotated 15 to 20 degrees. The feet should be secured in this position with tape and/or sandbags.
- The pelvis should not be rotated.
- Center midshaft, so that the femur is at isocenter.
- Instruct the patient to lie still and not move any part of their body.
- Instruct the patient to not cross their arms and legs.

SLICE ALIGNMENT AND SCAN RANGE

Coronal Sequence Acquisition

Slice Alignment

- On sagittal scout, slices are parallel to the shaft of the femur (Figure 54–1).
- Slices are parallel to a line extending from the femoral medial condyle to the lateral condyle.
- Resultant images should demonstrate the full shaft of the femur.
- The superior-to-inferior field of view should extend superior of the acetabulum to the proximal tibia (see Figure 54–3).
- The left-to-right field of view must include the musculature of the femur (Figure 54–2).

- The anteroposterior field of view should include the musculature of the femur.
- A coronal image of the femur is shown in Figure 54–3.

Phase and Frequency Orientation

- Phase: Right to left
- Frequency: Superior to inferior
- Phase and frequency orientations may be swapped to reduce motion artifact.

Saturation Band Placement

- A saturation band may be used to eliminate or reduce flow artifact.
- If used, the saturation band should be placed superior to the field of view.

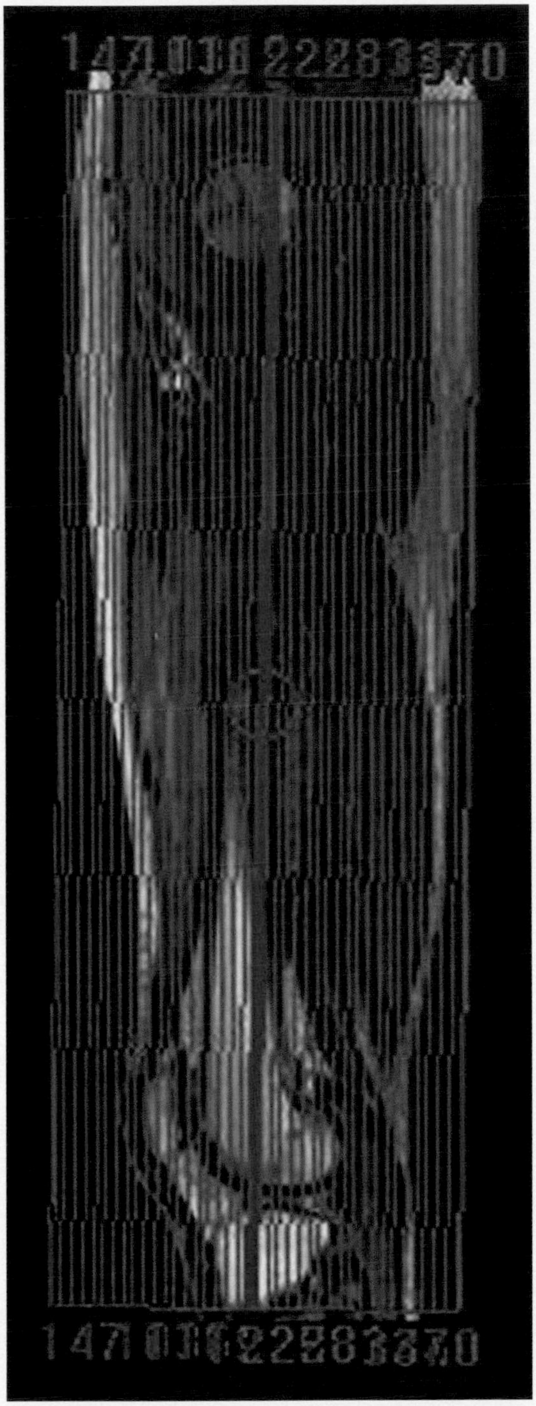

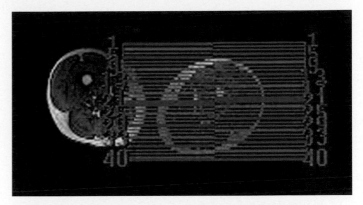

FIGURE 54–2. Axial scout image showing slice overlay for a coronal sequence of the left femur.

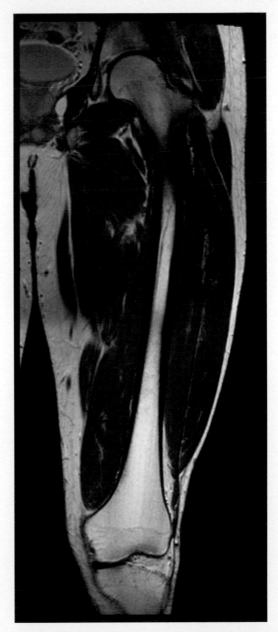

FIGURE 54–1. Sagittal scout image showing slice overlay for a coronal sequence.

FIGURE 54–3. Coronal T2-weighted image of the left femur. Note the anatomic structures such as the head of the femur, femoral neck, greater trochanter, femoral shaft, medical epicondyle, and medal condyle.

Sagittal Sequence Acquisition

Slice Alignment

- On coronal scout, slices are parallel to the shaft of the femur (Figure 54–4).
- Slices are parallel to a line extending from the femoral medial condyle to the lateral condyle.
- Resultant images should demonstrate the full shaft of the femur (Figure 54–6).
- The superior-to-inferior field of view should extend superior of the acetabulum to the proximal tibia (see Figure 54–6).
- The left-to-right field of view must include the musculature of the femur (Figure 54–5).
- The anteroposterior field of view should include the musculature of the femur.
- A sagittal image of the femur is shown in Figure 54–6.

Phase and Frequency Orientation

- Phase: Anteroposterior
- Frequency: Superior to inferior
- Phase and frequency orientations may be swapped to reduce motion artifact.

Saturation Band Placement

- A saturation band may be used to eliminate or reduce flow artifact.
- If used, the saturation band should be placed superior to the field of view.

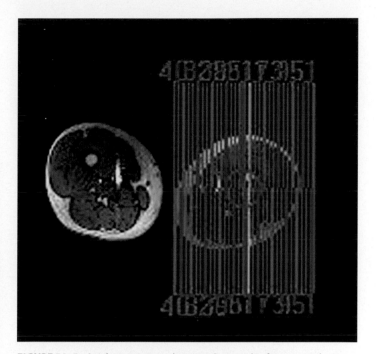

FIGURE 54–5. Axial scout image showing slice overlay for a sagittal sequence of the left femur.

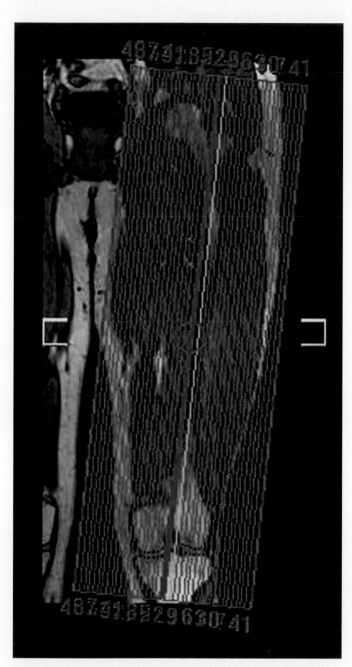

FIGURE 54–4. Coronal scout image showing slice overlay for a sagittal sequence of the left femur.

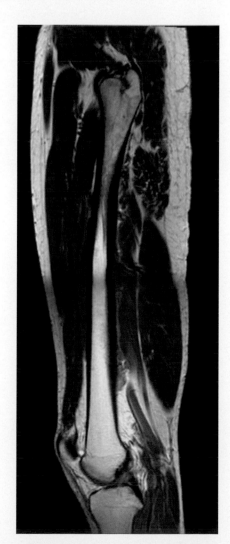

FIGURE 54–6. Sagittal T2-weighted image of the left femur.

Axial Sequence Acquisition

Slice Alignment

- On coronal and sagittal scouts, slices are perpendicular to the shaft of the femur (Figures 54–7 and 54–8).
- The superior-to-inferior field of view should extend superior to the acetabulum to the proximal tibia (see Figure 54–7).
- The left-to-right field of view must include the musculature of the femur.
- The anteroposterior field of view should include the musculature of the femur.
- An axial image of the femur is shown in Figure 54–9.

Phase and Frequency Orientation

- Phase: Anteroposterior
- Frequency: Right to left
- Phase and frequency orientations may be swapped to reduce motion artifact.

Saturation Band Placement

- A saturation band may be used to eliminate or reduce flow artifact.
- If used, the saturation band should be placed superior to the field of view.

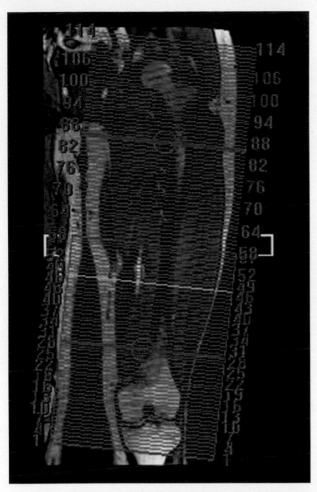

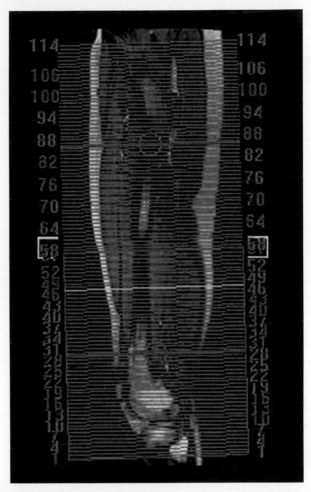

FIGURE 54–7. Coronal scout image showing slice overlay for an axial sequence of the left femur.

FIGURE 54–8. Sagittal scout image showing slice overlay for an axial sequence.

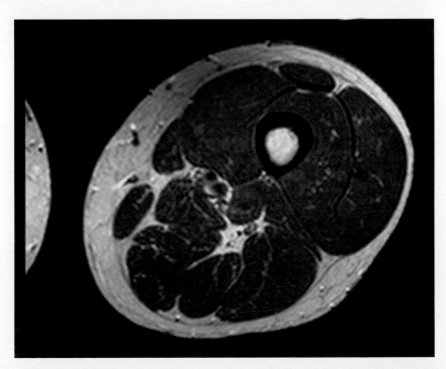

FIGURE 54–9. Axial T2-weighted image of the left femur. Note that this slice is at the midshaft level. Also notice the hypointense cortex and hyperintense medullary portion of the femur.

IMAGING APPLICATION

TABLE 54–1 • General Sequences												
General Sequences	**TR**		**TE**		**TI**		**FA (degrees)**		**NEX**		**SLT/GAP (in millimeters)**	
	1.5 T	3.0 T	1.5 T	3.0 T	1.5 T	3.0 T	1.5 T	3.0 T	1.5 T	3.0 T	1.5 T	3.0 T
T1 SE	500	500	15	20	N/A	N/A	90	90	3	3	4/1	4/1
T2 SE	4500	4000	70	70	N/A	N/A	90	90	3	3	4/1	4/1
PD	5000	3000	30	15	N/A	N/A	90	90	3	3	4/1	4/1
STIR	3000	4000	60	15	150	220	90	90	3	3	4/1	4/1
T1 SE post C+	500	500	15	20	N/A	N/A	90	90	3	3	4/1	4/1

Abbreviations: N/A, not applicable; PD, proton density; SE, spin echo; STIR, short tau inversion recovery.

SUGGESTED IMAGING APPLICATION VARIATIONS

Trauma

The attending radiologist and/or the requesting physician may ask for additional sequences or orthogonal planes depending on the traumatic injury.

Tumor

A tumor protocol may require sequences in addition to the routine femur protocol and a larger field of view to include the lesion. Additional pre- and postcontrast sequences may be included. Three-orthogonal-plane postcontrast sequences may be of benefit to the radiologist. The technologist should follow the protocol provided at their facility.

55

Knee

COIL SELECTION

- Primary coil: Extremity coil
- Secondary coil: Surface coil

PATIENT/PART POSITIONING AND CENTERING

- The patient is positioned supine and feetfirst on the MRI table or patient couch.
- Make the patient comfortable.

- The leg should be extended. The femoral epicondyles should be positioned parallel to the MRI table. This places the knee in true anatomic position.
- Support the patient's foot and lower leg. A supporting sandbag will help keep the leg in position and aid in patient comfort.
- Center on the patellar apex, so that the knee is at isocenter.
- Instruct the patient to lie still and not move any part of their body.
- Instruct the patient to not cross their arms and legs.

SLICE ALIGNMENT AND SCAN RANGE

Coronal Sequence Acquisition

Slice Alignment

- On axial scout, slices are parallel to a line extending from the posterior femoral medial condyle to the lateral condyle (Figure 55–1).
- Slices are parallel to the shafts of the femur and tibia (Figure 55–2).
- The superior-to-inferior field of view should extend from superior to the patella (including a distal portion of the quadriceps femoris tendon) to inferior to the tibial tuberosity.
- The left-to-right field of view should include the musculature of the knee.
- The anteroposterior field of view should extend anterior to the patella through the musculature posterior to the knee.
- A coronal image of the knee is shown in Figure 55–3.

Phase and Frequency Orientation

- Phase: Superior to inferior
- Frequency: Right to left
- Phase and frequency orientations may be swapped to reduce motion artifact.

Saturation Band Placement

- A saturation band may be used to eliminate or reduce motion artifact.
- If used, the saturation band should be placed superior to the field of view.

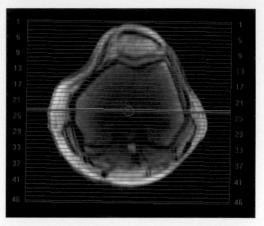

FIGURE 55–1. Axial scout image showing slice overlay for a coronal sequence.

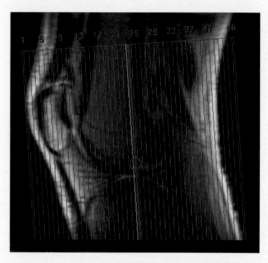

FIGURE 55–2. Sagittal scout image showing slice overlay for a coronal sequence. Note the good positioning of the knee.

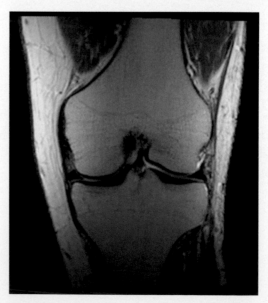

FIGURE 55–3. Coronal T2-weighted image. Note the anatomic structures such as the medial femoral condyle, lateral femoral condyle, medial tibial condyle, lateral tibial condyle, tibial spine, body of the medial meniscus, and body of the lateral meniscus.

Sagittal Sequence Acquisition

Slice Alignment

- On axial scout, slices are perpendicular to a line extending from the posterior femoral medial condyle to the lateral condyle (Figure 55–4.
- On coronal scout, slices are perpendicular to the tibial plateau (Figure 55–5).
- The superior-to-inferior field of view should extend from superior to the patella (including a distal portion of the quadriceps femoris tendon) to inferior to the tibial tuberosity (Figure 55–6).
- The left-to-right field of view should include the musculature of the knee.
- The anteroposterior field of view should extend anterior to the patella through the musculature posterior to the knee.
- A sagittal image of the knee is shown in Figure 55–7.

Phase and Frequency Orientation

- Phase: Superior to inferior
- Frequency: Anteroposterior
- Phase and frequency orientations may be swapped to reduce motion artifact.

Saturation Band Placement

- A saturation band may be used to eliminate or reduce motion artifact.
- If used, the saturation band should be placed superior to the field of view.

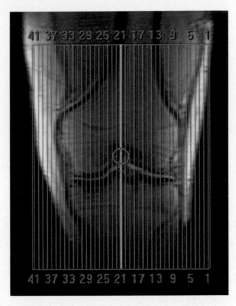

FIGURE 55–5. Coronal scout image showing slice overlay for a sagittal sequence.

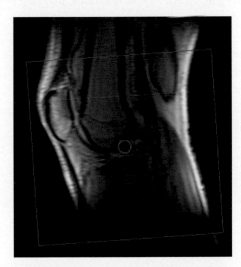

FIGURE 55–6. Sagittal scout image demonstrating the FOV, which is shown as a red perimeter box.

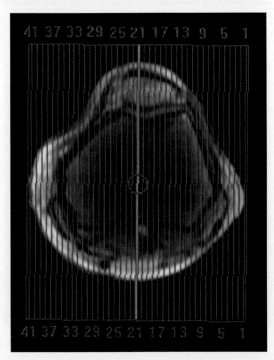

FIGURE 55–4. Axial scout image showing slice overlay for a sagittal sequence.

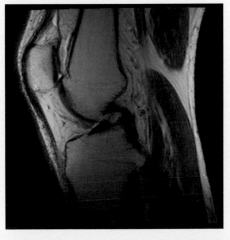

FIGURE 55–7. Sagittal T2-weighted image. Note the anatomic structures such as the quadriceps tendon, patellar tendon, posterior cruciate ligament (PCL), a portion of the anterior cruciate ligament (ACL), and patella.

Axial Sequence Acquisition

Slice Alignment

- On sagittal and coronal scouts, slices are parallel to the femoral condyles (Figures 55–8 and 55–9).
- The superior-to-inferior field of view should extend from superior to the patella (including a distal portion of the quadriceps femoris tendon) to inferior to the tibial tuberosity (see Figure 55–8).
- The left-to-right field of view should include the musculature of the knee.
- The anteroposterior field of view should extend anterior to the patella through the musculature posterior to the knee.
- An axial image of the knee is shown in Figure 55–10.

Phase and Frequency Orientation

- Phase: Anteroposterior
- Frequency: Right to left
- Phase and frequency orientations may be swapped to reduce motion artifact.

Saturation Band Placement

- A saturation band may be used to eliminate or reduce motion artifact.
- If used, the saturation band should be placed superior to the field of view.

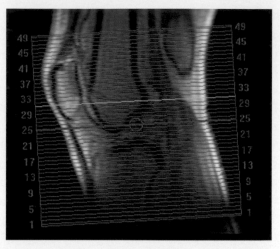

FIGURE 55–8. Sagittal scout image showing slice overlay for an axial sequence.

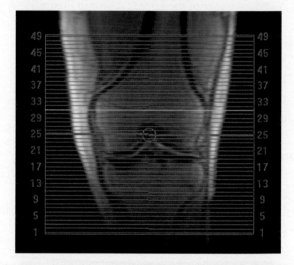

FIGURE 55–9. Coronal scout image showing slice overlay for an axial sequence.

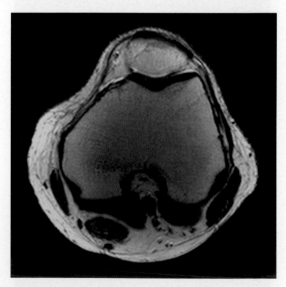

FIGURE 55–10. Axial T2-weighted image. Note the anatomic structures such as the medial condyle of the femur, lateral condyle of the femur, popliteal artery, and patella. Axial images are also beneficial in imaging the medial collateral ligament (MCL) and lateral collateral ligament (LCL).

IMAGING APPLICATION

	TR		TE		TI		FA (degrees)		NEX		SLT/GAP (in millimeters)	
General Sequences	**1.5 T**	**3.0 T**	**1.5 T**	**3.0 T**	**1.5 T**	**3.0 T**	**1.5 T**	**3.0 T**	**1.5 T**	**3.0 T**	**1.5 T**	**3.0 T**
T1 SE	500	500	15	20	N/A	N/A	90	90	3	3	3/0.3	3/0.3
T2 SE	4500	4000	70	70	N/A	N/A	90	90	3	3	3/0.3	3/0.3
PD	5000	3000	30	30	N/A	N/A	90	90	3	3	3/0.3	3/0.3
STIR	3000	4000	60	15	150	220	90	90	3	3	3/0.3	3/0.3
T1 SE post C+	500	500	15	20	N/A	N/A	90	90	3	3	3/0.3	3/0.3

TABLE 55–1 • General Sequences

Abbreviations: N/A, not applicable; PD, proton density; SE, spin echo; STIR, short tau inversion recovery.

SUGGESTED IMAGING APPLICATION VARIATIONS

Arthrogram

The injection of contrast media and/or gas in the capsular space may be requested. The requested media will be injected, usually under the guidance of fluoroscopy. The patient will then be imaged in MRI. Sequences in addition to the routine protocol may be requested by the radiologist.

Trauma

The attending radiologist and/or the requesting physician may ask for additional sequences or orthogonal planes depending on the traumatic injury.

Tumor

A tumor protocol may require sequences in addition to the routine knee protocol and a larger field of view to include the lesion. Additional pre- and postcontrast sequences may be included. Three-orthogonal-plane postcontrast sequences may be of benefit to the radiologist. The technologist should follow the protocol provided at their facility.

Lower Leg

56

COIL SELECTION

- Primary coil: Body coil
- Secondary coil: Surface coil

PATIENT/PART POSITIONING AND CENTERING

- The patient is positioned supine and feetfirst on the MRI table or patient couch.
- Make the patient comfortable.

- The leg should be extended. The femoral epicondyles should be positioned parallel to the MRI table. This places the knee in true anatomic position.
- Support the patient's foot and lower leg. A supporting sandbag will help keep the leg in position and aid in patient comfort.
- Center midshaft, so that the tibia and fibula are at isocenter.
- Instruct the patient to lie still and not move any part of their body.
- Instruct the patient to not cross their arms and legs.

SLICE ALIGNMENT AND SCAN RANGE

Coronal Sequence Acquisition

Slice Alignment

- On sagittal scout, slices are parallel to the shaft of the tibia (Figure 56–1).
- On axial scout, slices are parallel to a line extending from the tibial medial condyle to the lateral condyle.
- Resultant images should demonstrate the full shafts of the tibia and fibula
- The superior-to-inferior field of view should extend from the distal femur to calcaneus (see Figure 56–1).
- The left-to-right field of view must include the musculature of the lower leg.
- The anteroposterior field of view should include the musculature of the lower leg (Figure 56–2).
- A coronal image of the lower leg is shown in Figure 56–3.

Phase and Frequency Orientation

- Phase: Right to left
- Frequency: Superior to inferior
- Phase and frequency orientations may be swapped to reduce motion artifact.

Saturation Band Placement

- A saturation band may be used to eliminate or reduce flow artifact.
- If used, the saturation band should be placed superior to the field of view.

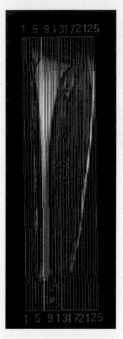

FIGURE 56–1. Sagittal scout image showing slice overlay for a coronal sequence.

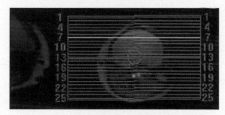

FIGURE 56–2. Axial scout image showing slice overlay for a coronal sequence.

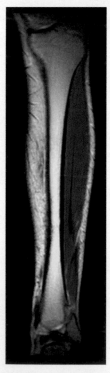

FIGURE 56–3. Coronal T2-weighted image.

Sagittal Sequence Acquisition

Slice Alignment

- On coronal scout, slices are parallel to the shaft of the tibia (Figure 56–4).
- On axial scout, slices are perpendicular to a line extending from the tibial medial condyle to the lateral condyle.
- Resultant images should demonstrate the full shafts of the tibia and fibula
- The superior-to-inferior field of view should extend from the distal femur to calcaneus (see Figure 56–6).
- The left-to-right field of view must include the musculature of the lower leg (Figure 56–5)
- The anteroposterior field of view should include the musculature of the lower leg.
- A sagittal image of the lower leg is shown in Figure 56–6.

Phase and Frequency Orientation

- Phase: Anteroposterior
- Frequency: Superior to inferior
- Phase and frequency orientations may be swapped to reduce motion artifact.

Saturation Band Placement

- A saturation band may be used to eliminate or reduce flow artifact.
- If used, the saturation band should be placed superior to the field of view.

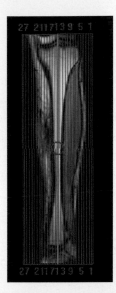

FIGURE 56–4. Coronal scout image showing slice overlay for a sagittal sequence.

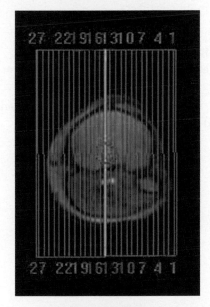

FIGURE 56–5. Axial scout image showing slice overlay for a sagittal sequence.

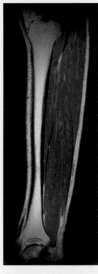

FIGURE 56–6. Sagittal T2-weighted image.

Axial Sequence Acquisition

Slice Alignment

- On sagittal and coronal scouts, slices are perpendicular to the shaft of the tibia (Figures 56–7 and 56–8.

- The superior-to-inferior field of view should extend from the distal femur to calcaneus (see Figure 56–8).

- The left-to-right field of view must include the musculature of the lower leg.

- The anteroposterior field of view should include the musculature of the lower leg.

- An axial image of the lower leg is shown in Figure 56–9.

Phase and Frequency Orientation

- Phase: Anteroposterior

- Frequency: Right to left

- Phase and frequency orientations may be swapped to reduce motion artifact.

Saturation Band Placement

- A saturation band may be used to eliminate or reduce flow artifact.

- If used, the saturation band should be placed superior to the field of view.

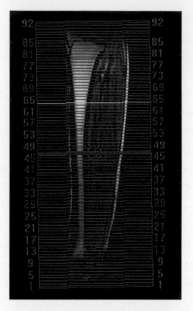

FIGURE 56–7. Sagittal scout image showing slice overlay for an axial sequence.

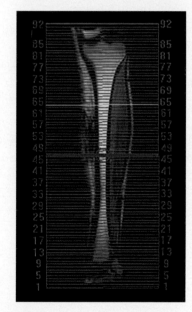

FIGURE 56–8. Coronal scout image showing slice overlay for an axial sequence.

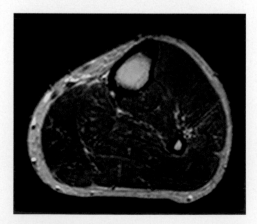

FIGURE 56–9. Axial T2-weighted image.

IMAGING APPLICATION

TABLE 56–1 • General Sequences

General Sequences	TR		TE		TI		FA (degrees)		NEX		SLT/GAP (in millimeters)	
	1.5 T	3.0 T	1.5 T	3.0 T	1.5 T	3.0 T	1.5 T	3.0 T	1.5 T	3.0 T	1.5 T	3.0 T
T1 SE	500	500	15	20	N/A	N/A	90	90	3	3	4/1	4/1
T2 SE	4500	4000	70	70	N/A	N/A	90	90	3	3	4/1	4/1
PD	5000	3000	30	15	N/A	N/A	90	90	3	3	4/1	4/1
STIR	3000	4000	60	15	150	220	90	90	3	3	4/1	4/1
T1 SE post C+	500	500	15	20	N/A	N/A	90	90	3	3	4/1	4/1

Abbreviations: N/A, not applicable; PD, proton density; SE, spin echo; STIR, short tau inversion recovery.

SUGGESTED IMAGING APPLICATION VARIATIONS

Trauma

The attending radiologist and/or the requesting physician may ask for additional sequences or orthogonal planes depending on the traumatic injury.

Tumor

A tumor protocol may require sequences in addition to the routine lower leg protocol and a larger field of view to include the lesion. Additional pre- and postcontrast sequences may be included. Three-orthogonal-plane postcontrast sequences may be of benefit to the radiologist. The technologist should follow the protocol provided at their facility.

57

Ankle

COIL SELECTION

- Primary coil: Extremity coil
- Secondary coil: Surface coil

PATIENT/PART POSITIONING AND CENTERING

- The patient is positioned supine and feetfirst on the MRI table or patient couch.
- Make the patient comfortable.
- The foot should be flexed so that the plantar surface is perpendicular to the MRI table. This places the foot in true anatomic position.

- The lower leg should form a 90-degree angle with the foot.
- Support the patient's foot and lower leg. A supporting sandbag will help keep the foot in position and aid in patient comfort.
- Center at the level of the lateral malleolus so that the ankle is at isocenter.
- Instruct the patient to lie still and not move any part of their body.
- Instruct the patient to not cross their arms.

SLICE ALIGNMENT AND SCAN RANGE

Coronal Sequence Acquisition

Slice Alignment

- On sagittal scout, slices are parallel to the shaft of the tibia (Figure 57–1).
- Slices are perpendicular to the tibiotalar joint (see Figure 57–1).
- On axial scout, slices are parallel to a line extending from the lateral malleolus to the medial malleolus (see Figure 57–2)
- The superior-to-inferior field of view should extend from the distal shaft of the tibia through the plantar fat pad (see Figure 57–1).
- The left-to-right field of view should include the musculature of the ankle (Figures 57–2 and 57–3).
- The anteroposterior field of view should extend from the metatarsals through the heel fat pad (see Figure 57–1).
- A coronal image of the ankle is shown in Figure 57–4.

Phase and Frequency Orientation

- Phase: Superior to inferior
- Frequency: Right to left
- Phase and frequency orientations may be swapped to reduce motion artifact.

Saturation Band Placement

- A saturation band may be used to eliminate or reduce motion artifact.
- If used, the saturation band should be placed superior to the field of view.

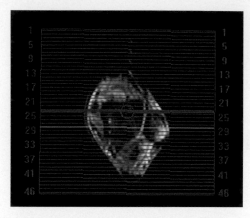

FIGURE 57–2. Axial scout image showing slice overlay for a coronal sequence.

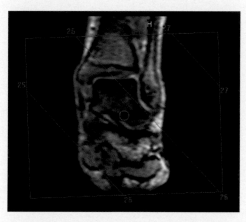

FIGURE 57–3. Coronal scout image demonstrating the FOV, which is shown as a red perimeter box.

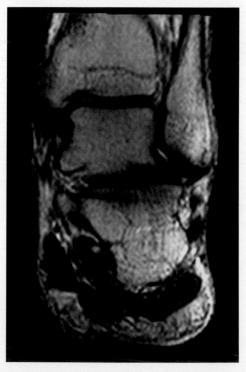

FIGURE 57–4. Coronal T2-weighted image. Note the anatomic structures such as the tibia, talus, fibula, tibiotalar joint, medial malleolus, lateral malleolus, talofibular joint, and calcaneus.

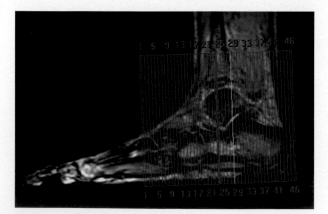

FIGURE 57–1. Sagittal scout image showing slice overlay for a coronal sequence. Note the good positioning of the foot so that the lower leg and foot form a 90-degree angle.

Sagittal Sequence Acquisition

Slice Alignment

- Slices are parallel to the shaft of the tibia (Figure 57–5).
- On coronal scout, slices are perpendicular to the tibiotalar joint (see Figures 57–5 and 57–6).
- On axial scout, slices are perpendicular to a line extending from the lateral malleolus to the medial malleolus (Figure 57–6).
- The superior-to-inferior field of view should extend from the distal shaft of the tibia through the plantar fat pad (Figure 57–7).
- The left-to-right field of view should include the musculature of the ankle (Figure 57–6).
- The anteroposterior field of view should extend from the metatarsals through the heel fat pad (see Figure 57–7).
- A sagittal image of the ankle is shown in Figure 57–8.

Phase and Frequency Orientation

- Phase: Superior to inferior
- Frequency: Anteroposterior
- Phase and frequency orientations may be swapped to reduce motion artifact.

Saturation Band Placement

- A saturation band may be used to eliminate or reduce motion artifact.
- If used, the saturation band should be placed superior to the field of view.

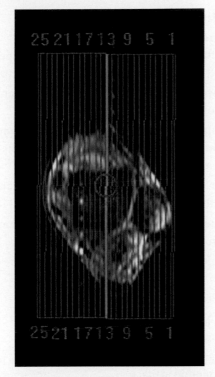

FIGURE 57–6. Axial scout image showing slice overlay for a sagittal sequence.

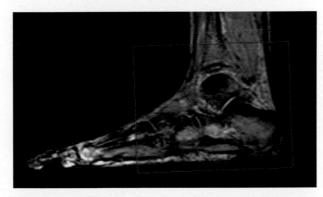

FIGURE 57–7. Sagittal scout image demonstrating the FOV, which is shown as a red perimeter box.

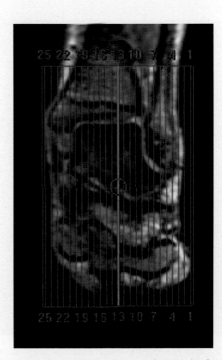

FIGURE 57–5. Coronal scout image showing slice overlay for a sagittal sequence.

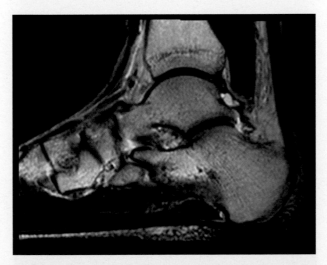

FIGURE 57–8. Sagittal T2-weighted image. Note the anatomic structures such as the Achilles tendon extending to the calcaneus, tibia, tibiotalar joint, talus, calcaneus, navicular, cuneiforms, and proximal metatarsals.

Axial Sequence Acquisition

Slice Alignment

- On sagittal and coronal scouts, slices are perpendicular to the shaft of the tibia. (Figures 57–9 and 57–10).

- As shown in Figures 57–9 and 57–10, slices are parallel to the tibiotalar joint.

- The superior-to-inferior field of view should extend from the distal shaft of the tibia through the plantar fat pad (see Figure 57–9).

- The left-to-right field of view should include the musculature of the ankle (see Figures 57–10 and 57–11).

- The anteroposterior field of view should extend from the metatarsals through the heel fat pad.

- An axial image of the ankle is shown in Figure 57–12.

Phase and Frequency Orientation

- Phase: Anteroposterior

- Frequency: Right to left

- Phase and frequency orientations may be swapped to reduce motion artifact.

Saturation Band Placement

- A saturation band may be used to eliminate or reduce motion artifact.

- If used, the saturation band should be placed superior to the field of view.

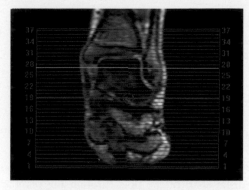

FIGURE 57–10. Coronal scout image showing slice overlay for an axial sequence.

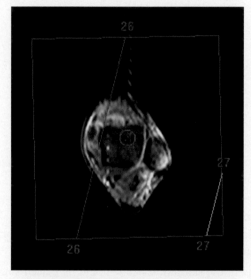

FIGURE 57–11. Axial scout image demonstrating the FOV, which is shown as a red perimeter box.

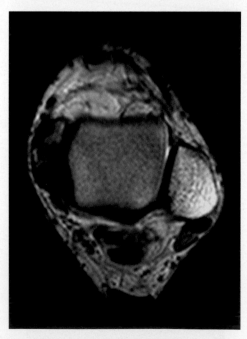

FIGURE 57–12. Axial T2-weighted image. Note that the anatomic structures such as the talus, medial malleolus, lateral malleolus, and talofibular joint.

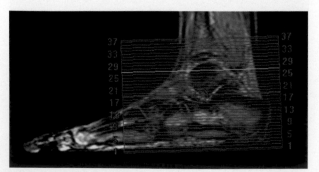

FIGURE 57–9. Sagittal scout image showing slice overlay for an axial sequence.

IMAGING APPLICATION

TABLE 57–1 • General Sequences

General Sequences	TR		TE		TI		FA (degrees)		NEX		SLT/GAP (in millimeters)	
	1.5 T	3.0 T	1.5 T	3.0 T	1.5 T	3.0 T	1.5 T	3.0 T	1.5 T	3.0 T	1.5 T	3.0 T
T1 SE	500	600	15	20	N/A	N/A	90	90	3	3	3/0.3	3/0.3
T2 SE	4500	4000	70	70	N/A	N/A	90	90	3	3	3/0.3	3/0.3
PD	3000	3000	30	25	N/A	N/A	90	90	3	3	3/0.3	3/0.3
STIR	3000	3000	60	15	150	200	90	90	3	3	3/0.3	3/0.3
T1 SE post C+	500	500	15	20	N/A	N/A	90	90	3	3	3/0.3	3/0.3

Abbreviations: N/A, not applicable; PD, proton density; SE, spin echo; STIR, short tau inversion recovery.

SUGGESTED IMAGING APPLICATION VARIATIONS

Arthrogram

The injection of contrast media and/or gas in the capsular space may be requested. The requested media will be injected, usually under the guidance of fluoroscopy. The patient will then be imaged in MRI. Sequences in addition to the routine protocol may be requested by the radiologist.

Trauma

The attending radiologist and/or the requesting physician may ask for additional sequences or orthogonal planes depending on the traumatic injury.

Tumor

A tumor protocol may require sequences in addition to the routine shoulder protocol and a larger field of view to include the lesion. Additional pre- and postcontrast sequences may be included. Three-orthogonal-plane postcontrast sequences may be of benefit to the radiologist. The technologist should follow the protocol provided at their facility.

Foot

COIL SELECTION

- Primary coil: Extremity coil
- Secondary coil: Surface coil

PATIENT/PART POSITIONING AND CENTERING

- The patient is positioned supine and feetfirst on the MRI table or patient couch.
- Make the patient comfortable.
- The foot should be flexed so that the plantar surface is perpendicular to the MRI table. This places the foot in true anatomic position.

- The lower leg should form a 90-degree angle with the foot.
- Support the patient's foot and lower leg. A supporting sandbag will help keep the foot in position and aid in patient comfort.
- Center on the tarsometatarsals so that the foot is at isocenter.
- Instruct the patient to lie still and not move any part of their body.
- Instruct the patient to not cross their arms.

SLICE ALIGNMENT AND SCAN RANGE

Sagittal Sequence Acquisition

Slice Alignment

- On coronal scout of the foot, slices are parallel with the long axis of the foot (Figure 58–1).
- On coronal scout of the ankle, slices are perpendicular to the tibiotalar joint (Figure 58–2).
- Slices are also perpendicular to the shafts of the tibia and fibula (see Figure 58–2).
- The superior-to-inferior field of view should extend from the distal shaft of the tibia through the plantar fat pad (Figure 58–3).
- The left-to-right field of view should include the musculature of the foot.
- The anteroposterior field of view should extend from the distal phalanges through the heel fat pad (Figure 58–4).
- A sagittal image of the foot is shown in Figure 58–4.
- Note: The radiologist at your imaging facility may allow the anteroposterior field of view to extend from the distal phalanges to the distal tarsal bones. If the smaller field of view is used, then the superior-to-inferior field of view would extend from the dorsal surface fat to the plantar surface fat.

Phase and Frequency Orientation

- Phase: Superior to inferior
- Frequency: Anteroposterior
- Phase and frequency orientations may be swapped to reduce motion artifact.

Saturation Band Placement

- A saturation band may be used to eliminate or reduce motion artifact.
- If used, the saturation band should be placed superior to the field of view.

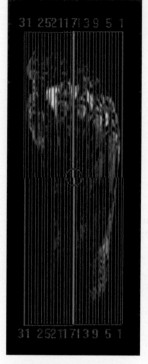

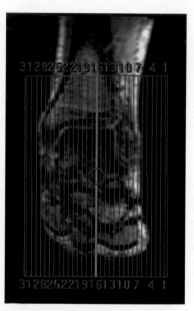

FIGURE 58–1. Coronal scout image of the foot showing slice overlay for a sagittal sequence.

FIGURE 58–2. Axial scout image of the foot showing slice overlay for a sagittal sequence.

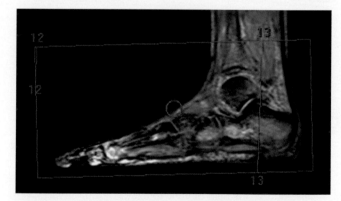

FIGURE 58–3. Sagittal scout image demonstrating the FOV, which is shown as a red perimeter box.

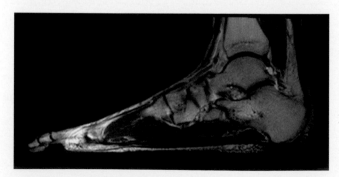

FIGURE 58–4. Sagittal T2-weighted image. Note the good positioning of the foot so that the lower leg and foot form a 90-degree angle. Also, notice the anatomic structures such as the Achilles tendon extending to the calcaneus, tibia, tibiotalar joint, talus, calcaneus, navicular, medial cuneiform, metatarsals, and phalanges.

Axial Sequence Acquisition

Option 1: Slices Aligned to the Plantar Surface

- On sagittal scout, slices are perpendicular with the plantar surface of the foot (Figure 58–5).
- On coronal scout, slices are perpendicular to the long axis of the foot (Figure 58–6).
- When the ankle joint is at 90 degrees, slices are parallel to the shafts of the tibia and fibula (see Figure 58–5).
- The superior-to-inferior field of view should extend from the distal shaft of the tibia through the plantar fat pad (see Figure 58–5).
- The left-to-right field of view should include the musculature of the foot (see Figure 58–7).
- The anteroposterior field of view should extend from the distal phalanges through the heel fat pad (Figure 58–6).
- An axial image alighted to the plantar surface is shown in Figure 58–8.
- Note: The radiologist at your imaging facility may allow the anteroposterior field of view to extend from the distal phalanges to the distal tarsal bones. If the smaller field of view is used, then the superior-to-inferior field of view would extend from the dorsal surface fat to the plantar surface fat.

Option 2: Slices Aligned to the Metatarsals

- On sagittal scout, slices are parallel with the metatarsals.
- On coronal scout, slices are perpendicular to the metatarsals.
- The superior-to-inferior field of view should extend from the distal shaft of the tibia through the plantar fat pad.
- The left-to-right field of view should include the musculature of the foot.
- The anteroposterior field of view should extend from the distal phalanges through the heel fat pad.
- Note: The radiologist at your imaging facility may allow the anteroposterior field of view to extend from the distal phalanges to the distal tarsal bones. If the smaller field of view is used, then the superior-to-inferior field of view would extend from the dorsal surface fat to the plantar surface fat.

Phase and Frequency Orientation

- Phase: Anteroposterior
- Frequency: Right to left
- Phase and frequency orientations may be swapped to reduce motion artifact.

Saturation Band Placement

- A saturation band may be used to eliminate or reduce motion artifact.
- If used, the saturation band should be placed superior to the field of view.

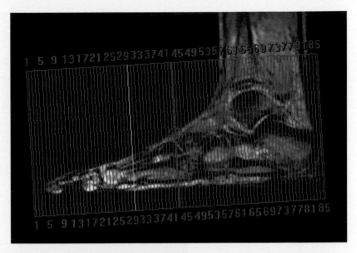

FIGURE 58–5. Sagittal scout image showing slice overlay for an axial sequence aligned with the plantar surface (option 1).

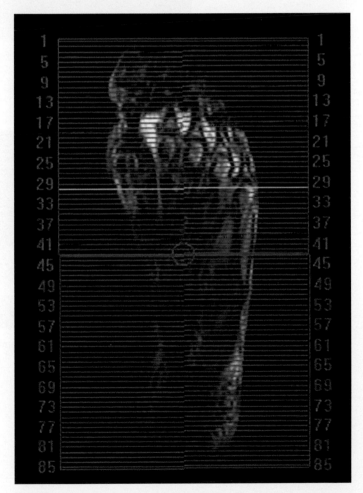

FIGURE 58–6. Coronal scout image showing slice overlay for an axial sequence.

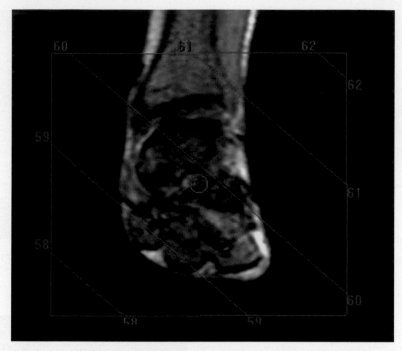

FIGURE 58-7. Axial scout image of the foot demonstrating the FOV, which is shown as a red perimeter box.

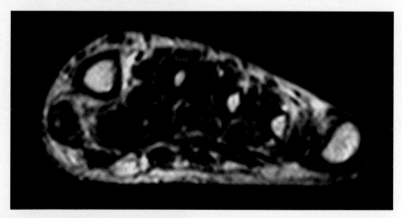

FIGURE 58-8. Axial T2-weighted image aligned with the plantar surface of the foot (option 1).

Coronal Sequence Acquisition

Option 1: Slices Aligned to the Plantar Surface

- On sagittal scout, slices are parallel with the plantar surface of the foot (Figure 58–9).
- When the ankle joint is at 90 degrees, slices are perpendicular to the shafts of the tibia and fibula (see Figure 58–10).
- The superior-to-inferior field of view should extend from the distal shaft of the tibia through the plantar fat pad (see Figure 58–9).
- The left-to-right field of view should include the musculature of the foot (Figure 58–11).
- The anteroposterior field of view should extend from the distal phalanges through the heel fat pad (Figure 58–11).
- A coronal image of the foot aligned to the plantar surface is shown in Figure 58–11.
- Note: The radiologist at your imaging facility may allow the anteroposterior field of view to extend from the distal phalanges to the distal tarsal bones. If the smaller field of view is used, then the superior-to-inferior field of view would extend from the dorsal surface fat to the plantar surface fat.

Option 2: Slices Aligned to the Metatarsals

- On sagittal scout, slices are parallel with the metatarsals (Figure 58–12).
- Slices are parallel with a line extending from the first metatarsal to the fifth metatarsal (Figure 58–13).
- The superior-to-inferior field of view should extend from the distal shaft of the tibia through the plantar fat pad.
- The left-to-right field of view should include the musculature of the foot (Figure 58–14).
- The anteroposterior field of view should extend from the distal phalanges through the heel fat pad (see Figure 58–14).
- A coronal image of the foot aligned to the metatarsals is shown in Figure 58–14.
- Note: The radiologist at your imaging facility may allow the anteroposterior field of view to extend from the distal phalanges to the distal tarsal bones. If the smaller field of view is used, then the superior-to-inferior field of view would extend from the dorsal surface fat to the plantar surface fat.

Phase and Frequency Orientation

- Phase: Superior to inferior
- Frequency: Right to left
- Phase and frequency orientations may be swapped to reduce motion artifact.

Saturation Band Placement

- A saturation band may be used to eliminate or reduce motion artifact.
- If used, the saturation band should be placed superior to the field of view.

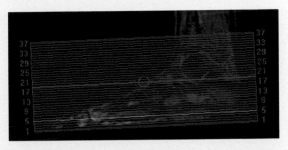

FIGURE 58–9. Sagittal scout image showing slice overlay for a coronal sequence aligned with the plantar surface (option 1). Note the good positioning of the foot so that the lower leg and foot form a 90-degree angle.

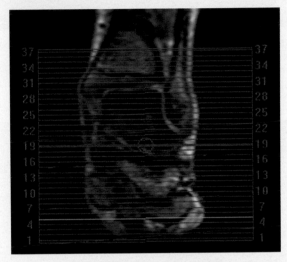

FIGURE 58–10. Axial scout image of the foot showing slice overlay for a coronal sequence aligned with the plantar surface (option 1).

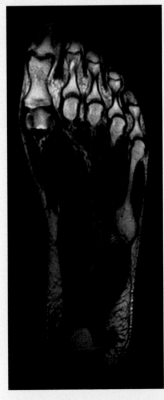

FIGURE 58–11. Coronal T2-weighted image aligned with the plantar surface of the foot (option 1).

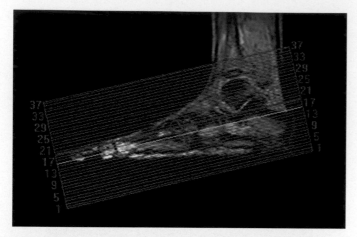

FIGURE 58–12. Sagittal scout image showing slice overlay for a coronal sequence aligned with the metatarsals (option 2). Note the good positioning of the foot so that the lower leg and foot form a 90-degree angle.

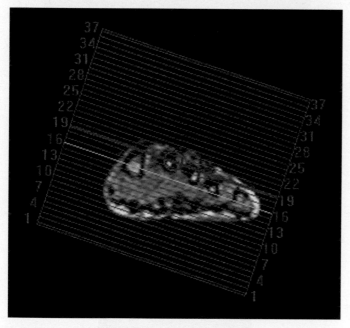

FIGURE 58–13. Axial scout image of the foot showing slice overlay for a coronal sequence aligned with the metatarsals (option 2).

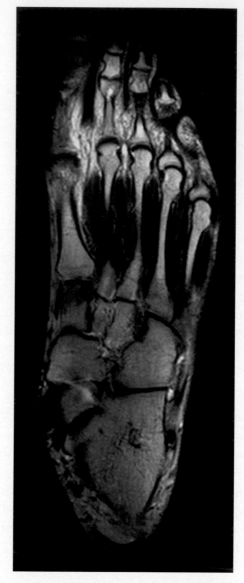

FIGURE 58–14. Coronal T2 image of the foot aligned with the metatarsals (option 2). Compare Figures 58–11 and 58–14 and notice how the metatarsals are better visualized.

IMAGING APPLICATION

TABLE 58-1 • General Sequences												
General Sequences	**TR**		**TE**		**TI**		**FA (degrees)**		**NEX**		**SLT/GAP (in millimeters)**	
	1.5 T	**3.0 T**	**1.5 T**	**3.0 T**	**1.5 T**	**3.0 T**	**1.5 T**	**3.0 T**	**1.5 T**	**3.0 T**	**1.5 T**	**3.0 T**
T1 SE	500	500	15	20	N/A	N/A	90	90	3	3	3/0.3	3/0.3
T2 SE	4500	4000	70	70	N/A	N/A	90	90	3	3	3/0.3	3/0.3
PD	3000	2500	30	30	N/A	N/A	90	90	3	3	3/0.3	3/0.3
STIR	3000	3000	60	15	150	220	90	90	3	3	3/0.3	3/0.3
T1 SE post C+	500	500	15	20	N/A	N/A	90	90	3	3	3/0.3	3/0.3

Abbreviations: N/A, not applicable; PD, proton density; SE, spin echo; STIR, short tau inversion recovery.

SUGGESTED IMAGING APPLICATION VARIATIONS

Arthrogram

The injection of contrast media and/or gas in the capsular space may be requested. The requested media will be injected, usually under the guidance of fluoroscopy. The patient will then be imaged in MRI. Sequences in addition to the routine protocol may be requested by the radiologist.

Trauma

The attending radiologist and/or the requesting physician may ask for additional sequences or orthogonal planes depending on the traumatic injury.

Tumor

A tumor protocol may require sequences in addition to the routine shoulder protocol and a larger field of view to include the lesion. Additional pre- and postcontrast sequences may be included. Three-orthogonal-plane postcontrast sequences may be of benefit to the radiologist. The technologist should follow the protocol provided at their facility.

59

Lower Extremity Arthrogram

The injection of contrast media in to the capsular space (direct method) may be requested. The requested media will be injected, usually under the guidance of fluoroscopy. The patient will then be imaged in MRI. Sequences in addition to the routine protocol may be requested by the radiologist. As the arthrogram may be performed on a variety of joints, use the guidelines for the specific joint of interest.

This is an example of a hip arthrogram (Figures 59–1 to 59–3).

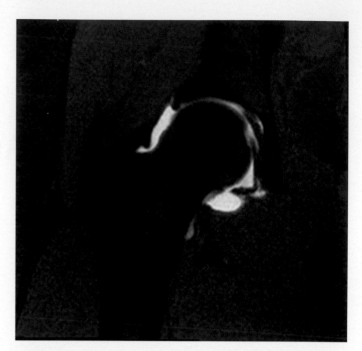

FIGURE 59–2. Coronal image of a hip arthrogram. Note the hyperintense contrast injected into the joint space.

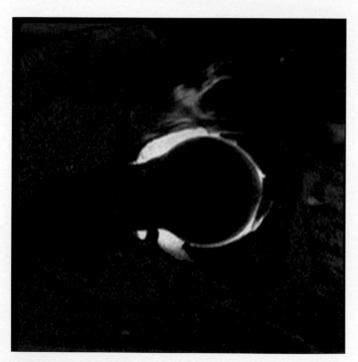

FIGURE 59–1. Axial image of a hip arthrogram. Note the hyperintense contrast injected into the joint space.

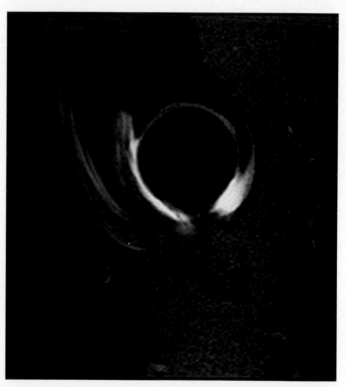

FIGURE 59–3. Sagittal image of a hip arthrogram. Note the hyperintense contrast injected into the joint space.

PART III

Registry Review

MR Review Questions

1. **What orientation are the vectors of the ¹H protons pointing in if they are in random alignment?**

   A. Mz

   B. Mxy

   C. M-z

   D. All directions

2. **What is the status of the protons when they are in the antiparallel orientation?**

   A. Low energy

   B. Mid-range energy

   C. High energy

   D. In the Mxy

3. **What role do the protons that are aligned antiparallel to the main magnetic field play?**

   A. They contribute to signal for image detail and contrast.

   B. They do not contribute signal.

   C. They contribute most of the signal.

   D. Their high-energy signal appears in the outer area of k-space.

4. **What is the mass number the sum of?**

   A. Protons

   B. Protons and electrons

   C. Protons and neutrons

   D. Protons, neutrons, and electrons

5. **What causes resonance to occur?**

   A. Main magnetic field

   B. Larmor frequency

   C. Gradient magnetic field

   D. Shim coils

6. **What best defines the time required for the longitudinal magnetization to recover 63%?**

   A. Spin-lattice relaxation

   B. Spin-spin lattice

   C. T2* relaxation

   D. Net magnetization

7. **Where does the dephasing of the net magnetization occur?**

   A. Mz

   B. Mxy

   C. M-z

   D. Along the Gpe

8. **What is the gyromagnetic ratio used for?**

   A. To determine magnetic field homogeneity

   B. Magnetic shielding requirements

   C. To determine the 5-gauss line

   D. To calculate the Larmor frequency

9. **What is another name for the sum of the individual magnetic moments?**

   A. Diamagnetic magnetization

   B. Net magnetization

   C. Precession

   D. Resonance

10. **What percentage of the protons will return to the longitudinal magnetization in 5 T1 relaxation times?**

    A. 100%

    B. 63%

    C. 42%

    D. 37%

11. **What is another name for T2 decay?**

    A. Spin-lattice relaxation time

    B. Spin-spin relaxation

    C. Free-induction decay

    D. Longitudinal magnetization

12. **How should the protons in the main magnetic field be described?**

    A. In random alignment with the main magnetic field

    B. Orientated in the transverse plane

    C. Aligned with the main magnetic field

    D. Positioned along the Mz axis

13. **What is the gyromagnetic ratio for ^{1}H?**

    A. 42.58 MHz/T

    B. 63% of 1 T1 relaxation time

    C. 23 mT/M

    D. Depends on the main magnetic field strength

14. **What is the magnetic field strength in tesla for a 5000-gauss magnet?**

    A. 10 T

    B. 5 T

    C. 1 T

    D. 0.5 T

15. **How will a tissue that is considered to have a long T2 appear on a T2-weighted pulse sequence?**

    A. Bright

    B. Intermediate

    C. Dark

    D. Isointense

16. **How will fat appear on a T1-weighted pulse sequence?**

    A. Bright

    B. Intermediate

    C. Dark

    D. Isointense

17. **What is the Larmor frequency for ^{1}H in a 10,000 Gauss MRI unit?**

    A. 42.58 MHz/T

    B. Depends on the gyromagnetic ratio of ^{1}H

    C. 42.58 MHz

    D. Depends on the main magnetic field strength

18. **Of the following, which is the strongest T1-weighted pulse sequence?**

    A. TR = 500 ms; TE = 40 ms

    B. TR = 350 ms; TE = 40 ms

    C. TR = 500 ms; TE = 30 ms

    D. TR = 350 ms; TE = 30 ms

19. **How will cerebrospinal fluid appear on a T1-weighted pulse sequence?**

    A. Bright

    B. Intermediate

    C. Dark

    D. Isointense

20. **How are the spin-spin relaxation and the intrinsic inhomogeneities of the main magnetic best referenced?**

    A. T1

    B. Spin density

    C. T2

    D. T2*

21. **What type of information is stored in the central portion of k-space?**

    A. Low signal, contrast

    B. Low signal, detail

    C. High signal, contrast

    D. High signal, detail

22. **What unit of measurement is the homogeneity of the main magnetic field measured in?**

    A. mT/M

    B. βo

    C. M

    D. ppm

23. **How should the radiofrequency (RF) receiver coil be positioned to the static magnetic field?**

    A. Transverse

    B. Parallel

    C. Oblique

    D. Horizontal

24. Of the following components, which is used to develop homogeneity of the magnetic field?

    A. Shim coils
    B. Gradient coils
    C. Magnetic shielding
    D. RF coils

25. What term is used to define the slope of the gradient field?

    A. Gradient strength
    B. Slew rate
    C. Maximum amplitude
    D. Rise time

26. What component is the term *fill factor* best associated with?

    A. Cryostat
    B. RF coil
    C. Shim coil
    D. Magnetic shielding

27. What is used to cool a resistive magnet?

    A. Liquid helium
    B. Air
    C. Water
    D. Both liquid helium and nitrogen

28. What component is used to restrict stray RF signals from entering the MRI suite?

    A. RF coils
    B. Shim coils
    C. RF shielding
    D. Active shielding

29. What are the units of measurement G/cm and mT/m best associated with?

    A. Specific absorption rate
    B. Larmor frequency
    C. Tissue heating
    D. Gradient strength

30. Where are the current-carrying wire windings of a superconductive magnet located?

    A. Liquid hydrogen cryostat
    B. Liquid nitrogen cryostat
    C. Liquid helium cryostat
    D. Water bath

31. What effect might occur if the door to the MRI suite is left open?

    A. The homogeneity of the magnet will be compromised.
    B. The magnetic fringe field will extend outside the suite.
    C. RF energy may enter the suite.
    D. The magnet will overheat.

32. Which component is used to encode the RF signal into the patient?

    A. RF transmit coil
    B. RF receive coil
    C. Gradient coils
    D. Shim coils

33. What would 1 L of liquid helium equal in a gaseous state?

    A. 820 L
    B. 760 L
    C. 720 L
    D. 695 L

34. What perimeter around an MRI unit is considered safe to the public?

    A. 5-gauss line
    B. RF field
    C. Outside the MRI suite
    D. A nearby hallway

35. What produces the noise in an MRI unit?

    A. Main magnetic field turning on/off
    B. Liquid cryogen pumps
    C. Shim coils adjusting the homogeneity of the magnetic field
    D. Gradient coils turning on/off

36. What is the temperature of liquid helium?

    A. −317°F
    B. −320°F
    C. −452°F
    D. −460°F

37. **Which of the following definitions best defines signal-to-noise ratio?**

    A. Ability to differentiate between small structures

    B. Difference between high and low signal

    C. Difference between the signal and graininess of the image

    D. Calculating the signal difference between 2 different points of reference

38. **What effect does decreasing the slice thickness have on spatial resolution?**

    A. Increases

    B. Decreases

    C. No effect

39. **What effect does increasing the magnetic field strength have on the signal-to-noise ratio?**

    A. Increases

    B. Decreases

    C. No effect

40. **What effect does decreasing the receiver bandwidth have on the signal-to-noise ratio?**

    A. Increases

    B. Decreases

    C. No effect

41. **What effect does decreasing the echo time have on the signal-to-noise ratio?**

    A. Increases

    B. Decreases

    C. No effect

42. **What effect does increasing the repetition time have on the signal-to-noise ratio?**

    A. Increases

    B. Decreases

    C. No effect

43. **What effect does decreasing the echo time have on scan time?**

    A. Increases

    B. Decreases

    C. No effect

44. **What effect does doubling the number of signal excitations have on the signal-to-noise ratio?**

    A. Increases

    B. Decreases

    C. No effect

45. **Which method will increase the signal-to-noise ratio by approximately 40%?**

    A. Reducing the receiver bandwidth by one-half

    B. Increasing the echo time

    C. Increasing the slice thickness

    D. Increasing the number of signal excitations

46. **How does noise appear in an image?**

    A. Signal loss

    B. Undetectable

    C. Bright

    D. Grainy

47. **What effect does using a smaller RF receiver coil have on the signal-to-noise ratio?**

    A. Increases

    B. Decreases

    C. No effect

48. **How would an increase in TE affect T1-weighted contrast?**

    A. Increased

    B. Decreased

    C. Not affected

    D. Increased by the $\sqrt{2}$

49. **What does the term *flip angle* best refer to?**

    A. Rephasing of the ^{1}H protons

    B. Tipping the protons away from the longitudinal plane

    C. Reorientation of the protons as a result of the T2 effect

    D. Regrowth of the ^{1}H protons along the longitudinal axis

50. **How should magnets operating in the range of 1.0 to 2.0 T be referred to?**

    A. Ultra-high field

    B. High field

    C. Mid-field

    D. Low field

51. **Which of the following types of magnets would best be used for MR spectroscopy?**

    A. Resistive

    B. Superconductive

    C. Permanent

    D. A and B only

52. **What device is used to either excite or detect the MR signal?**

    A. Magnetic shielding

    B. Gradient coils

    C. Shim coils

    D. RF coils

53. **Which of the following would best define a quench?**

    A. A sudden loss of superconductivity

    B. A power failure

    C. A reduced homogeneity

    D. Something that only occurs in resistive magnets

54. **What causes the precession of the protons?**

    A. RF signal

    B. T2 relaxation

    C. Main magnetic field

    D. Gradient field

55. **Where are the data collected?**

    A. Along the Gss

    B. Along the Gpe

    C. Along the Gro

56. **In which axis is an RF artifact best seen?**

    A. Slice selection axis

    B. Frequency encoding axis

    C. Phase encoding axis

    D. All of the above

57. **How much of a gap is recommended to reduce the effects of cross-talk?**

    A. 10%

    B. 20%

    C. 30%

    D. 40%

58. **How can susceptibility artifacts best be limited?**

    A. Spin echo pulse sequences

    B. Presaturation bands

    C. Gradient echo pulse sequences

    D. Gating

59. **What is another name for a Gibbs artifact?**

    A. Chemical shift

    B. Aliasing

    C. Ghosting

    D. Truncation

60. **Of the following, which method would be recommended to correct for phase mismapping?**

    A. Increasing the FOV

    B. Gating

    C. Presaturation

    D. Decreasing NEX

61. **What artifact may result due to the difference in the precessional frequencies of fat and water?**

    A. Chemical shift artifact

    B. Wraparound artifact

    C. Gibbs artifact

    D. Zipper artifact

62. **What characteristic is apparent when identifying a ghost artifact?**

    A. Appears in the phase-encoding direction

    B. Appears along the slice-selection axis

    C. Results as a misfiring of the gradients

    D. Appears along the readout gradient

63. **How can flow-related ghosting artifacts be reduced?**

    A. Increasing the FOV

    B. Increasing the number of signal averages

    C. Presaturation

    D. Aliasing

64. **What causes a wraparound artifact?**

    A. Readout gradient error

    B. Small FOV

    C. Pulsatile motion

    D. None of the above

65. **What type of artifact would a loss of signal/signal void best represent?**

    A. Metal artifact

    B. Chemical shift artifact

    C. Truncation artifact

    D. Ghosting

66. **What type of artifact could be described as a misregistration of signal between fat and water?**

    A. Truncation artifact

    B. Chemical shift artifact

    C. Wraparound artifact

    D. Aliasing

67. **How can partial voluming be compensated?**

    A. Increasing the FOV

    B. Increasing the number of signal averages

    C. Changing the phase- and frequency-encoding directions

    D. Decreasing the slice thickness

68. **Of the following artifacts, which may result from (1) RF signals entering the scanning suite, (2) interference in electronic devices in the MRI suite, (3) a material producing static electricity, or (4) an interference caused by AC fluctuations?**

    A. Truncation

    B. Wraparound

    C. RF

    D. Chemical shift

69. **If a presaturation pulse is positioned outside of the FOV and placed over the blood vessels entering into the scanning volume, how would the blood appear in the scanned tissue?**

    A. Hyperintense

    B. Isointense to blood in an adjacent blood vessel

    C. Hypointense

70. **What term is used when referring to the flow of blood that is in the opposite direction to the slice selection?**

    A. In phase

    B. Co-current flow

    C. Slice phenomenon

    D. Countercurrent flow

71. **What is used to trigger a pulse sequence in a cardiac gating sequence?**

    A. QRS peak

    B. T wave

    C. R-to-R interval

    D. None of the above

72. **Which of the following best describes laminar flow at the center of the lumen of a normal vessel?**

    A. Fluctuates and is erratic across the diameter of the vessel

    B. Spirals

    C. Is faster than at the vessel wall

    D. Appears bright due to slow flow

73. **According to the entry slice phenomenon, how would the signal from blood appear in the initial slice in the countercurrent direction?**

    A. Nulled

    B. Isointense

    C. Hypointense

    D. Hyperintense

74. **How do gadolinium-based contrast agents primarily enhance central nervous system–type pathologies?**

    A. Normal blood flow

    B. Breakdown in the blood-brain barrier

    C. The volume of contrast agent used

    D. Delayed timing in imaging after injection

75. **What is a chelation bond used to bind?**

    A. Two chemicals together

    B. Heavy metals to other chemicals

    C. Rare-earth metal to a ligand

    D. Two ligands together

76. **What is the chelate component used in Gd-DTPA?**

    A. Gadolinium

    B. Sodium

    C. Dimeglumine

    D. DTPA

77. **How do gadolinium-based contrast agents affect tissue weighting?**

    A. Lengthen T1

    B. Shorten T1

    C. Lengthen T2

    D. None of the above

78. **What are gadolinium-based contrast agents considered to be?**

    A. Superparamagnetic

    B. Paramagnetic

    C. Diamagnetic

    D. Ferromagnetic

79. **What pulse sequence is recommended to be used in conjunction with gadolinium-based contrast agents?**

    A. T1 weighted

    B. Spin density weighted

    C. T2 weighted

    D. Inversion recovery

80. **Of the following, which is a false statement regarding the requirements for designing an intravenous (IV) gadolinium-based MRI contrast agent?**

    A. It must be able to be absorbed in the villi of the large colon and excreted via the gastrointestinal tract.

    B. It must have low toxicity.

    C. It must be able to alter the T1 and T2 imaging parameters.

    D. It must demonstrate tissue-specific distribution.

81. **Which of the following is a contraindication when administering gadolinium-based contrast agents?**

    A. Pregnancy

    B. Anemia

    C. Lactation

    D. All the above

82. **Which component is used to encode the RF signal into the patient?**

    A. RF transmit coil

    B. RF receive coil

    C. Gradient coils

    D. Shim coils

83. **Which of the following pulse sequences is best represented by a 90-degree RF pulse followed by a 180-degree pulse?**

    A. Spin echo

    B. T1 weighted

    C. Gradient echo

    D. Inversion recovery

84. **Which of the following pulse sequences is best represented by a 180-90-180–degree pulse sequence?**

    A. Spin echo

    B. T1 weighted

    C. Gradient echo

    D. Inversion recovery

85. **Which gradient coil is activated as the slice selection gradient coil when imaging in the coronal axis?**

    A. Gx

    B. Gy

    C. Gz

86. **What additional component is activated during the excitation pulse in a spin echo sequence?**

    A. Gss

    B. Gpe

    C. Gfe

    D. Both B and C

87. **Which of the following pulse sequences is best represented by a 90-degree RF pulse and then followed by a gradient reversal?**

    A. Spin echo

    B. T1 weighted

    C. Gradient echo

    D. Inversion recovery

88. **Which component is active during the rephasing of the transverse magnetization in a spin echo pulse sequence?**

    A. Gpe

    B. Gss

    C. Gro

    D. ADC

89. **What term is used to define the time in which 69% of the T1 relaxation of a given tissue crosses the Mxy?**

    A. Spin-lattice relaxation

    B. Null point

    C. Spin-spin lattice relaxation

    D. Dephasing of the transverse magnetization

90. **The time between the initial RF pulse and the activation of the RF receive coil is referred to as which of the following?**

    A. TR

    B. TE

    C. TI

    D. Flip angle

91. What is the term used to define the time between the initial 90-degree pulses?

    A. TR
    B. TE
    C. TI
    D. Flip angle

92. In a spin echo pulse sequence, what axis are the data collected along?

    A. Slice selection
    B. Longitudinal
    C. Phase encoding
    D. Readout

93. In a gradient echo pulse sequence, what rephases the protons?

    A. TR
    B. 180-degree pulse
    C. Flip angle
    D. Gro

94. What is the image weighting if obtained with a 70- to 110-degree flip angle and short TE value?

    A. T1 weighted
    B. Proton density weighted
    C. Inversion recovery weighted
    D. T2* weighted

95. What purpose does the initial 180-degree pulse serve?

    A. Uses the protons aligned in the antiparallel orientation to collect data for imaging
    B. Increases signal
    C. Decreases scan time
    D. Provides additional time for 2 tissues with similar relaxation times to separate as they return to the Mz

96. What is the extent of the TR for an inversion recovery pulse sequence?

    A. Initial 180-degree inversion pulse to the next 180-degree inversion pulse
    B. Initial excitation pulse to the next inversion pulse
    C. Rephasing pulse to the next inversion pulse
    D. Excitation pulse to the readout pulse

97. Which pulse sequence acquires all phase-encoding lines in a single repetition time?

    A. Conventional spin echo
    B. Rapid acquisition with relaxation enhancement

    C. Echo planar imaging
    D. Gradient echo

98. With which pulse sequence are the terms *echo train length* and *turbo factor* best associated?

    A. RARE
    B. Inversion recovery
    C. Gradient echo
    D. Conventional spin echo

99. What component is used to restrict stray RF signals from entering the MRI suite?

    A. RF coils
    B. Shim coils
    C. RF shielding
    D. Active shielding

100. Of the following, which may be used when referring to the ^{1}H protons aligned with the βo?

    A. Transverse plane
    B. Mxy
    C. Longitudinal axis
    D. M-z

101. What symbol is used to best refer to the oscillating magnetic field produced by the RF coil?

    A. M
    B. βo
    C. β_1
    D. M-z

102. How does an increase in the effective TE affect scan time?

    A. Increased
    B. Decreased
    C. Not affected

103. Which of the following weighted sequences would be produced with a TR of 1200 milliseconds (ms) and a TE of 25 ms?

    A. T1 weighted
    B. T2 weighted
    C. Proton density weighted
    D. T2* weighted

104. **Which parameter is used to define the time between the initial 180-degree pulse and the excitation pulse in an inversion recovery sequence?**

    A. TI
    B. TR
    C. TE
    D. TE/2

105. **What is the scan time for a data acquisition of:**

TR = 4000 ms	NEX = 2
TE = 90 ms	Phase-encoding steps = 256
FOV = 25 cm	Frequency-encoding steps = 128
ETL = 4	Slice thickness = 10 mm

    A. 4.2 minutes
    B. 8.5 minutes
    C. 12.4 minutes
    D. 34.1 minutes

106. **What is the gyromagnetic ratio for the hydrogen proton in a 1.5-T MRI system?**

    A. 1-to-1
    B. 63.87 MHz/T
    C. 42.58 MHz/T
    D. 63.87 MHz

107. **Of the following, which is used to denote the Larmor frequency for a 1.5-T MRI unit?**

    A. Mz
    B. MHz/T
    C. MHz
    D. mT/m

108. **What is another name for the protons that are aligned parallel with the main magnetic field?**

    A. Spin up
    B. High energy
    C. Spin down
    D. Both A and B

109. **What is the following calculation used for: $\omega_o = \beta_o \times \gamma$?**

    A. Magnetic field strength
    B. Larmor frequency
    C. SAR
    D. Gyromagnetic ratio

110. **What term is used to describe the spinning (gyrating motion) of the hydrogen proton around the main magnetic field?**

    A. Precession
    B. Magnetic moment
    C. Alignment
    D. Net magnetization vector

111. **What causes resonance to occur?**

    A. Net magnetization
    B. Magnetic field strength
    C. Gradient field
    D. Larmor frequency

112. **Where would the net magnetization vector be oriented if a 90-degree pulse is applied?**

    A. Mz
    B. Transverse plane
    C. Longitudinal plane
    D. M-z

113. **What amount of time is required for *all* of the net magnetization to return to the Mz?**

    A. 1 T1 relaxation time
    B. TR = 1000 ms
    C. TE = 90 ms
    D. 5 T1 relaxation times

114. **Where does the dephasing of the net magnetization occur?**

    A. Mz
    B. Transverse plane
    C. Longitudinal plane
    D. M-z

115. **Of the following, which is an example of an intrinsic contrast parameter?**

    A. TR
    B. TE
    C. Flip angle
    D. Proton density

116. **What structures compose the brainstem from superior to inferior order?**

    A. Midbrain, pons, and medulla oblongata
    B. Pond, midbrain, and medulla oblongata
    C. Medulla oblongata, midbrain, and pons
    D. Midbrain, pons, and medulla oblongata

117. **Of the following, which would demonstrate a short T1 relaxation?**

    A. Fat

    B. CSF

    C. Ligaments

    D. Menisci

118. **What is another name for the initial RF pulse?**

    A. Rephasing

    B. TR

    C. Excitation

    D. T1

119. **Of the following statements, which are true regarding what effect a short TE will have on image weighting?**

    1. Dephasing of the net magnetization is reduced

    2. TE controls T2 weighting

    3. Used for T1-weighted imaging

    A. 1 and 2 only

    B. 2 and 3 only

    C. 1 and 3 only

    D. 1, 2, and 3

120. **Where in k-space are the low spatial frequencies that produce contrast located?**

    A. Center

    B. Periphery

    C. Top half

    D. Bottom half

121. **What effect will result if the voxel volume (slice thickness) is increased?**

    A. Decreased partial volume averaging

    B. Increased signal

    C. Increased spatial resolution

    D. Increased number of pixels

122. **Of the following, which will increase signal?**

    1. Increase TR

    2. Decrease the receiver bandwidth

    3. Increase NEX

    A. 1 and 2 only

    B. 2 and 3 only

    C. 1 and 3 only

    D. 1, 2, and 3

123. **Of the following, which are correct about high magnetic field strength?**

    1. Increases the net magnetization

    2. Increases signal-to-noise ratio

    3. Decreases chemical shift artifact

    A. 1 and 2 only

    B. 2 and 3 only

    C. 1 and 3 only

    D. 1, 2, and 3

124. **Of the following, which will reduce the signal-to-noise ratio?**

    1. Short TR

    2. Low flip angle (20 degrees)

    3. Increasing the NEX or NSA

    A. 1 and 2 only

    B. 2 and 3 only

    C. 1 and 3 only

    D. 1, 2, and 3

125. **In a conventional spin echo pulse sequence, what components are activated during the encoding of the signal?**

    A. 90-degree RF and Gss

    B. Gpe and Gro

    C. Gro and ADC

    D. 180-degree RF and Gss

126. **If using an ETL or TF of 10, how many times will the Gpe be turned on/off during each TR cycle?**

    A. 1

    B. 2

    C. 10

    D. 20

127. **What is the purpose of the second 180-degree pulse in an inversion recovery pulse sequence?**

    A. Invert the net magnetization into the M-z

    B. Dephase the M

    C. Encode the signal

    D. Rephase

128. **In a fast spin echo or turbo spin echo pulse sequence, what is the purpose of the additional 180-degree pulses within each TR cycle?**

    A. Invert the net magnetization into the M-z

    B. Dephase the M

C. Encode the signal

D. Rephase

129. **The term *null point* is best applied to which of the following pulse sequence?**

A. Conventional spin echo

B. Gradient echo

C. Fast or turbo spin echo

D. Inversion recovery

130. **Where does the TE in an inversion recovery pulse sequence extend?**

A. Initial 180-degree pulse to when the receiver RF coil is activated

B. Initial 180-degree pulse until the second 180-degree pulse

C. Initial 180-degree pulse to the 90-degree pulse

D. Excitation pulse to when the receiver RF coil is activated

131. **In a gradient echo pulse sequence, which component is responsible for rephasing?**

A. RF

B. Gss

C. Gpe

D. Gro

132. **When acquiring a coronal image of the shoulder, where would a presaturation pulse most likely be positioned to control for vascular ghosting?**

A. Above

B. Anterior

C. Medial

D. Posterior

133. **Of the following MRA techniques, which manipulates the longitudinal magnetization by saturating the stationary spins so that the inflowing spins produce a bright signal?**

A. Time of flight

B. Phase contrast

C. Velocity encoding

D. Contrast enhanced

134. **The use of RF pulses outside the FOV best describes which of the following methods used to control phase mismapping?**

A. Swapping phase and frequency

B. Presaturation

C. Respiratory compensation

D. Cardiac gating

135. **Techniques such as anti-aliasing and no phase wrap may be used to control for which of the following artifacts?**

A. Chemical shift

B. Cross-talk/excitation

C. Truncation

D. Wraparound

136. **What artifact is produced when adjacent slices receive energy from an RF excitation pulse?**

A. Cross-talk/excitation

B. Wraparound

C. Truncation

D. Chemical shift

137. **Of the following pulse sequences, which would be the best to control for a magnetic susceptibility–type artifact?**

A. Spin echo

B. Gradient echo

C. Inversion recovery

138. **What artifact may be produced by the frequent opening and closing of the door entering into the MRI suite?**

A. Truncation

B. RF

C. Cross-talk/excitation

D. Magnetic susceptibility

139. **Of the following artifacts, which would *not* appear along the frequency axis?**

A. Chemical shift

B. Aliasing

C. Motion

D. Zipper

140. **Which of the following components would be responsible for encoding the signal in the patient's body?**

A. RF transit coil

B. Gradient coils

C. Shim coils

D. RF receiver coil

141. Which of the following components is responsible for maintaining magnetic field homogeneity?

    A. Magnetic shielding

    B. Shim coils

    C. RF shielding

    D. Gradient coils

142. *Rise time*, *slew rate*, and *duty cycle* are terms used to describe which of the following components?

    A. Magnetic field

    B. RF coils

    C. Magnetic shielding

    D. Gradient coils

143. How are the current-carrying windings in a superconducting magnet cooled?

    A. Air conditioning

    B. Water

    C. Liquid helium

    D. Magnet cooling is not required.

144. Which of the following components uses the term *parts per million* (ppm) to define the quality?

    A. Magnetic field

    B. Gradient coils

    C. Magnetic shielding

    D. RF shielding

145. What does the term *fringe field* most commonly refer to?

    A. 5-gauss

    B. Gradient field

    C. Magnetic field

    D. RF receiver coil

146. What effect does increasing the magnetic field strength have on the SNR?

    A. Increase

    B. Decrease

    C. No effect

147. Of the following, which would probably *not* be associated with nonferromagnetic implants such as those used in the hip?

    A. Torque and attraction

    B. Heating

    C. Artifact production

    D. None of the above

148. What is the maximum SAR level for the whole body?

    A. 3

    B. 4

    C. 8

    D. 12

149. Which of the following pulse sequences would most likely produce the greatest SAR?

    A. Gradient echo

    B. Fast/turbo spin echo

    C. Inversion recovery

    D. Conventional spin echo

150. How are most gadolinium-based contrast agents primarily excreted from the body?

    A. Kidneys

    B. Liver

    C. Gastrointestinal tract

    D. Lungs

151. What effect will gadolinium have on areas of the brain if the blood-brain barrier has been disrupted?

    A. Hyperintense (bright)

    B. Isointense to white matter

    C. Hypointense (low signal)

    D. Magnetic susceptibility effect will suppress the signal in the surrounding tissue

152. How will CSF appear in a patient with hydrocephalus following an injection of a gadolinium-based contrast agent?

    A. Dark

    B. Intermediate to bright

    C. Bright

    D. Very bright

153. Of the following structures, which would not normally enhance with gadolinium?

    A. Tumors

    B. Infection

    C. Active multiple sclerosis

    D. Edema

154. Of the following, which may be a contradiction to the use of gadolinium?

    A. Pregnancy

    B. Follow-up post radiation therapy

    C. Infections

    D. Postoperative diskectomy

155. **The attraction force of an object when exposed to a magnetic field depends on which of the following factors?**

    1. Mass of the object
    2. Ferromagnetic properties of the object
    3. Magnetic field strength

    A. 1 and 2 only
    B. 2 and 3 only
    C. 1 and 3 only
    D. 1, 2, and 3

156. **What do hydrogen protons tend to do when exposed to a strong homogenous magnetic field?**

    A. They align perpendicular to the magnetic field.
    B. They align parallel to the magnetic field.
    C. Slightly more than half align parallel and the remaining align antiparallel.
    D. Equal amounts align parallel and antiparallel.

157. **Why does CSF appear bright on a T2-weighted image?**

    A. CSF has a long T1 relaxation.
    B. CSF has a short T1 relaxation.
    C. CSF has a long T2 relaxation.
    D. CSF has a short T2 relaxation.

158. **For an axial image, which gradient coil axis is assigned for slice selection?**

    A. Gx
    B. Gy
    C. Gz

159. **A patient weighing 220 lb weighs how much in kilograms?**

    A. 22
    B. 44
    C. 100
    D. 110

160. **What term best describes the ^{1}H protons outside of the main magnet?**

    A. Parallel alignment
    B. Random orientation
    C. Precession
    D. Phase

161. **How are the ^{1}H protons oriented when the patient is moved into the main magnetic field?**

    A. Longitudinal magnetization
    B. Mxy

    C. Random alignment
    D. M

162. **What does the symbol Mz indicate?**

    A. Net magnetization
    B. Transverse magnetization
    C. Longitudinal magnetization
    D. Static magnetic field

163. **What other term can be used to depict the protons that align in the antiparallel orientation?**

    A. High energy
    B. Transverse energy
    C. Longitudinal magnetization
    D. Net magnetization

164. **What do the ^{1}H protons precess around?**

    A. βo
    B. Mz
    C. Mxy
    D. M

165. **Where is the net magnetization following a 90-degree RF pulse?**

    A. Mz
    B. Mxy
    C. M-z
    D. βo

166. **What is the sensitivity of ^{1}H?**

    A. 100
    B. 10
    C. 1
    D. 42.5 MHz

167. **What does 1 T equal?**

    A. 42.58 MHz
    B. 42.58 MHz/T
    C. 1000 Gauss
    D. 10,000 Gauss

168. **What information does a vector used to indicate the magnetic field or net magnetization as applied in MR provide?**

    A. Orientation and strength
    B. Speed and contrast
    C. Time and distance
    D. Frequency and magnetization

169. **What is the Larmor frequency used for?**

    A. To adjust the main magnetic field

    B. To align the protons with the magnetic field

    C. To move the net magnetization away from the Bo

    D. To be received by the RF receiver coil

170. **What term is used to describe the motion of the M in the βo?**

    A. Magnetic moment

    B. Parallel alignment

    C. Relaxation

    D. Precession

171. **What do the cruciate ligaments best relate to?**

    A. Shoulder

    B. Hip

    C. Wrist

    D. Knee

172. **What does 1 T1 relaxation time equal?**

    A. 37% dephased

    B. 63% recovery along the Mz

    C. 37% regrowth

    D. 100% return of the longitudinal magnetization

173. **When used properly, what amount of noise reduction have earplugs been proven to reduce during an MRI exam?**

    A. 5-10 dB

    B. 10-18 dB

    C. 10-30 dB

    D. 20-25 dB

174. **Of the following factors, which does *not* contribute to the SAR?**

    A. βo

    B. TR

    C. TE

    D. Volume of tissue within the RF coil

175. **How many electrons are needed to balance Gd^{3+}?**

    A. 0

    B. 1

    C. 2

    D. 3

176. **What type of a chemical bond is specifically used for gadolinium-based contrast agents?**

    A. Covalent

    B. Chelate

    C. Ionic

    D. Metallic

177. **What is Gd^{3+} considered to be?**

    A. A chelating agent

    B. A ligand

    C. A metallic ion

    D. An organic molecule

178. **Of the following, which is *not* required in the design of RF coils?**

    A. Positioning of the coil so the signal from the protons can be received along thelongitudinal axis of the magnetic field

    B. Homogeneity across the volume of the coil

    C. Fill factor

    D. "Q"

179. **What is the name of the vessel that houses the magnetic windings and liquid helium?**

    A. Dewar

    B. Tank

    C. Bucket

    D. Cryostat

180. **What is the term for the rapid loss of a superconductive magnet's superconductivity?**

    A. Boil-off rate

    B. Quench

    C. Fringe field

    D. Gauss line

181. **How much gadolinium-based contrast agent would you administer to an adult weighting 235 lb at 0.2 mL/kg?**

    A. 4.4 mL

    B. 4.7 mL

    C. 20.0 mL

    D. 21.2 mL

182. **Which best controls for the T1 weighting of an image?**

    A. TR

    B. TE

    C. Gro

    D. 20-degree FA

183. **Which of the following is improved as an RF receiver coil is better filled?**

    A. Spatial resolution
    B. Contrast-to-noise
    C. Signal-to-noise
    D. Patient comfort

184. **What effect would doubling the NEX have on the SNR?**

    A. SNR would remain the same
    B. Increase by a factor of 1.4
    C. Increase by a factor of 1.5
    D. Increase by a factor of 2

185. **What happens if the echo time is increased?**

    A. T1 weighting is increased.
    B. T2 weighting is increased.
    C. Proton density weighting is increased.
    D. T1 weighting is decreased.

186. **What MR exam might be indicated if the patient is complaining of pain and numbness in their left lower foot?**

    A. Lumbar spine
    B. Thoracic spine
    C. Cervical spine
    D. Brain

187. **How is the effect of magnetic field inhomogeneity on the FID best expressed?**

    A. T1 relaxation time
    B. T2 decay time
    C. T2* decay

188. **What is the ligand in gadopentetate dimeglumine (Gd-DTPA)?**

    A. Gadolinium
    B. DTPA
    C. DO3A
    D. Diamagnetic

189. **What is achieved when equal resolution in all reformatted planes is performed?**

    A. Isotropic imaging
    B. Rectangular pixel imaging
    C. Anisotropic imaging
    D. Switching the Gpe and Gro orientations

190. **Which of the following sequences is best depicted with a TR of 600 ms and a TE of 30 ms?**

    A. T1-weighted sequence
    B. Spin density–weighted sequence
    C. T2-weighted sequence
    D. Inversion recovery sequence

191. **Which of the following responses best characterizes a spin echo pulse sequence?**

    A. TR followed by the TE
    B. 90-degree excitation pulse followed by the 180-degree rephasing pulse
    C. TE is within the TR recovery
    D. Flip angle RF excitation pulse followed by the gradient reversal

192. **What specific parameter around the MR scanner is considered safe for individuals to stay outside of until they have been screened?**

    A. 0.5-gauss line
    B. 5-gauss line
    C. 5-T line
    D. 0.5-T line

193. **The measure of power absorbed per unit mass (W/kg) best describes which of the following?**

    A. SAR
    B. RF
    C. Gradient field strength
    D. Main magnet field strength

194. **Of the following, which would most likely *not* be a contraindication for performing an MRI examination?**

    A. Orthopedic implants
    B. Aneurysm clip
    C. Cardiac pacemaker
    D. Cochlear implants

195. **Which of the following best depicts the rotating frame of reference used to simplify the complex motion of precessing spins?**

    A. M_z
    B. β_0
    C. B_1
    D. M_{xy}

196. Which statement is correct regarding RF cable positioning?

    A. RF cables can be looped safely.

    B. RF cables can touch the patient's skin.

    C. It is acceptable to place a blanket over the patient and RF cable.

    D. It is advised to position the RF cable to exit the center of the bore.

197. Who was awarded the Nobel Prize in Physics in 1952 for their contributions in studying the chemical structure of substances?

    A. Felix Bloch and Edward Purcell

    B. Nicola Tesla

    C. Erwin Hahn

    D. Raymond Damadian

198. What was Isidor Rabi given credit for discovering?

    A. Gadolinium-based contrast agents

    B. RF coils

    C. Shim coil design

    D. Nuclear magnetic resonance

199. Who won a Nobel Prize in 2003 for their contribution in introducing gradients in the magnetic field to determine the origin of the radio waves emitted from the nuclei of the object of study?

    A. Paul Bottomley

    B. Raymond Damadian

    C. Paul Lauterbur

    D. Erwin Hahn

200. Who is given credit for performing the first scan of the human body?

    A. Raymond Damadian

    B. Paul Bottomley

    C. Paul Lauterbur

    D. Peter Mansfield

201. In Figure III–1A, what does 1A best represent?

    A. Body of the corpus callosum

    B. Rostrum

    C. Genu of the corpus callosum

    D. Splenium of the lateral ventricle

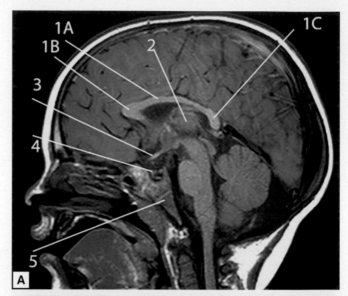

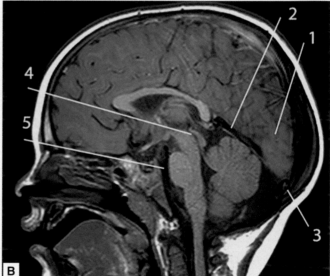

FIGURE III-1

202. In Figure III–1A, what does 2 best represent?

    A. Third ventricle

    B. Midbrain

    C. Massa intermedia

    D. Temporal lobe

203. In Figure III–1A, what does 3 best represent?

    A. Carotid artery

    B. Pituitary stalk

    C. Olfactory nerve

    D. Optic nerve

204. In Figure III–1A, what does 4 best represent?

A. Carotid artery

B. Infundibulum

C. Middle cerebral artery

D. Pituitary gland

205. In Figure III–1A, what does 5 best represent?

A. Sphenoid sinus

B. Clivus

C. Nasopharynx

D. Sella turcica

206. In Figure III–1B, what does 1 best represent?

A. Temporal lobe

B. Parietal lobe

C. Occipital lobe

D. Cerebellum

207. In Figure III–1B, what is the vascular structure 2?

A. Superior sagittal sinus

B. Straight sinus

C. Inferior sagittal sinus

D. Posterior cerebral artery

208. In Figure III–1B, what does 3 best represent?

A. Confluence of sinuses

B. Internal occipital protuberance

C. Sigmoid sinus

D. Internal jugular vein

209. In Figure III–1B, what does 4 best represent?

A. Inferior sagittal sinus

B. Quadrigeminal cistern

C. Great cerebral vein

D. Cerebral aqueduct

210. In Figure III–1B, what does 5 best represent?

A. Circle of Willis

B. Carotid artery

C. Basilar artery

D. Jugular vein

211. In Figure III–2, what does 1 best represent?

A. Central sulus

B. Lateral sulcus

C. Convolution

D. Longitudinal fissure

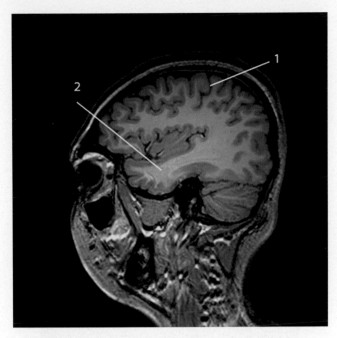

FIGURE III-2

212. In Figure III–2, what does 2 best represent?

A. Frontal lobe

B. Temporal lobe

C. Parietal lobe

D. Occipital lobe

213. In Figure III–3, what does 1 best represent?

A. Pontine blood vessels

B. Mastoid air cells

C. Seventh and eighth cranial nerves

D. 10th cranial nerve

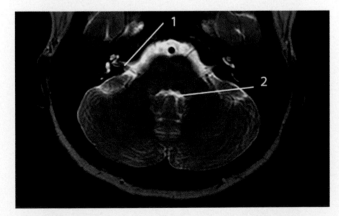

FIGURE III-3

214. In Figure III–3, what does 2 best represent?

A. Quadrigeminal cistern

B. Third ventricle

C. Fourth ventricle

D. Spinal canal

215. **In Figure III–4A, what does 1 best represent?**

    A. Optic nerve

    B. Anterior commissure

    C. Optic chiasm

    D. Optic track

216. **In Figure III–4A, what does 2 best represent?**

    A. Circle of Willis

    B. Basilar artery

    C. Lateral sinus

    D. Middle cerebral artery

217. **In Figure III–4B, what does 1 best represent?**

    A. Superior sagittal sinus

    B. Inferior sagittal sinus

    C. Straight sinus

    D. Basilar artery

218. **In Figure III–4B, what does the hypointense structure 2 best represent?**

    A. Tentorium cerebelli

    B. Posterior cerebral artery

    C. Quadrigeminal cistern

    D. Fourth ventricle

219. **In Figure III–4C, what does 1 best represent?**

    A. Pons

    B. Midbrain

    C. Temporal lobe

    D. Medulla oblongata

220. **In Figure III–4C, what does 2 best represent?**

    A. Cerebral aqueduct

    B. Straight sinus

    C. Basilar artery

    D. Straight sinus

221. **In Figure III–5, what does this image best represent?**

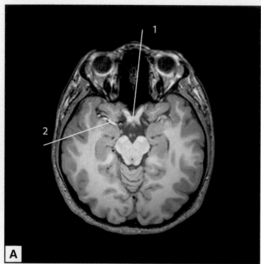

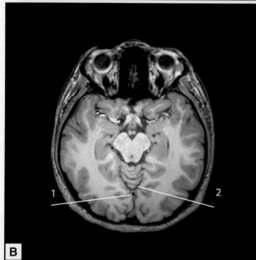

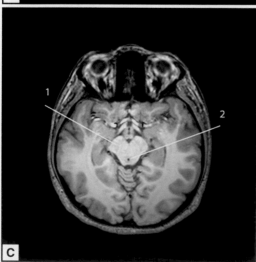

FIGURE III-4

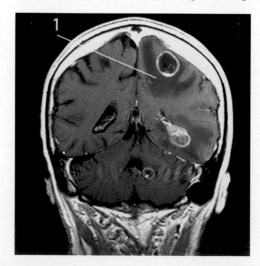

FIGURE III-5 Reprinted from Grey M.L., Alinani J.M. (2018). CT & MRI Pathology: A Pocket Atlas, 3rd ed. New York: McGraw-Hill, with permission from The McGraw-Hill Professional.

A. T1 weighted

B. Proton density weighted

C. T1 weighted with contrast

D. T2 weighted

222. In Figure III–6, what does this image best represent?

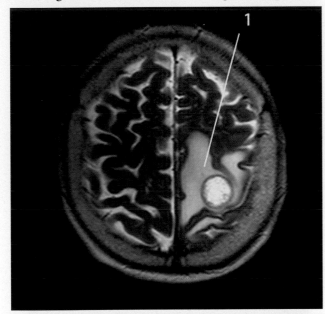

FIGURE III-6 Reprinted from Grey M.L., Alinani J.M. (2018). CT & MRI Pathology: A Pocket Atlas, 3rd ed. New York: McGraw-Hill, with permission from The McGraw-Hill Professional.

A. T1 weighted

B. Proton density weighted

C. T1 weighted with contrast

D. T2 weighted

223. In Figures III–5 and III–6, what does 1 best represent?

A. Edema

B. Infection

C. Tumor

D. CSF

224. In Figure III–7, what does 1 best represent?

A. Third ventricle

B. Foramen of Monro

C. Lateral ventricle

D. Middle cerebral artery

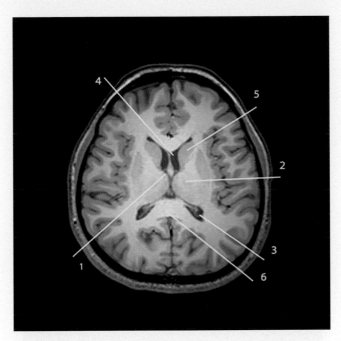

FIGURE III-7

225. In Figure III–7, what does 2 best represent?

A. Thalamus

B. Parietal lobe

C. Midbrain

D. Caudate nucleus

226. In Figure III–7, what does 3 best represent?

A. Lateral ventricle

B. Trigone of the lateral ventricle

C. Frontal horn

D. Body of the lateral ventricle

227. In Figure III–7, what does 4 best represent?

A. Temporal horn of the lateral ventricle

B. Body of the lateral ventricle

C. Trigone of the lateral ventricle

D. Frontal horn of the lateral ventricle

228. In Figure III–7, what does 5 best represent?

A. Head of the caudate nucleus

B. Thalamus

C. Massa intermedia

D. Internal capsule

229. In Figure III–7, what does 6 best represent?

A. Genu

B. Splenium

C. Thalamus

D. Massa intermedia

230. In Figure III–8, what does 1 best represent?

A. Posterior sinus

B. Lateral sinus

C. Free blood

D. Occipital vein

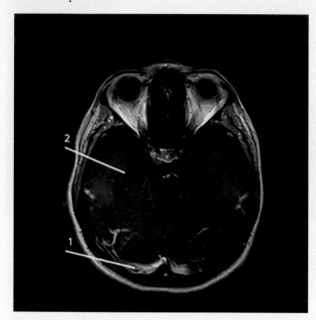

FIGURE III-8

231. In Figure III–8, what does 2 best represent?

A. Middle cerebral artery

B. Sylvian fissure

C. Inferior horn

D. Part of the sphenoid bone

232. In Figure III–9, what does the torn tendon 1 best represent?

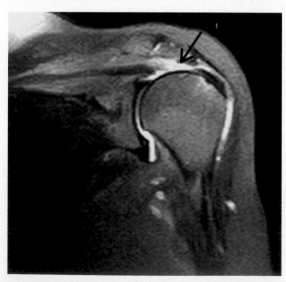

FIGURE III-9 Reprinted from Grey M.L., Alinani J.M. (2018). CT & MRI Pathology: A Pocket Atlas, 3rd ed. New York: McGraw-Hill, with permission from The McGraw-Hill Professional.

A. Supraspinatus tendon

B. Teres minor

C. Infraspinatus

D. Subscapularis

233. In Figure III–10, what does 1 best represent?

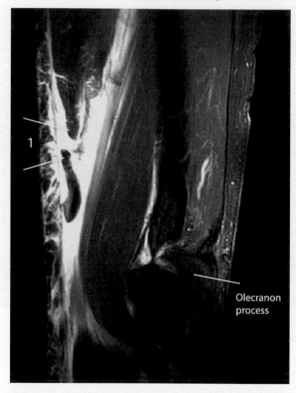

FIGURE III-10 Reprinted from Grey M.L., Alinani J.M. (2018). CT & MRI Pathology: A Pocket Atlas, 3rd ed. New York: McGraw-Hill, with permission from The McGraw-Hill Professional.

A. Brachial artery

B. Quadriceps tendon

C. Biceps tendon

D. Triceps tendon

234. In Figure III–11, what does the concave surface 1 best represent?

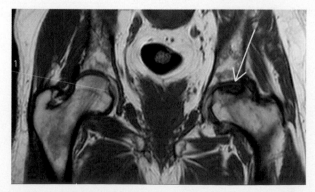

FIGURE III-11 Reprinted from Grey M.L., Alinani J.M. (2018). CT & MRI Pathology: A Pocket Atlas, 3rd ed. New York: McGraw-Hill, with permission from The McGraw-Hill Professional.

A. Acetabulum

B. Head of the femur

C. Lesser trochanter

D. Fovea capitis

235. In Figure III–12, what does the hypointense structure (arrow) best represent?

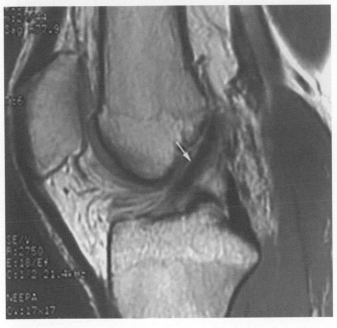

FIGURE III-12

A. Patella tendon

B. ACL

C. PCL

D. Collateral ligament

236. In Figure III–13, what does the hypointense structure (larger arrow) best represent?

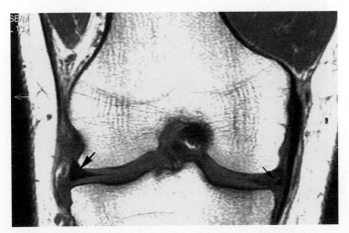

FIGURE III-13 Reprinted from Grey M.L., Alinani J.M. (2018). CT & MRI Pathology: A Pocket Atlas, 3rd ed. New York: McGraw-Hill, with permission from The McGraw-Hill Professional.

A. Meniscus

B. Collateral ligament

C. Articular cartilage

D. Patellar ligament

237. In Figure III–14, what does the hypointense structure 1 best represent?

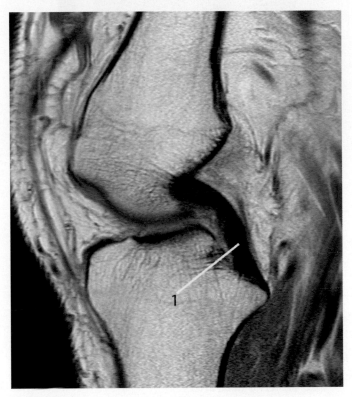

FIGURE III-14

A. ACL

B. Popliteal artery

C. Patellar ligament

D. PCL

238. In Figure III–15, what does the torn structure (arrow) best represent?

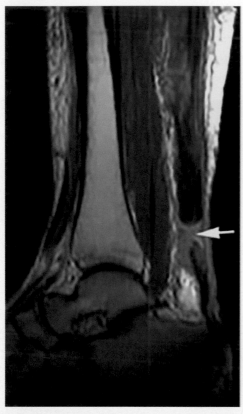

FIGURE III-15 Reprinted from Grey M.L., Alinani J.M. (2018). CT & MRI Pathology: A Pocket Atlas, 3rd ed. New York: McGraw-Hill, with permission from The McGraw-Hill Professional.

A. Posterior tibial artery

B. Peroneal tendon

C. Soleus tendon

D. Achilles tendon

239. In Figure III–16, what does 1 best represent?

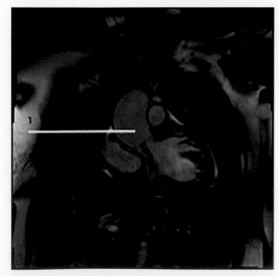

FIGURE III-16

A. Aortic arch

B. Ascending aorta

C. Descending aorta

D. Superior vena cava

240. In Figure III–17, what does 1 best represent?

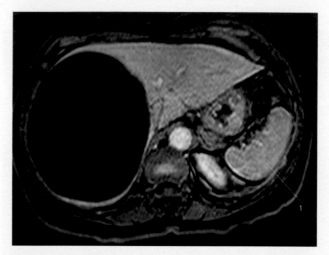

FIGURE III-17 Reprinted from Grey M.L., Alinani J.M. (2018). CT & MRI Pathology: A Pocket Atlas, 3rd ed. New York: McGraw-Hill, with permission from The McGraw-Hill Professional.

A. Spleen

B. Kidney

C. Adrenal gland

D. Stomach

241. In Figure III–18, what does 1 best represent?

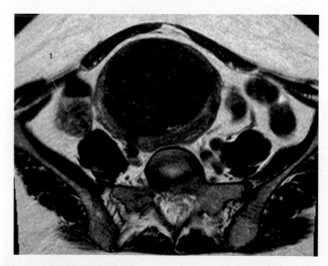

FIGURE III-18 Reprinted from Grey M.L., Alinani J.M. (2018). CT & MRI Pathology: A Pocket Atlas, 3rd ed. New York: McGraw-Hill, with permission from The McGraw-Hill Professional.

A. Uterus

B. Ascending colon

C. Ileum of the small bowel

D. Ovary

242. In Figure III–19, what abnormality is best represented?

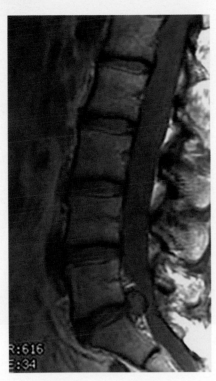

FIGURE III-19 Reprinted from Grey M.L., Alinani J.M. (2018). CT & MRI Pathology: A Pocket Atlas, 3rd ed. New York: McGraw-Hill, with permission from The McGraw-Hill Professional.

A. Compression fracture of L4

B. Spondylolisthesis

C. Spinal tumor (meningioma)

D. Herniated disk

243. In Figure III–20, what does 1 best represent?

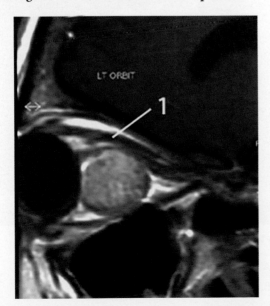

FIGURE III-20 Reprinted from Grey M.L., Alinani J.M. (2018). CT & MRI Pathology: A Pocket Atlas, 3rd ed. New York: McGraw-Hill, with permission from The McGraw-Hill Professional.

A. Optic nerve

B. Medial rectus muscle

C. Superior oblique muscle

D. Superior rectus muscle

244. In Figure III–21, what is this artifact?

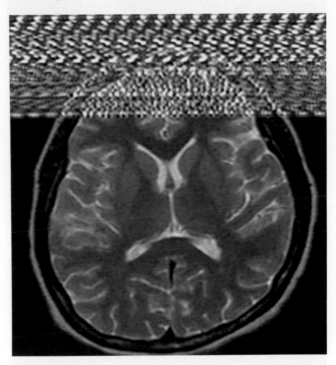

FIGURE III-21

A. RF

B. Ghosting

C. Wraparound

D. Magnetic susceptibility

245.   Based on Figure III–22A, what artifact will occur on the axial image of Figure III–22B?

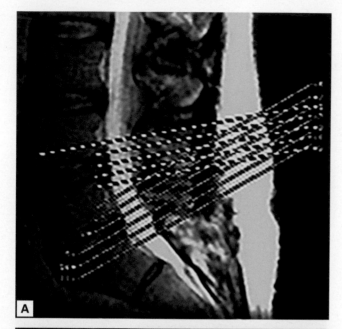

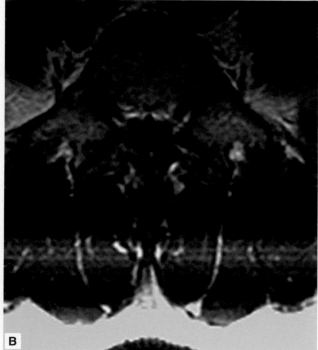

FIGURE III-22

A. RF leak

B. Ghosting

C. Cross-talk

D. Magnetic susceptibility

246.   In Figure III–23, what is the name of this artifact?

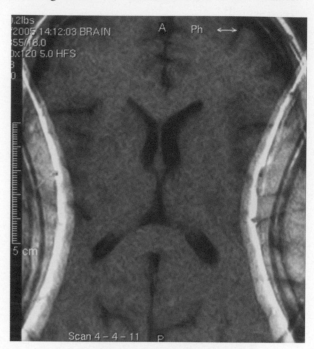

FIGURE III-23

A. Cross-talk

B. Magnetic susceptibility

C. Ghosting

D. Wraparound

247.   In Figure III–24, what is the name of this artifact?

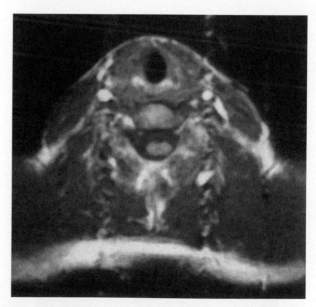

FIGURE III-24

A. Wraparound

B. Magnetic susceptibility

C. Cross-talk

D. Ghosting

248. **In Figure III–25, what does 1 best represent?**

    A. Straight sinus

    B. Great cerebral vein

    C. Superior sagittal sinus

    D. Interhemispheric fissure

249. **In Figure III–25, what structure does 2 best represent?**

    A. Longitudinal fissure

    B. Falx cerebri

    C. Tentorium cerebri

    D. Dura

250. **In Figure III–25, what does 3 best represent?**

    A. Diploe

    B. Cranial muscle

    C. Subcutaneous tissue

    D. CSF

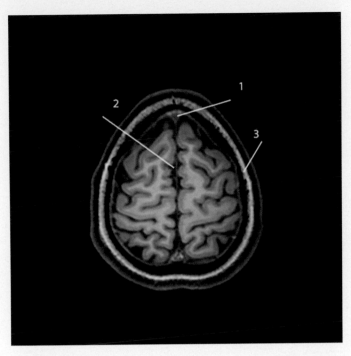

FIGURE III-25

MR Answer Explanations

1. **D** – Without the influence of the main magnetic field, the protons are not aligned with any specific orientation.

2. **C** – Protons aligned in the antiparallel orientation are in the high-energy state.

3. **B** – Only the protons in the parallel orientation contribute to the signal.

4. **C** – The mass number is the total number of protons and neutrons in an atomic nucleus.

5. **B** – Magnetic resonance occurs when the protons are exposed to a radiofrequency (RF) pulse that is at the Larmor frequency. For example, a 90-degree RF pulse would move the protons from the Mz (longitudinal magnetization) to the Mxy (transverse magnetization).

6. **A** – T1 relaxation (spin-lattice relaxation time) is the time it takes the spins to regain equilibrium by returning back to the Mz following a 90-degree pulse. The RF energy imparted to the protons has moved the net magnetization from the Mz into the Mxy. There is no longitudinal magnetization; it has all been moved into the transverse magnetization. When the RF is turned off, then the protons begin to "relax" and return back to the Mz, thus allowing recovery of the longitudinal magnetization. In one T1 relaxation time, 63% of the protons return back to the Mz.

7. **B** – Following a 90-degree RF pulse, the net magnetization is in the Mxy (transverse magnetization). While some of the protons are returning back to the Mz (T1 relaxation), others are dephasing in the Mxy.

8. **D** – The gyromagnetic ratio is a constant used to calculate the Larmor frequency. What is the gyromagnetic ratio for ^{1}H? What about other elements, such as ^{23}Na? Calculate for a magnetic field strength of 1.0 T and then 1.5 T. Note the difference? Hint: The gyromagnetic ratio for ^{23}Na is 11.26 MHz/T.

9. **B** – Once the patient has been moved inside the bore of the magnet, their hydrogen protons align either parallel or antiparallel. Thus, the hydrogen protons are aligned in the parallel orientation with the main magnetic field are considered to be the net magnetization.

10. **A** – Following 5 T1 relaxation times, all the protons have relaxed back to the Mz.

11. **B** – T2 decay or T2 relaxation is also called spin-spin relaxation. The phase "spin-spin relaxation" may also be described as "spin-spin lattice" and refers to the dephasing of the (M) in the Mxy or transverse plane.

    Macroscopically, each proton acts as an individual magnetic moment affecting their surrounding protons. This effect results in a pushing and pulling of the protons based on the orientation (vector) of their individual magnetic fields. In spin-spin lattice, the first "spin" refers to the longitudinal regrowth of the (M), whereas the second "spin" refers to the dephasing that occurs because of T2*. The asterisk (*) in T2* is used to indicate the inherent inhomogeneities in the main magnetic field. The asterisk (*) is also used to indicate the T2*-weighted gradient echo pulse sequence.

12. **C** – Hydrogen protons will be aligned with the main magnetic field, either parallel (M) or antiparallel (M-z).

13. **A** – This gyromagnetic ratio is specific for ^{1}H. Each element with spin potential has its own gyromagnetic ratio. See earlier answer explanation for Question 8.

14. **D** – Tesla and gauss are units used to define magnet strength. One tesla is equal to 10,000 Gauss. So, 5000 Gauss would be equal to 0.5 T. In the early development of MRI, there were a variety of field strengths available. To resource this information, remember that MRI was initially referred to as nuclear magnetic resonance imaging (NMRI) or just NMR.

15. **A** – The intensity of the signal from a tissue having a long T2 decreases less than that from a tissue having a short T2. Review a T2 relaxation curve comparing short T2 and long T2 tissues.

16. **A** – Fat has a shorter T1 than gray or white matter. The protons realign quickly after an RF pulse, and the signal appears brighter. Review a T1 relaxation curve comparing short T1 and long T1 tissues.

17. **C** – The question is asking for the Larmor frequency of a 1-T system. First, convert gauss to tesla. In this example, we know 10,000 gauss equals 1 tesla. Likewise, the gyromagnetic ratio for hydrogen (^1H) is 42.58 MHz/T. Multiply 42.58 MHz by 1 T to find the answer. Note: The Larmor frequency would be different if imaging a different element at 1 T. See earlier answer explanation for Question 8.

18. **D** – The shortest TR value and the shortest TE value produce the strongest T1-weighted image.

19. **C** – This question simply asks how cerebrospinal fluid (CSF) would appear. To better understand how this occurs, review T1-weighted imaging, TR values, TE values, and T1 relaxation values for tissue.

20. **D** – Every manmade magnet has inhomogeneities that affect the main magnetic field. Magnetic shim coils help to correct these imperfections. The asterisk (*) is used to symbolize these magnetic inhomogeneities. Note: One quality control test used to measure the signal-to-noise ratio of the main magnet is the water bottle phantom test. In this test, the higher the signal-to-noise ratio, the better the homogeneity of the magnet. For more information, see Grey ML, Coffey CW. Methods for evaluating image quality in magnetic resonance imaging. *J Am Soc Radiol Technol.* 1987;58(4):339-344.

21. **A** – The central portion of k-space stores low signal frequencies and image contrast. The outer portion stores high frequencies and image detail.

22. **D** – Parts per million (ppm). The lower the ppm, the more homogeneous is the magnet.

23. **A** – The RF receiver coil is positioned so it can detect the electrical voltage of the net magnetization (M) in the transverse plane.

24. **A** – Shimming the magnet eliminates inhomogeneities within the main magnet field. Passive shimming uses iron inside the magnet, whereas active magnetic shimming uses current-carrying windings to further improve field homogeneity. Magnetic field homogeneity is measured in parts per million (ppm).

25. **B** – The slew rate is the slope of the linear ramp section of the gradient waveform that indicates the maximum amplitude (strength) of the gradient to the rise time. Fast gradient coils require faster rise times, which demonstrate a steeper slew rate

26. **B** – The better the RF receiver coil is filled with tissue, the greater is the amount of signal for imaging.

27. **C** – Of the 3 types of magnets developed, only the superconductive used liquid cryogens for cooling. The resistive magnets were developed at lower field strengths and cooled by water.

28. **C** – External and unwanted RF signals are restricted from entering into the MRI suite through the use of RF shielding in the walls, ceiling, flooring, windows, doors, and areas where cables enter into the MRI suite.

29. **D** – Gradient strength can be measured in either G/cm or mT/m.

30. **C** – Initially, superconductive magnetics used dual liquid cryostats. The outer cryostat (dewar) was for liquid nitrogen, whereas the inner cryostat (dewar) contained liquid helium. The current-carrying windings were submerged in the liquid helium (–452°F) to allow the magnets to operate at a higher field strength and operate at near the state of superconductivity. Historically, cryogens would "boil off" and need to be replaced by refilling the dewars with their respective cryogen, commonly called cryogenic transfer. Newer superconductive magnets only have a liquid helium cryostat due to cryogenic refrigerator systems (cold head) used to reliquify helium.

31. **C** – Securing the MRI suite from stray RF signals reduces the chance of RF artifact interference.

32. **C** – The gradient coils (ie, Gx, Gy, and Gz) are responsible for phase and frequency encoding along a given slice plane.

33. **B** – One liter of liquid helium would produce 760 L of gaseous helium. This could be an asphyxiation safety concern if a superconductive magnet were to quench and the gaseous helium was unable to leave (evacuate) the environment.

34. **A** – Before magnetic shielding, the 5-gauss line would be clearly visible. After the development of magnetic shielding, the 5-gauss line was ideally within the MRI suite. Today, magnetic safety is indicated by zone markers.

35. **D** – The turning on and off of the current-carrying gradient coils produces the noise associated with MRI. The knocking noise is heard during imaging.

36. **C** – The temperature of liquid helium is –452°F. Liquid helium begins to boil as the temperature rises. The state of superconductivity is –460°F. At this temperature, there is no resistance to electricity.

37. **C** – Signal-to-noise ratio is useful in determining image quality. It is a ratio between the signal produced in the area being imaged and the graininess (noise) or unwanted signal. The higher the number, the better is the quality.

38. A – Decreasing the slice thickness increases spatial resolution and reduces partial volume averaging.

39. A – Increasing the main magnetic field moves more protons into parallel alignment. This allows for an increase in signal.

40. A – Decreasing the receiver bandwidth decreases unwanted frequencies (noise) that do not benefit the image quality from being collected (received) at time TE. For example, if the signal from the unwanted frequencies (noise) is reduced and the signal from the frequencies that are beneficial is collected, the signal-to-noise ratio (SNR) has increased.

41. A – Decreasing the TE allows the signal to be collected while more protons are in the Mxy.

42. A – Longer TR will allow more time for all the protons to move into the Mxy.

43. C – Because TE is not a factor in calculating scan time, it has no impact on scan time. In addition, TE is shorter than TR.

44. A – Doubling the number of excitations (NEX) or number of signal acquisitions (NSA) increases the signal-to-noise ratio (S/N) by a factor of 1.4. Expressed as a percentage, this would result in a 41% increase in the signal without any increase in noise. However, it would double the scan time. Interestingly, to notice any difference in image quality, the signal would need to be doubled.

45. A – While increasing the NEX would increase the signal, the amount of NEX was not mentioned. Decreasing the receiver bandwidth by half would increase the signal-to-noise ratio by reducing the noise only.

46. D – Noise appears as a grainy image.

47. A – The smaller the RF receiver coil, the better is the signal-to-noise ratio. Unfortunately, smaller RF receiver coils are limited to the area they can cover. Phase-array coils are multiple small RF receiver coils connected together to cover a larger body area.

48. B – T1-weighted pulse sequences consist of a short TR time and a short TE time. The shorter the TR and TE values, the heavy is the T1-weighted image. See earlier answer explanation for Question 18.

49. B – The term *flip angle* (FA), also referred to as tip angle, applies to gradient echo pulse sequences. In gradient echo imaging, the FA is listed along with the TR and TE values. It indicates how far the net magnetization (M) is moved away from the Mz and toward the Mxy. Spin echo–type pulse sequences do not use the term flip angle because it is always implied that the (M) is moved into the Mxy transverse plane.

50. B – Historically, the magnetic field has been grouped according to field strength.

Ultra-low	≤0.1 T
Low	0.2-0.35 T
Midfield	0.5-1.0 T
High	1.0-2.0 T
Ultra-high	>2.0 T

51. B – Only superconductive magnets can reach field strengths high enough to perform MR spectroscopy (MRS).

52. D – RF transmitting and receiving coils will excite and detect the MR signal.

53. A – The loss of superconductivity "quench" can only affect superconductive magnets.

54. A – An RF signal at the Larmor frequency will cause the protons to precess around the βo.

55. C – Data are collected along the frequency-encoding gradient (Gfe). The frequency-encoding gradient can also be symbolized as (Gro).

56. B – An RF artifact is seen along the frequency-encoding axis.

57. C – Minimally, a 30% gap between adjacent slices will help eliminate RF signal interference.

58. A – These artifacts are most prominent with high-field systems and on images acquired with gradient echo sequences, rather than spin echo sequences. Presaturation bands assist with reducing ghosting artifacts.

59. D – Some artifacts have more than one name. It is important to be familiar with all the names that apply to an artifact. Gibb's artifact may also be referred to as truncation or edge ringing. Being able to identify the artifact by its specific characteristics and knowing how to correct the artifact as best as possible are beneficial.

60. A – Mismapping, wraparound, and just wrap are names commonly used to describe this artifact. The most common method to correct this problem is to increase the field of view (FOV).

61. A – Fat protons resonate at a frequency approximately 3.5 ppm lower than that of water protons. At 1.5 T, there is a frequency difference of 225 Hz.

62. A – This is a type of motion artifact associated with cardiac motion, pulsatile flow of blood or CSF, and respiration. This artifact is usually referred to as ghosting.

63. **C** – Using a presaturation pulse outside the FOV can eliminate the unwanted pulsatile signal from affecting the area of interest. For example, adding a presaturation pulse modifies the pulse sequence diagram, increases the scan time, and increases the specific absorption rate (SAR).

64. **B** – Wraparound or aliasing occurs when the FOV is too small. During image reconstruction, the computer is confused as to where to place the frequencies outside the FOV and wraps them over to the opposite side of the image. This gives the image an overlapping appearance and is why this artifact is called "wraparound."

65. **A** – In CT, a metal artifact would appear with streaks. In MR, however, a metal susceptibility artifact would appear as an area with a loss of signal.

66. **B** – See answer explanation for Question 61.

67. **D** – Reducing the slice thickness can correct for partial volume averaging artifact. Note: To better understand, review the full width at half maximum (FWHM) of the slice sensitivity profile.

68. **C** – RF artifacts may be caused by different circumstances.

69. **C** – The blood will appear dark due to the RF saturation of the protons in the blood entering into the FOV.

70. **D** – Co-current flow is in the same direction as the slice selection. Countercurrent flow is the blood coming in the opposite direction as the slice selection.

71. **C** – In spin echo sequences, the R-to-R interval is used to determine the TR.

72. **C** – The center of laminar flow moves at a faster rate than flow along the wall of the vessel due to resistance. Other types of flow include vortex, which has a spiraling motion; turbulent flow, which consists of different velocities or fluctuates erratically; and stagnant or plug-type flow, which indicates a blockage.

73. **D** – The blood will appear bright since the protons have not been saturated.

74. **B** – Gadolinium contrast agents do not cross the intact blood-brain barrier (BBB). If the BBB is disrupted by a disease process, the contrast agent diffuses into the interstitial space and shortens the T1 relaxation time of the tissue, resulting in increased signal intensity on T1-weighted images.

75. **C** – A chelation bond forms a stronger bond necessary for gadolinium-based contrast agents (GBCAs). This type of bond reduces dissociation of the contrast agent.

76. **D** – DTPA is the ligand used to bond with gadolinium (Gd^{3+}) to create gadopentetate dimeglumine (Gd-DTPA), also known as Magnevist.

77. **B** – Gadolinium shortens T1 and T2 relaxation time in tissues; however, gadolinium has a greater influence on T1 relaxation than T2 relaxation. Shortening the T1 relaxation results in increased signal intensity on T1-weighted images.

78. **B** – GBCAs are paramagnetic. This refers to the unpaired electrons (eg, gadolinium ions, Gd^{3+}) used in many MRI contrast agents. Diamagnetic is slightly repelled by a magnet, paramagnetic has slight magnetic susceptibility, superparamagnetic has strong magnetic susceptibility, and ferromagnetic is strongly attracted to the magnet.

79. **A** – See answer explanation for Question 77.

80. **A** – GBCAs are excreted mostly through the kidneys and to a lesser extent the hepatobiliary system. Free gadolinium ion is toxic. This is the primary reason why a chelation bond is used. See answer explanation for Question 75.

81. **B** – GBCAs administered to patients with sickle cell anemia specifically and any other type of anemia in general may cause complications. Although gadolinium may be excreted in low concentrations in human milk, it is recommended that nursing mothers express their milk prior to the exam and not breastfeed for 36 to 48 hours after the administration of an MR contrast agent to ensure that the nursing child does not receive the drug in any notable quantity by mouth. In pregnant patients, GBCAs have been shown to cross the blood-placenta barrier and appear in the urinary bladder of the fetus. The contrast agent would then be excreted into the amniotic fluid and then subsequently swallowed by the fetus. This will then be filtered and excreted in the urine of the fetus, with the entire cycle being repeated innumerable times.

82. **C** – Gradient coils are used to encode the RF signal into the patient. The signal is encoded with the slice selection (Gss) gradient and then the frequency-encoding (Gfe or Gro) gradient and the phase-encoding (Gpe) gradient.

83. **A** – Conventional spin echo (CSE) pulse sequence is commonly known as a 90-degree excitation pulse followed by a 180-degree rephasing pulse. A fast spin echo (FSE) or turbo spin echo (TSE) has an initial 90-degree excitation pulse followed by several 180-degree rephasing pulses. FSE and TSE are manufacturer terms for the same type of pulse sequence, which is known as rapid acquisition with relaxation enhancement (RARE). As an interesting point, Siemens and Philips use the term TSE, whereas GE, Picker, Toshiba, and Hitachi use the term FSE. Do you know how to calculate the scan time for CSE and RARE sequences?

84. **D** – In the inversion recovery (IR) pulse sequence, the initial 180-degree pulse is an inversion pulse that moves the net magnetization from the M + z to the M − z. Then the 90-degree pulse is the excitation pulse followed by a rephasing pulse. Short tau IR (STIR) and fluid attenuation IR (FLAIR) are common current sequences.

85. **B** – The Gy gradient is perpendicular to the coronal plane. Gx would be the Gss for a sagittal image, whereas Gz would be the Gss for an axial image. Orthogonal imaging would require 2 gradients to be used for slice selection.

86. **A** – In addition to the 90-degree RF excitation pulse, the Gss is also activated.

87. **C** – Gradient echo pulse sequences use a gradient reversal for rephasing the net magnetization in the Mxy, whereas spin echo pulse sequences use a 180-degree RF rephasing pulse.

88. **B** – During the excitation and rephasing pulses, the Gss is activated.

89. **B** – The null point refers to the time after the 180-degree inversion pulse when the magnetic moment of a group of precessing hydrogen molecules is at 90 degrees to the main magnetic field. The null point occurs at 69% of the T1 relaxation value of a given tissue. The inversion time (TI) used will depend on the tissue signal that is selected to be nulled. A short TI is used to null fat signal, and a long TI is used to null fluid such as CSF.

90. **B** – The echo time (TE) is selected depending on the weighting of the desired image. Short TE times are used for proton density–weighted and T1-weighted images. Long TE times are used for T2-weighted images.

91. **A** – The repetition time (TR) is the time between the initial 90-degree excitation pulses.

92. **D** – The data are collected along the frequency-encoding gradient (Gfe or Gro). The receiver RF coil and ADC (analog to digital converter) are also activated during this time.

93. **D** – Unlike the spin echo pulse sequence, the protons are rephased using the frequency-encoding gradient coil. The Gfe is also known as the readout gradient (Gro). The process is called a gradient reversal.

94. **A** – This is a gradient echo pulse sequence. The main give-away is the use of the term *flip angle* (FA). A T1-weighted gradient echo sequence uses a large FA with a short TR and short TE.

95. **D** – In addition, following the TI, an RF excitation pulse is applied to move all the protons 90 degrees. Those that have aligned back along the longitudinal magnetization (M + z) move into the transverse (Mxy) and provide signal for the image. Those that were somewhere else other than the M + z likewise move 90 degrees but are not in the Mxy for signal readout; thus, they do not contribute signal to the image because they were nulled.

96. **A** – The inversion pulse is different from the excitation or rephasing pulses. In addition, the inversion pulse (TI) is only used when performing IR pulse sequences like STIR or FLAIR.

97. **C** – Echo planar imaging (EPI) pulse sequence acquires data for an image in less than a second.

98. **A** – Rapid Acquisition with Relaxation Enhancement (RARE) is the correct term when referring to FSE or TSE sequences.

99. **C** – RF shielding is in the walls, ceiling, floor, windows, door, and cable outlets. Note: Cell phones and walkie-talkies cannot be used within the MRI suite due to RF shielding. Fire fighters should know that they will not be able to communicate with these devices if they go inside the suite.

100. **C** – The terms *longitudinal axis* and *z-axis* may be used interchangeably. The symbol (Mxy) is used to indicate the (M) in the transverse plane following a 90-degree RF pulse. The (M-z) symbol could be used to indicate the (M) following a 180-degree RF pulse in an IR pulse sequence.

101. **C** – The (M) represents the net magnetization, the (βo) represents the main magnetic field, and the (M-z) represents the net magnetization following a 180-degree RF pulse.

102. **B** – The effective TE (ETE) is an imaging parameter in RARE sequences. As the number of ETE increases, so does the echo train length (ETL). Thus, the greater the ETL, the shorter is the scan time. Review the calculation for scan time.

103. **C** – A proton density–weighted sequence would have a long TR with a short TE.

104. **A** – The inversion time (TI) is the time between the initial 180-degree inversion pulse and the 90-degree excitation pulse.

105. **B** – The formula to calculate the scan time for RARE is as follows:

$$TR \times Gpe \times NEX \div ETL$$
$$4000 \times 256 \times 2 \div 4 = 2,048,000 \div 4$$
$$= 512,000 \text{ milliseconds}$$

Now convert from milliseconds to seconds = 512 seconds

Now convert from seconds to minutes = 8.5 minutes

All the other information indicates the imaging parameters used in the example. Remember, it is important to know what information is needed to solve a problem!

106. **C** – The gyromagnetic ratio for the hydrogen proton is 42.58 MHz/T.

107. **C** – The question is asking how to state the frequency.

108. **A** – The terms *spin up* and *spin down* date back to the original magnets. These first units were vertical field; thus, the βo was vertical and pointing up.

109. **B** – The βo is the unit symbol for main magnetic field strength in tesla. The γ is the unit symbol for the gyro-magnetic ratio.

110. **A** – Precession is the cone-shaped (spinning top–like) motion around the magnetic field. This happens to the patient's protons when they are moved into the magnetic field.

111. **D** – Turning on the RF (Larmor frequency) signal causes the hydrogen protons to resonate. If the frequency is not correct, there will be no resonances of the protons.

112. **B** – Once the patient is in the magnet, their hydrogen protons either align parallel or antiparallel to the main magnetic field. The majority of the protons will align in the parallel orientation Mz or longitudinal plane. If a 90-degree RF pulse is applied, the (M) will move into the Mxy or transverse plane.

113. **D** – After 5 T1 relaxation times, all the net magnetization has returned to the Mz longitudinal axis.

114. **B** – As an example, after a 90-degree RF pulse, the net magnetization has moved from the Mz into the Mxy (transverse plane). Dephasing occurs after the RF has been turned off.

115. **D** – The number of hydrogen protons in the anatomic structure will vary. Consider the difference between the gray matter and white matter of the brain.

116. **D** – The structures, from superior to inferior, are the midbrain, pons, and medulla oblongata.

117. **A** – The hydrogen protons in fat realign faster after the RF pulse, and their signal appears bright.

118. **C** – The excitation pulse is the pulse that moves the (M) into the Mxy. Names for 2 common types of pulses include the inversion pulse (180 degrees) used in IR sequences and the rephasing pulse (180 degrees) used to rephase the protons that are in the Mxy.

119. **D** – All 3 statements are correct.

120. **A** – This question is similar to Question 21 (see answer explanation). It is just asked in a different way.

121. **B** – As the slice thickness increases, the number of protons providing signal increases.

122. **D** – Increasing TR allows more time for all the (M) to move into the (Mxy). Likewise, increasing the NEX or NSA will increase signal and be noticeable if doubled (see answer explanation for Question 44). While decreasing the receiver bandwidth may not add signal, it will reduce unwanted frequencies (noise) and, as a result, increase the signal-to-noise ratio.

123. **A** – Chemical shift increases as the magnetic field increases. See answer explanation for Question 61.

124. **A** – A short TR and low flip angle (FA) does not allow all the (M) to move into the Mxy for signal readout. Increasing the NEX or NSA, especially if doubled, will increase the signal

125. **A** – The 2 components active during the encoding of the signal would be the Gpe and the Gro or Gfe. The gradient readout (Gro) and the gradient frequency encoding (Gfe) are the same.

126. **C** – In the RARE spin echo pulse sequence, the speed of this fast-imaging sequence is corrected by the number of rows of phase encoding that can be acquired per TR cycle. In the example in this question, having an echo train length (ETL) or turbo factor (TF) of 10 would imply that this technique would be 10 times faster than the CSE sequence. See answer explanation for Question 105 for calculation.

127. **D** – The IR pulse sequence has 3 RF pulses, 180 degrees (inversion pulse), 90 degrees (excitation pulse), and 180 degrees (rephasing pulse).

128. **D** – In the RARE sequence, each 180-degree pulse is set at time echo (TE) from the initial 90-degree excitation pulse. The average of the TE values is the effective TE (ETE).

129. **D** – The purpose of the null point is to allow time for 2 tissues with similar relaxation times to relax further, resulting in greater separation of the signal of the 2 tissues. See answer explanation for Question 95.

130. **A** – The TE extends from the initial 180-degree inversion pulse to the readout of the signal. During the readout portion of the sequence, the components that are active include (1. the RF receiver coil, (2) the ADC, and (3) the Gfe.

131. **D** – The frequency-encoding gradient (Gfe), also known as the readout gradient (Gro), performs the function of rephasing. Compare this with the SE pulse sequence.

132. **C** – Placing the saturation band medial to the shoulder would saturate the signal of blood in the subclavian artery entering into the FOV covering the shoulder. This would reduce motion artifact, specifically, ghosting artifact.

133. **A** – In this MR angiography technique, the enhancement of the blood signal results from flow-related phenomena, more specifically, in-flow enhancement.

134. **B** – This helps to control for ghosting-related artifacts. See answer explanation for Question 132 above.

135. **D** – These techniques automatically adjust the FOV.

136. **A** – Providing a gap of at least 30% between adjacent slices will reduce this artifact.

137. **A** – CSE and RARE are beneficial in reducing magnetic susceptibility–type artifacts.

138. **B** – Frequent use of the door over an extended period of time may wear out or deteriorate the spring clips positioned along the edge of the door. These should be inspected to ensure they are functional and in good working order as they are used to keep stray RF energy from entering the MR suite.

139. **C** – Motion artifacts appear along the Gpe.

140. **B** – Once the RF transmit coil has transmitted the Larmor frequency into the patient, the 3 pairs of gradient coils are used to encode the signal. The signal is encoded according to the slice selection, frequency encoding, and phase encoding.

141. **B** – Passive and active shimming are used to eliminate the magnetic field inhomogeneities.

142. **D** – These terms define the quality of a gradient coil system. The information can be used to compare the quality of various manufacturer gradient systems for purchasing decision making.

143. **C** – The windings are submerged in liquid helium near the state of superconductivity.

144. **A** – The lower the ppm of the main magnet, the better is the field homogeneity.

145. **C** – The term *fringe field* refers to extension of the magnetic field into the surrounding environment. What is the fringe field (x-axis, y-axis, and z-axis) of your MRI unit? The units should be expressed in gauss. The term *5-gauss line* indicates the fringe field measured from the isocenter of the magnetic field to the point where a magnetic strength of 5 gauss is measured.

146. **A** – As the magnetic field strength increases, more hydrogen protons will align in the parallel orientation and are able to contribute signal.

147. **A** – Nonferromagnetic material is not affected by magnetic attraction or torque forces. However, heating and artifact production may be possible. Screening all who are planning to enter the MRI suite is important.

148. **B** – The maximum specific absorption rate (SAR) for the whole body is not to exceed 4 W/kg averaged over 15 minutes.

149. **B** – The ETL in the RARE sequence uses multiple 180-degree rephasing pulses. Gradient echo does not use RF to rephase the (M).

150. **A** – GBCAs are primarily excreted through the renal system. Some excretion may occur through the hepatobiliary system and, to a lesser extent, through lactation.

151. **A** – Contrast can pass through the BBB if there is a disruption in the membrane.

152. **A** – The CSF will appear dark.

153. **D** – Edema does not enhance. Edema would appear dark (hypointense) on a T1-weighted sequence and bright (hyperintense) on a T2-weighted sequence.

154. **A** – See answer explanation for Question 81.

155. **D** – Torque and artifact will also be affected.

156. **C** – The (M) is parallel to the βo.

157. **C** – CSF has a long T2 relaxation. This is seen with a long TR and a long TE.

158. **C** – The Gz axis (gradient) is perpendicular to the slice.

159. **C** – One kilogram equals 2.2 lb.

160. **B** – Without the effect of a stronger magnetic field, each ^{1}H proton will orient itself based on its own magnetic moment and the influence of neighboring ^{1}H protons.

161. **A** – The ^{1}H protons are aligned along the longitudinal axis of the magnetic field. The (M) is parallel with the βo (M + z). The remaining ^{1}H protons in the high-energy state are aligned antiparallel in the (M – z).

162. **C** – The symbol (Mz) indicates the (M) is aligned along the z-axis; thus, (Mz) indicates longitudinal magnetization. If the symbol were only (M), then it would imply the net magnetization.

163. **A** – Other terms that can be used to describe the antiparallel ^{1}H protons include high-energy state and spin down. The term *spin down* dates back to the vertical field initial NMR units, and the βo was oriented up. Thus, with the βo vertical and pointing up, the (M) is also oriented up. Parallel ^{1}H protons are referred to as low-energy-state and spin-up protons.

164. **A** – The main magnetic field is what the ^{1}H protons precess around, similar to Earth precessing around the Sun.

165. **B** – The net magnetization is moved from the (Mz) longitudinal magnetization into the (Mxy) transverse magnetization when the Larmor frequency is turned on for a specific period of time. This is called a 90-degree RF pulse.

166. **A** – All of the ^{1}H protons align with the main magnetic field. The majority (M) align parallel (Mz), with the remaining aligning (M – z) antiparallel.

167. **D** – One tesla equals 10,000 Gauss. The question is not asking about frequency (answer A; gyromagnetic ratio) or Larmor frequency (42.58 MHz/T; answer B).

168. **A** – The use of a vector conveys (1) orientation or direction and (2) strength or magnitude of the main magnetic field (βo) along with the net magnetization (M).

169. **C** – The Larmor frequency is used to move the protons.

170. **D** – Precession is the spinning top–like motion of the ^{1}H protons (M + z and M – z) in the βo.

171. **D** – The anterior cruciate and posterior cruciate ligaments are associated with the knee.

172. **B** – Five T1 relaxation times equal 100% recovery of the magnetization to the (Mz).

173. **C** – Earplugs can help reduce the noise by 10 to 30 dB.

174. **C** – The TE is the time between the initial RF pulse and signal readout. The βo is used to calculate the

Larmor frequency. The TR indicates how often the RF is turned on. The greater the amount of tissue within the RF coil, the greater is the deposit of SAR.

175. **D** – For Gd^{3+}, the 3+ indicates that this is an ion and 3 electrons are needed to balance it.

176. **B** – A chelation type of bond is needed to bind a metallic ion to a ligand and to reduce the chance of dissociation. Gadolinium is toxic; however, if the bond is intake, it is not toxic.

177. **C** – Gd^{3+} is a metallic ion. It has a valance of 3+. See answer explanation for Question 175.

178. **A** – The RF receiver coil is designed to be positioned so the signal cuts across the coils in the transverse axis. Tuning the RF coil improves the homogeneity of the coil. The better the RF coil is filled, the better the signal-to-noise ratio (SNR). The Q is an overall measure of the performance of the coil. The higher the Q, the better is the coil. RF receiver coils can be compared using their Q values.

179. **D** – Historically, there were 2 cryostats. The liquid nitrogen cryostat was the other cryostat used to reduce the boil-off rate of liquid helium in the liquid helium cryostat.

180. **B** – The sudden loss of the magnet's superconductivity is called a quench. This also results in the rapid evaporation of the liquid helium.

181. **C** – It is recommended not to exceed 20 mL of a GBCA. A 220-lb patient would receive the maximum dose. A 235-lb patient would receive 20 mL, not the calculated dose.

182. **A** – The peak in the contrast-to-noise ratio, in general, occurs at about one-half the average T1 relaxation. From this, the best T1 contrast is obtained by choosing a TR somewhat less than the T1 values of the tissues involved.

183. **C** – The more tissue within the receiver coil, the better is the signal-to-noise ratio because there is less space for background noise (noise is the space surrounding the tissue within the coil).

184. **B** – Doubling the NEX or NSA would result in an increase in the signal-to-noise ratio (SNR) by a factor of 1.4. When converted to a percentage, this would be a 41% increase.

185. **B** – The TE primarily controls T2 weighting. Given that the TR is long, as the TE increases, T2 weighting increases.

186. **A** – The nerves coming from the lumbar spine branch into the lower extremities. Likewise, the nerves of the cervical spine branch into the upper extremities.

187. **C** – T2 decay or T2 relaxation is the dephasing (Free Induction Decay (FID)) that occurs in the Mxy (transverse plane). The (*) symbol in T2* relaxation represents the effects of the inhomogeneities of the main magnetic field βo. Question: What component is used to help reduce the inhomogeneities? Answer: Passive shimming

for the magnet and active shimming to help account for the patient.

188. **B** – The gadolinium is the metallic ion that needs to be bound to a ligand to be a chelate bond. The DTPA is the ligand. It helps maintain the bond so the gadolinium does not dissociate.

189. **A** – With advancements in technology, the pixel/voxel size has decreased to a point where all 3 axes can be equal. This is called isotropic imaging. If only the x-axis and y-axis are equal and the z-axis (slice thickness (SLT)) is greater, then this is called anisotropic imaging. The same principle applies to CT.

190. **A** – Short TR and TE values are used for T1-weighted imaging. Question: What are the TR and TE values for T1 weighting, proton density weighting, and T2 weighting?

191. **B** – A 90-degree excitation RF pulse followed by a 180-degree rephasing RF pulse is a classic spin echo pulse sequence. Question: What is the sequence for excitation and rephasing for other types of pulse sequences?

192. **B** – Historically, the 5-gauss line has been the standard. In today's MRI environment, all individuals must stay outside of zone IV until they have been properly screened.

193. **A** – The specific absorption rate (SAR) is a measure of exposure to RF. The main effect is an increase in body temperature. Federal guidelines set limits on RF exposure.

194. **A** – Each implant should be taken as a case-by-case review and discussed with your radiologist.

195. **C** – The B_1 field represents the rotating magnetic field represented by the ^1H protons following the RF transmitted at the Larmor frequency.

196. **D** – Daily quality control (QC) should be performed to evaluate the integrity of the RF cable. This is a simple process of checking for cracks along the length of the cable.

197. **A** – Felix Bloch (1905-1983) and Edward Purcell (1912-1997) were awarded the Nobel Prize in 1952 for their development of new ways and methods for nuclear magnetic precision measurements. Nuclear magnetic resonance spectroscopy (NMRS) was used to advance chemistry.

198. **D** – Isidor Rabi (1898-1988) was awarded the Nobel Prize in Physics in 1944 for his discovery of nuclear magnetic resonance (NMR), which is used in MRI.

199. **C** – In 2003, Paul Lauterbur (1929-2007) shared the Nobel Prize in Physiology or Medicine with Peter Mansfield. Paul is credited with introducing gradient coils used to encode spatial information.

200. **A** – Raymond Damadian (born 1936) is credited with inventing the first MRI scanner. He also performed the first image of a human in an MRI unit. Damadian discovered that tumors and normal tissue can be distinguished

in vivo by nuclear magnetic resonance (NMR) because of their prolonged relaxation times, both T1 (spin-lattice relaxation) and T2 (spin-spin relaxation). Unfortunately, he was not awarded a Nobel Prize for his contributions but was considered at the time along with Paul Lauterbur and Peter Mansfield. Damadian was the owner of FONAR, a company that manufactured MRI scanners.

201. **A** – The corpus callosum is composed of 4 parts: (1) the rostrum (not indicated); (2) genu (1B); (3) body (1A); and (4) splenium (1C). This is the largest white matter tract connecting the 2 hemispheres of the brain. The other 2 white matter connection points are the anterior commissure and the posterior commissure. In sectional imaging such as with CT and MRI, neuroanatomy is seen in a 2-dimensional perspective. However, neuroanatomy is 3 dimensional and should be learned that way. Notice structures according to being anterior/posterior, superior/inferior, and medial/lateral. In this midline section, many neuroanatomic structures are seen.

202. **C** – The massa intermedia is also referred to as the interthalamic adhesion. It connects the 2 lobes of the thalamus together by passing through the third ventricle.

203. **D** – The optic nerve is also known as the second cranial nerve.

204. **D** – The pituitary gland is in the sella turcica. The infundibulum or pituitary stalk is not shown.

205. **B** – The clivus is formed by contributions from the body of the sphenoid bone and from the basilar part of the occipital bone.

206. **C** – The occipital lobe is 1 of the 4 lobes of the cerebral hemisphere.

207. **B** – The straight sinus drains venous blood into the confluence of sinuses (3). The tentorium cerebelli can also be seen separating the occipital lobes from the cerebellum.

208. **A** – The superior sagittal sinus (SSS) and the straight sinus (2) join to form the confluence of sinuses (3). The venous blood then moves laterally in the left and right lateral sinus, also known as the transverse sinus.

209. **D** – The cerebral aqueduct, also known as the aqueduct of Sylvius, is a passageway for CSF from the third ventricle to the fourth ventricle. It passes through the midbrain.

210. **C** – The basilar artery is found along the midline just anterior to the pons. The arterial supply of blood to the brain and the venous drainage can be identified by the location of the vessel.

211. **A** – The central sulcus separates the frontal lobe from the parietal lobe of the cerebrum. Note: The precentral gyrus is the motor cortex, whereas the postcentral gyrus is the sensory cortex.

212. **B** – This is a parasagittal image showing the temporal lobe. Note: Just superior is the Sylvian fissure.

213. **C** – The seventh cranial nerve (slightly more anterior) and the eighth cranial nerve are shown here. Thin section imaging is needed to reduce partial volume average and better show these thin structures.

214. **C** – The fourth ventricle is midline and posterior to the pons. Note: The basilar artery is anterior to the pons and along the midline.

215. **C** – The optic chiasm has an X-shaped appearance. As the optic nerves enter the chiasm, some optic nerve fibers from each eye cross and continue posteriorly along the optic tracts. The optic tracts continue posteriorly as the optic radiata until they reach the occipital lobes known as the vision centers of the brain.

216. **D** – The middle cerebral artery is part of the circle of Willis. The middle cerebral arteries move laterally along the Sylvian fissure.

217. **C** – The straight sinus is part of the venous drainage network of the brain. Along with the SSS, it drains blood into the confluence of sinuses. From here, the blood moves laterally through the lateral or transverse sinuses.

218. **A** – The hypointense U-shaped structure is the tentorium cerebelli. It separates the occipital lobes of the cerebrum from the cerebellum. It is similar to the falx cerebri.

219. **B** – The brainstem is comprised of 3 parts. Beginning superiorly and moving inferiorly, there are the midbrain, pons, and medulla oblongata. Each section has a unique shape and size. Note: There are adjacent structures that can be helpful in identifying the specific section of the brainstem.

220. **A** – The cerebral aqueduct, or aqueduct of Sylvius, connects the third ventricle to the fourth ventricle and passes through the midbrain. See Figure III-1B (4) sagittal image and answer explanation for Question 209.

221. **C** – On a T1-weighted image with intravenous (IV) contrast, the CSF and edema will be dark and the tumor bright.

222. **D** – On a T2-weighted image, the tumor and edema will be bright. It can be difficult to separate the edema from the tumor. IV contrast and T1-weighted sequence are helpful.

223. **A** – Edema is hypodense on T1-weighted sequences and hyperintense on T2-weighted sequences. However, on T1-weighted sequences with IV contrast, the tumor is better seen separate of the surrounding edema.

224. **B** – The foramen of Monro is also known as the interventricular foramen. It connects and provides a passageway for CSF to flow from the 2 lateral ventricles into the third ventricle.

225. **A** – The thalamus is located on both sides of the third ventricle. The interthalamic adhesion passes through the third ventricle to connect the 2 lobes of the thalamus together.

226. **B** – The trigone or atrium is triangular in shape and is part of the lateral ventricles. It is where the occipital and temporal horns of the lateral ventricles meet. It is also where the largest accumulation of the choroid plexus is most easily seen. The choroid plexus is located in all 4 of the ventricles.

227. **D** – This is the left frontal (anterior) horn of the lateral ventricle. Note the 2 foramina of Monro exiting the frontal horns to allow the CSF to flow into the third ventricle seen in the midline.

228. **A** – The caudate nucleus is divided into 3 sections: (1) the head; (2) the body; and (3) the tail. The largest part is the head, seen in this image. As the caudate nucleus moves posteriorly just under the body of the ventricles, it decreases in size. The body and tail of the caudate nucleus are better seen in the coronal plane.

229. **B** – The corpus callosum is composed of 3 sections: (1) the genu; (2) the body; and (3) the splenium. See Figures III–1A to III–1C and answer explanation for Question 201.

230. **B** – The lateral (transverse) sinus is part of the venous drainage system. It drains venous blood from the confluence of sinuses bilaterally into the sigmoid sinuses and then into the jugular veins.

231. **C** – This is the inferior (temporal) horn of the right lateral ventricle. Compare it with the left side.

232. **A** – The supraspinatus tendon is located under the acromion and is seen well on this coronal image. The bright (hyperintense) area is fluid (arrow). The torn tendon has a darker signal and is retracted.

233. **C** – The torn bicep tendon is low signal and retracted. The bright (hyperintense) signal surrounding the tendon is fluid from the full tear.

234. **D** – The fovea capitis on the head of the femur is where the ligamentum teres (more commonly known as the ligament of the head of the femur) attaches. Along with the ligament of the head of the femur is the blood supply coming from the acetabulum to the head and neck of the femur. When this blood supply is hindered, avascular necrosis of the head of the femur occurs. Note the avascular necrosis of the left head of the femur.

235. **B** – The anterior cruciate ligament attaches to the anterior part of the intercondylar of the tibia and ascends posteriorly to attach to the back of the lateral wall of the intercondylar fossa of the femur. There are 2 cruciate ligaments; the other is the posterior cruciate ligament (PCL).

236. **A** – The meniscus appears triangular in this coronal plane and has a hypointense signal. The small arrow shows a torn meniscus.

237. **D** – The structure represents the posterior cruciate ligament (PCL). Compare with Figure III–12, and see answer explanation for Question 235.

238. **D** – This is a full tear of the Achilles tendon. The Achilles tendon may also be known as the calcaneal tendon because this tendon attaches to the calcaneus (heel) of the foot. Compare signal patterns of torn tendons and free fluid with Figure III–10, and see answer explanation for Question 233.

239. **B** – The aortic arch is divided into the ascending portion, the arch portion, and the descending portion. Knowing the boundaries of each is helpful in identifying cardiac anatomy.

240. **A** – The spleen is located on the left side of this image. There is a large cystic structure in the liver.

241. **D** – The ovary as seen in this image is a mixed-signal structure lateral to the uterus. The pathology seen is a leiomyoma.

242. **D** – This is a herniated disk at the level of L5/S1.

243. **D** – On this oblique sagittal image of the orbit, the superior rectus muscle is seen along its length. Just beneath is the optic nerve (second cranial nerve) being displaced by a mass. The inferior rectus muscle is also seen along its length. This imaging plane does not show the medial or lateral rectus muscles very well. The retro-orbital fatty tissue is seen as hyperintense signal on this T1-weighted sequence with IV contrast. The mass is a benign cavernous hemangioma.

244. **A** – This artifact is seen along the frequency-encoding axis. The frequencies entering from the outside are interfering with the RF signal coming from the MRI unit. Each row going across the image represents a frequency.

245. **C** – Cross-talk artifact results from signal interference that occurs between adjacent slices in a multislice data acquisition. Note the close proximity of the 2 slice overlay groups, especially over the pertinent anatomic structures.

246. **D** – Wraparound occurs when the FOV is smaller than the object being imaged.

247. **D** – This type of motion artifact is more commonly called ghosting. It results from the pulsatile motion of the carotid arteries (in this example) along the phase-encoding axis.

248. **C** – The superior sagittal sinus is seen anteriorly (1) and posteriorly in cross section. The SSS is part of the venous drainage system.

249. **B** – The falx cerebri separates the 2 cerebral hemispheres. The space on both sides of the falx is the longitudinal fissure. The longitudinal fissure may also be referred to as the interhemispheric fissure.

250. **A** – The diploe is the cancellous marrow-filled portion of the bone, in this example, the skull. The diploe separates the outer table (hypointense) of the calvarium and the inner table (hypointense) of the calvarium.

Index

Note: Page numbers followed by *f* indicate figures; and page numbers followed by *t* indicate tables.